CARING
FOR
OLDER
ADULTS
HOLISTICALLY

THIRD EDITION

Mary Ann Anderson, Ph.D., APRN, BC
Fellow, National Gerontological Nursing Association
College of Health Professions
Weber State University
Ogden, Utah

F.A. DAVIS COMPANY • Philadelphia

F. A. Davis Company
1915 Arch Street
Philadelphia, PA 19103
www.fadavis.com

Printed in the United States of America

Last digit indicates print number: 10 9 8 7 6 5 4 3

The painting used on the front cover is "The Prophecy - Sleep Suite 2," 1955, by Stanton MacDonald-Wright (1890-1973). Courtesy of Goldfield Galleries, 8380 Melrose Ave., Los Angeles, CA 90069, (323) 651-1122.

Acquisitions Editor: Lisa Deitch
Developmental Editor: Michelle Clarke
Cover Designer: Louis J. Forgione

As new scientific information becomes available through basic and clinical research, recommended treatments and drug therapies undergo changes. The author(s) and publisher have done everything possible to make this book accurate, up to date, and in accord with accepted standards at the time of publication. The author(s), editors, and publisher are not responsible for errors or omissions or for consequences from application of the book, and make no warranty, expressed or implied, in regard to the contents of the book. Any practice described in this book should be applied by the reader in accordance with professional standards of care used in regard to the unique circumstances that may apply in each situation. The reader is advised always to check product information (package inserts) for changes and new information regarding dose and contraindications before administering any drug. Caution is especially urged when using new or infrequently ordered drugs.

Library of Congress Cataloging-in-Publication Data

Caring for older adults holistically / [edited by] Mary Ann Anderson–3rd ed.
    p. ; cm.
  Rev. ed. of: Caring for the elderly client. 2nd ed. c1999.
  Includes bibliographical references and index.
  ISBN 0-8036-1053-X
  1. Geriatric nursing. 2. Holistic nursing. I. Anderson, Mary Ann, 1946- II. Caring for the elderly client.
  [DNLM: 1. Geriatric Nursing. 2. Aging–physiology. 3. Ethics, Clinical–Aged. 4. Health Promotion–Aged. 5. Health Services for the Aged. 6. Nursing Diagnosis–methods. 7. Nursing, Practical. WY 152 C27708 2003]
  RC954.A53 2003
  610.73'65–dc21

                                                    2002041562

This book is dedicated to the courageous licensed practical and vocational nurses who continue on in the best practice model of the profession.

Thank you.

FOREWORD

The increasing median age and total number of older adults in our society present numerous challenges for the health care system. Persons over age 65 are more frequently hospitalized than other age groups and have longer lengths of stay. More than half of the intensive care unit (ICU) beds and nearly all nursing home beds are filled by older persons. The elderly comprise most of home health caseloads.

In addition to adequate and competent health-care services in general, high-quality nursing services for the older population are and will continue to be required. Nursing is a unique discipline in its ability to address the physical, psychological, and social elements of care and to provide comprehensive, coordinated services that not only treat illness but also promote health and restore optimum function. When the health care needs of older adults are examined, most can be identified as appropriately falling within the realm of nursing practice.

As health care has become increasingly high tech, attention must be paid to ensuring that the importance of "high touch" (physical, emotional, and spiritual) is not overlooked. This is particularly important in the nursing care of older adults. Caring, support, and continued development, so important to the health and well-being of older adults, are best afforded through human contact.

Licensed practical nurses have long contributed to direct nursing care in a high-touch manner. Practicing under the direction of registered nurses (RNs) and others with statutory authority, licensed practical nurses (LPNs) bridge expanding medical and nursing technologies with the most human elements of direct care. The long tradition of direct "hands-on" care associated with practical nursing will have even greater importance in an increasingly complex, sophisticated, and technological health care system. To effectively and competently meet present and future demands, LPNs must mesh the caring aspects of direct nursing services with new knowledge and skills.

Caring for Older Adults Holistically is a much-needed resource to assist LPNs in meeting the new challenges of providing high-quality services to older adults. Throughout this book, a positive view of aging and the aged is conveyed. Recognizing the individuality of each person and promoting optimal function are recurrent themes.

Many fine chapters review a wide range of clinical practice topics basic to gerontological nursing. These are well-written and easy to absorb. Practical guidelines and case studies bridge theory and practice on a level appropriate for the LPN. From wellness promotion to restorative care, theory and practice skills are offered to guide LPNs in assessing, planning, delivering, and evaluating care.

In addition to the wealth of clinical information provided, this book offers insights into the managerial responsibilities assumed by LPNs. This inclusion is most refreshing and relevant. Despite the arguments by some colleagues that LPNs *should not* assume management roles, the reality is that some *do*. Fortunately, the authors recognize the actual roles LPNs must fill and review the essentials of managerial activities on a level appropriate for LPN nursing.

Great strides have been made in the educational, research, and practice components of gerontological nursing. *Caring for Older Adults Holistically* translates these advancements into a practical level appropriate for LPNs and offers guidance to this important group of nurses as they secure their niche in a dynamic health care system.

Charlotte Elliopoulos, RNC, MPH
Specialist in Geriatric and
Long-Term Nursing

PREFACE TO THIRD EDITION

The face of nursing care and how it is delivered has changed significantly from the initial writing of this book in 1995 and this, the third edition. One change is that of increased respect for elderly people. Because of that trend, the title of the book has changed. Older adults are being recognized more and more as just that—older adults. This is in concert with the term *younger adults*. The terms *elderly, old*, and *geriatric* are not in the respectful vernacular. What a delightful change in the care of older persons. A positive aspect of this growing trend is that nurses who give care to older adults receive more respect as well. I know it is a small change, but it is in the right direction.

This edition of *Caring for Older Adults Holistically* has focused on meeting the increasingly higher demands made on licensed practical and vocational nurses (LPNs) to give older persons care. The demands of downsizing and the employment of more care technicians and fewer licensed nurses require the nurse to function on a higher level than ever before in nursing history. Therefore, this edition has even more information on the scope of LPN management responsibilities, with a special section on working with nursing assistants.

LPNs need to know how to perform their skills in hospitals, nursing homes, and home health agencies. The new chapter on communicable diseases is an effort to give them information about current and common diseases across facilities. There is up-to-the-minute information on the growing numbers of cases of human immunodeficiency virus (HIV)/acquired immunodeficiency syndrome (AIDS) in older adults as well as the remote, but ever-spreading West Nile fever (a case was reported in my home state last year!).

Because more and more people are living to be older, there are more deaths in the older population. That is what prompted the chapter on end-of-life issues. This topic also has become an item for the national nursing agenda. This chapter, written by an experienced social worker, blends practical and factual knowledge with the caring concepts that are prevalent throughout the book.

Each chapter has been reviewed and appended in order to keep the content current. Some new pictures have been added for the same reason. In addition, each chapter has critical thinking exercises that can be used as homework to be submitted to the faculty person, or as "think" pieces to stimulate interest and discussion in the class. The case studies at the end of each chapter, as well as the sample test questions, have been retained.

The instructor's guide has been updated with interesting teaching suggestions that promote critical thinking, diverse learning activities, and a diversified test bank. The third edition has retained its personality of being easily readable and immediately useful to students.

PREFACE TO SECOND EDITION

Welcome to the second edition of *Caring for the Elderly Client*. The response to the first edition was gratifying and prompted this writing. This text apparently meets a need for students and educators, which was the goal for writing it. With the aging population of this country increasing at an ever more rapid rate, it is critical for all nurses to be prepared to care for the aging population in a caring and knowledgeable way. That is the purpose of this text.

The opportunity to prepare a second edition has allowed for an additional effort to meet the learning needs of the student. This has been done in several ways. The size of the book has been changed. The new format leaves more margin space for students to take notes or highlight concepts that have special meaning for them. The space should be especially helpful when the student is working with the case studies. Color has been added to strengthen the visual appeal of the book, and the new cover enhances the concept of caring with its pleasant visual appeal.

The second edition has retained the strong critical thinking aspect of the book with some enhancements. The case studies provide a strong component of the critical thinking aspects of the text as well. The instructor's guide is an excellent strength of this book. It provides the faculty person with learning activities as well as a diversified test bank. The second edition has retained its personality of being easily readable and immediately useful for students.

PREFACE TO FIRST EDITION

Most nurses in the workforce today, regardless of practice setting, are caring for older persons. With the exception of labor and delivery, the client population in health care environments is composed predominantly of persons age 65 or older. Whether they refer to themselves as gerontological nurses or not, nurses in today's health care settings must possess and use knowledge unique to caring for older clients.

Caring for an older person is not the same as caring for a middle-aged person with gray hair and wrinkles. It requires knowledge related to normal aging changes, altered responses to illness, environments of care, and a host of other topics specific to the aging individual. Thus, gerontological nursing is as specialized a field as pediatric nursing.

Many schools of nursing have recognized the need to prepare nursing students for their practice roles in caring for elderly clients. Courses on gerontological nursing are offered separately or integrated into curricula in most schools preparing licensed practical/vocational nurses (LPN) and registered nurses (RN). Continuing education courses and seminars on issues in gerontological nursing are offered widely throughout the country. Although numerous textbooks and articles on gerontological nursing are in print, few comprehensive textbooks are specifically geared to the LPN.

This book was compiled in response to the need for a clear, concise, basic text on caring for older clients that includes information pertinent to any practice setting. Although it is written at the licensed practical/vocational nurse level and makes frequent reference to LPNs throughout, its content is also relevant to registered nurses seeking basic information. It can be used as a required or supplemental text in gerontological nursing courses offered in LPN and LPN-RN ladder programs, as well as other levels of nursing education. Because of its readability and its broad focus on multiple and diverse issues, it can also be used as a refresher or reference manual for practicing nurses.

The role of the LPN varies significantly from setting to setting. Although she may provide direct patient care in the hospital, she may be the supervisor or even director of nursing in the long-term care facility. Some may question the appropriateness of this range in roles and responsibilities for the LPN. The need exists, however, to educate and prepare practical nurses for the roles they are currently asked to assume in the practice arena. This book was written to address the multifaceted roles and significant responsibilities of the LPN in various health care settings. These responsibilities range from health promotion to medication administration and evaluation of side, toxic, and desired effects; to collection of physical and psychological assessment data; to making assignments for nursing assistants.

This book includes several features that set it apart from other gerontological texts. Its overall approach is health and wellness oriented, rather than sickness oriented. It includes chapters on health promotion and restorative care that are pertinent, not only in the community and rehabilitative settings but in hospitals, nursing homes, and day-care centers.

Written with an emphasis on the humanistic aspects of caring, this book attempts to blend the gentle nurturing components of nursing with the technological knowledge necessary for caregiving. The pictures throughout the text are added to remind the reader that the information contained in the chapter pertains to human beings. Thus, it must be applied in a manner that recognizes individual differences, frailties, fears, and strengths.

The diversity of topics and the range of expertise among the contributors is another unique feature of this text. Nursing experts with sound, practical experience were chosen from all over the United States and asked to condense their knowledge on a particular topic into basic, relevant information with practical application. The result is a textbook addressing clinical topics such as lab values, pharmacology, health problems, and psychological assessment, as well as health and wellness topics and management and environmental topics. Each chapter, whether clinical, management, or otherwise, is presented in a framework that lends itself to application in the practice setting.

Case studies are included in every chapter to enhance the applicability of the chapter content. The reader is given an opportunity to review a real-life situation and answer pertinent questions. Such case studies represent practice situations that the gerontological nurse frequently faces. The questions are written in a format that gives the reader experience in answering standardized test questions similar to those on licensing exams.

As a final note, it is important to recognize the gender references throughout this text. The authors acknowledge that nurses and clients are both male and female. For ease of readability, however, nurses are referred to as female and clients as male throughout the content of this text.

ACKNOWLEDGMENTS

I enjoyed working on this book and welcomed the opportunity to do a third edition. The process reunites me with other gerontological nurses who I would like to acknowledge for their professional and useful contributions. Their work is what makes the book so valuable to read.

Gratitude also needs to be expressed to Emily Ravsten for her ability to understand the beauty in older adults and photograph it. I appreciate the knowledgeable assistance I received from Michelle Clarke at F. A. Davis.

I sincerely want to acknowledge the patient tutoring of all older adults who have received care from the nurses involved in preparing this book. They have taught us much, and without their timely instruction in the lessons of life and living, this book would not be possible.

CONTRIBUTORS

Sister Rose Therese Bahr, ASC
Provincial Councilor
Adorers of the Blood of Christ
Wichita, Kansas

Colleen Brill, RN, MSN
Mental Health Nurse Manager
Phelps County Medical Center
Rolla, Missouri

Kyle Cannon, RN, BSN
Communicable Disease Nurse Supervisor
Salt Lake Valley Health Department
Salt Lake City, Utah

Tamara Chase, MSN, RN
Assistant Professor
Weber State University
Ogden, Utah

Kathleen R. Culliton, APRN, MS, GNP
Associate Professor
Weber State University
Ogden, Utah

Kay Martin Grott, RNC, MS, GNP
Vanderbilt Hospital Intensive Care Unit
Nashville, Tennessee

Pamela E. Hugie, MSN, RN
Outreach Coordinator
Weber State University
Ogden, Utah

Vivian J. Koroknay
Director of Rehabilitation and Restorative
  Care Services
Asbury Methodist Village
Gaithersburg, Maryland

Mary Ann Johnson, PhD, RNC, GNP
Retired

Mary Lou Long, RNC, MSN
Clinical Director, Nursing
St. Luke's Regional Medical Center
Boise, Idaho

Judith Pratt
Associate Professor
Weber State University
Ogden, Utah

Emily Ravsten, MSW
Denver Department of Human Services
Denver, Colorado

Jeanne Robertson Samter
Assistant Professor of Nursing
North Georgia College & State University
Dahlonega, Georgia

Yvonne A Sehy, PhD, RN, GNP
Gerontology Center
University of Utah
Salt Lake City, Utah

Mary McCarthy Slater
Long-Term Care Manager
Christian Health Center
Lexington, Kentucky

Elaine Tagliareni, RNC, MS
Associate Professor, Nursing
Community College of Philadelphia
Philadelphia, Pennsylvania

Verle Waters, RN, MA
Dean Emerita
Ohlone College
Fremont, California

CONSULTANTS

Tamara D. Espejo, RN, BS, MS (C)
Instructor
Baldy View R.O.P.
Claremont, California
(Vocational education)

Colleen Magee, RN, BSN, Med
Teacher
Rockford Public Schools
Rockford, Illinois
(LPN program)

Rozann M. Reyerson, RN,
MSEd, MS
Assistant Professor in Nursing
University of South Dakota
Watertown, South Dakota
(ADN program)

Marilyn J. Vontz, PhD, MSN, MA,
BS, RN
Nurse Educator
Bryan College of Health Sciences
Lincoln, Nebraska
(DI program, which will become a BSN
program)

Stephanie Whitaker, MSN,
RN, CDE
Field Services Coordinator
Physician's Choice Home Health Services
Kissimmee, Florida
(In-service education)

CONTENTS

UNIT II • CLINICAL PRACTICE

Foundations of Care
for the Older Adult

Elaine Tagliareni
Verle Waters
Mary Ann Anderson

chapter 1

The Aging Experience

Learning Objectives

After completing this chapter, the student will be able to:

1. Describe the demographics of people older than 65 years of age in the United States.
2. Define the term "ageism."
3. Identify age-related changes in the following body systems:
   Cardiovascular
   Respiratory
   Musculoskeletal
   Integumentary
   Gastrointestinal
   Genitourinary
   Neurological
   Special senses

▶ INTRODUCTION

Welcome to the exciting specialty of gerontological nursing. This is a relatively new nursing specialty and has within it certified nurses, clinical specialists, and geriatric nurse practitioners who give care only to people who are older than age 65 years. There are nurses who have a great deal of experience as well as novice (or new) nurses just like you. Together, all of us, experienced and novice, make a valuable team to care for the frail and vulnerable older adults who come to us for nursing care. In addition, many nurses have the opportunity of working with well elderly persons who are focused on health promotion. Gerontological nursing is exciting and varied, and I compliment you for being interested in this area of health care.

Old age is new. I find that simple statement to be true because, at my age, I actually feel the consequences of aging. I am sure many of you reading this book do not notice from week to week or month to month that you are aging. I am 56 years old, have some chronic diseases, and I feel it. Growing older is new for every person who experiences it and for our society as well. In the history of this country, there have never been so many people older than age 65. The composition of the American population is different today from that of any previous generation. Of course, there were old people before, but their numbers were small compared with the number of people older than age 65 today.

In 1776, when the Declaration of Independence was signed, a child born in the United States had a life expectancy of 35 years. In 1930, it was 59.7 years; 1965 it was 70.2 years and today, the average life expectancy is 76.4 years, with 34.8 million people over the age of 65 in the United States (Eliopolous, 2001). That is a large number of older adults, and as a licensed practical nurse (LPN), you need to learn the skills and techniques that will allow you to give older people excellent care. It is the challenge of your generation of nurses.

Throughout most of human history, only 1 in 10 people could expect to live to the age of 65 years. Today, 80% of Americans can anticipate reaching that age or older (Eliopolous, 2001). In fact, two-thirds of all men and women who have lived beyond the age of 65 in the entire history of the world are alive today. Sometimes called "the Graying of America," this dramatic change in our population has many ramifications in politics, economics, health care, recreation, and entertainment. All facets of life, not just health care, are affected by the fact that many more older adults are living today than in the past.

▶ DEMOGRAPHICS

People aged 65 years and older comprise 12.7% of the population in this country, that is, more than one in every eight Americans. There are many numbers I could share with you in this section of the chapter, but I find most students do not want to read demographic data unless they have to in order to pass a test. I would prefer you learn the importance of the numbers rather than just memorize them.

Here are two important pieces of demographic information that will impact your practice as an LPN.

1. The older, white population will grow more slowly than before, and in the next 40 years, it will begin to decline by comparison with African-American and other ethnic minority groups. Current minority populations are projected to represent 25% of the elderly population in 2030.
2. The fastest-growing segment of the population in this country are people older than 85 years of age.

POINT OF INTEREST

The increased numbers of elderly people in the United States have resulted in new definitions of aging. The term "young-old" is used for people 65 to 74 years old; the term "middle-old" is used for people 75 to 84 years old; "old-old" is used for people 85 to 100; and the term "elite old" is used for persons older 100 years of age. It is necessary to define the differences for each age group because their health needs, medication dosages, and frailty relate specifically to their age category.

CRITICALLY EXAMINE THE FOLLOWING:

Before reading the next section, take the time necessary to complete this critical thinking exercise. You will find similar exercises in every chapter throughout this book. They are designed to assist you in preparing for class discussion by asking you to think about the questions and make interesting and creative comments. Critical thinking is an essential component of nursing. These exercises are a positive way to begin to develop that all-important skill.

How Will It Impact Your Nursing Practice to Have:

1. Increasing numbers of old-old people as your clients?
2. Increasing numbers of nonwhite, older adults as your clients?

Because this is your first critically thinking exercise, I am going to answer the questions as though I were a student. It is hoped that this will assist you in considering how you will answer the questions. Your faculty person may request this assignment to be turned in at the next class session, or it may be used as a point for class discussion. However it is used, it is an opportunity for you to critically think and then compare your thinking with your classmates. Here are my responses.

1. When I planned on going to nursing school, I wanted to be an obstetrical nurse. I was excited to think about working in labor and delivery, and I cannot imagine anything nicer than working in the newborn nursery. However, if the population of older people, especially the very old, is growing, I need to consider working in gerontology. If that is where I am going to be because of the need for nurses, I am going to become very good at taking care of fragile old-old or elite old people. They sound like my type of challenge!
2. I live in Utah where 95% of the population is white. I will have an adjustment to make when my patients are not mostly white and of the same working class, emigrant society. What I need to learn about are the cultures of other ethnic groups so I can be an effective nurse and meet their needs on a high level.

Projections indicate that the size of this age group will double between 2000 and 2040. At present there are more people having their 85th birthday every day in this country than babies being born.

▶ THE IMPACT OF AGING ON NURSING

The great increase in the number of older people means that nursing practice must be different from what it has been in the past. Dr. Robert Butler (1969), a geriatric specialist, said that all graduates going into health-care work today will spend 75% of their working lives caring for older people. Current national statistics state that 65% of all patients in acute care hospitals are age 65 or older, as are 83% of those in home care and 92% of those in nursing homes. Tim Porter O'Grady, a nursing futurist, said in the year 2000, that if a nurse was not preparing for a job in gerontology, that nurse was not preparing for the nursing jobs of the future. The graying of America calls for gerontologically qualified nurses who can work in diverse health-care settings. The purpose of this book is to assist you to meet that objective.

Health care has changed in various ways because of the number of people who are aging. As a group, older citizens are a very powerful political force; they have influenced the actions of Congress and the President on health-related issues and will continue to do so. A few yeas ago, Congress passed legislation providing insurance coverage for catastrophic medical events for those under Medicare, which added a relatively small amount to the cost of Medicare insurance paid by recipients. The new plan was, however, unacceptable to older adults, and as a result of numerous calls and letters, Congress was persuaded to rescind its legislation.

Older adults want and expect to have a say in the kind of health care they receive, where they receive it, and from whom. They are better educated than any other generation of older adults, and therefore, have the knowledge to make more sophisticated demands on the health-care system. For instance, demand is growing for home-care services from older people who need assistance and nursing care but prefer to be cared for at home.

This population of new clients in the health-care system requires you, the nurse, to consider them in a new way. Never before have nurses had to care for such a large number of older adults who have survived the Holocaust, two World Wars, the Korean and Vietnam Wars, the Great Depression, and rock and roll! Because the survival experiences and life skills of these elderly people are new to health care, they require society to address them in a new way.

▶ ATTITUDES TOWARD AGING

The study of aging is a very important part of nursing. Many myths, stereotypes, and prejudices about old age exist in our culture, and nurses need to be able to separate myths and prejudices from fact. Modern researchers are intently studying the aging experience (another indication of the importance of this topic in today's world). This chapter draws from their findings to represent a realistic picture of the processes and effects of aging. Myths and prejudices about old age are pervasive in our society. Browsing through a greeting card display reveals some very good examples of the stereotypes and fables of aging:

"I won't say you're old," reads one greeting card, "But in horse years, you'd be glue on this envelope."

"Happy birthday, Hot Stuff! Who says people our age can't still live in the fast lane?" reads another. The inside message: "Voila! Adult diapers with racing stripes."

As the contents of many of the cards imply, old age conjures up images of rocking chairs, dentures, memory loss, and incontinence. People laugh at the humor in the birthday cards, but a serious societal danger lurks in such negative and prejudicial images. Stereotypes, myths, and distortions concerning aging and old people lead to actions that discriminate against the aged. American culture glorifies youth. Print and television advertising, clothing fashions, and other expressions of the desirable norm all push the image of zestful youth. Because today's adults have grown up in this culture, they pick up its values and prejudices without realizing it.

One of the authors of this chapter joined a tour group led by a sincere, well-intentioned young man. He tried to exchange a friendly word with every person in the group. He spoke to a healthy-looking man, who may have been in his late 70s, in a raised voice as though he assumed that the man was hard of hearing. "What did you used to be?" he asked. After a pause, the older man replied, "I still am." The behavior exhibited by the young tour guide is an example of ageism.

▶ AGEISM

The term "ageism" was coined in 1968 by Butler (1969) to describe negative attitudes and practices that were directed toward the aged. He defined ageism as a systematic stereotyping of and discrimination against people simply because they are old. Ageism is very similar to racism and sexism, which discriminate against people because of skin color and gender. As a society we are outraged by acts of racism and sexism, but we seem to accept ageism as a norm for behavior. Old people are categorized as confused, rigid in thought and manner, and old-fashioned in morality and skills. Yet, older adults are as individual and unique as are people of all other age groups. It simply seems easier to place them in a negative category and ignore them. Ageism allows the younger generation to see older people as different; thus, they subtly cease to identify with their elders as human beings.

In the decades since Dr. Butler first wrote about ageism, a steady improvement in attitudes toward the aged has been seen. This change partly resulted from general public education, increased attention in the media, and broadening of education about gerontology in colleges and universities. Seriously negative attitudes toward the aged still exist. They appear subtly, covertly, and even unconsciously. Like racism and sexism, ageism is still persistent.

An example is the cosmetic industry which thrives on the sale of products that eliminate age spots, smooth away wrinkles, conceal gray hairs, and make one look younger than one's actual age. Growing old is represented as a calamity, and being old as having a dreaded disease. The last years of life are pictured as time spent in death's waiting room.

In reality, elderly people do not offer a panorama of doom and death. Many senior citizens live well into their 80s, and 90s with "youthful vigor," in relative physical comfort and safety, and in good health. Many others do have chronic health problems, but because the problems are well managed and well controlled, such people consider themselves healthy and lead active, fulfilling lives. Still others have significant limitations that affect their independence and activity, but they are able to enjoy a rich and varied existence because they live with family members or in other protected environments.

Negative images of the nursing home, envisioned by some people, are in part an expression of ageism. Most nursing homes give excellent care to a frail and vulnerable population that cannot be cared for elsewhere. Another point of information, unknown by many people, is that only 5% of those older than 65 years of age are in nursing homes at any one time (Eliopolous, 2001). Today's nursing home is characterized by a concept of *rehabilitative*, not *custodial* care, a perspective that calls for nursing interventions intended to support the highest possible level of independence despite physical and cognitive limitations.

It is easy for society to judge, criticize, and ignore an older person. Do an internal examination to determine if you are ageist. Do you get impatient when an older person is in front of you driving on the freeway? I tell my gerontology students that they will not pass the class until they have mastered that type of patience. I give them assignments to sit down and unhurriedly talk to a well elderly person. I suggest they go to lunch or shopping, even at the grocery store. The students are encouraged to ask the person about living with ration cards, going to war, or being left a widow or widower after 50 to 60 years of marriage. The ageism in our society has kept most of us from knowing about the aging process and respecting those who survive it. It is time for that to change!

An important concept to remember is that of the uniqueness of the individual. Just as every child or every middle-aged adult is, in some way unique, so is the older adult. The mistaken belief that one old person is just like another is an expression of ageism, and this perception can lead to potentially harmful treatment. Doctors and nurses sometimes treat older patients as they might treat a child, calling them by their first names without asking how they wish to be addressed or, worse yet, calling them "honey" or "dearie." Caregivers often are guilty of "infantilizing" the elderly. It is easy to see how such treatment increases dependence and frailty, rather than fostering independence even for a person with limitations. Not all old people are cranky and gloomy, although the man or woman who was cranky and gloomy at age 40 is probably more so at 80. People tend to become more and more like themselves as they age. All who work in the health-care field need to examine their own attitudes and biases about older adults in general and about frail or ill older adults in particular in order to successfully battle ageism.

▶ THE NORMAL AGING PROCESS

Since the early 1950s, much research has taken place in both Europe and the United States on identifying and classifying common physiological and psychosocial changes that occur as people grow older. These changes have been termed *normal* because they represent alterations in body structure and function that occur gradually throughout life. In this context, aging is seen as a natural process, and the changes associated with it are considered to be expected and continuous. If you are curious about your potential normal aging changes, you need to look at your grandparents. What acute and chronic diseases do they have? At what age do people in your family die? Do the men go bald; do the women develop osteoporosis? We all will age until we die. To me, that comment makes aging the desirable choice between the two. I would sooner grow old than die young.

To fully understand the normal aging process, nurses must realize that aging is a normal developmental event and that patterns of aging vary dramatically among older adults. Although the profession studies normal age changes that are universal, every person ages in a particular, individualized way. No two individuals are alike; in fact, the number of ways people age may be seen as

equal to the number of people who have lived into old age. As individuals age, they become more diverse, not more alike. Thus, the range of "normal" aging characteristics is wide, and each individual exhibits a unique interplay of physical, social, and environmental influences that define the personal aging experience.

Often, older adults do have a chronic or acute illness superimposed on age-related changes, but development of disease is not a normal part of aging. It is essential for you, the LPN, to understand this perspective and develop a positive approach to normal aging. It also is important to remember that most older adults live actively and independently in the community, and cope successfully with age-related changes and chronic illnesses (remember that only 5% of them are in nursing homes). Health, then, for older adults, might well be defined as the ability to function at an individual's highest potential, despite the presence of age-related changes and risk factors.

Essential facts about the normal aging process can be summarized as follows:

- As individuals age, they become more diverse, not more alike.
- Age-related changes develop in each individual in a unique way.
- Normal aging and disease are separate entities.
- Normal aging includes both gains and losses and does not necessarily indicate decline.
- Successful adaptation to the aging process is accomplished by most older adults.

▶ NORMAL PHYSIOLOGICAL CHANGES ACCORDING TO BODY SYSTEMS

Specific age-related changes are described in terms of the body systems with which they are associated. Common functional changes experienced by older adults, as a result of physiological alterations, also are discussed. The term *function* refers to the older adult's ability to perform activities of daily living (ADLs) and independent activities of daily living (IADLs), and takes into consideration the quality of life of the individual. As the older adult experiences an increase in the number and intensity of age-related

changes, functional independence is often
jeopardized. Nursing approaches to prevent
losses and promote self-care in light of age-
related changes also are considered in this
section.

THE CARDIOVASCULAR SYSTEM

The cardiovascular system loses its efficiency
with age, but because older adults require less
oxygen both at rest and during exercise, many
people effectively compensate for changes in
circulatory function. However, the high incidence of cardiovascular disease in the older
population often makes it difficult to distinguish normal age-related changes from those
related to sickness. One of the "good news"
facts about cardiovascular disease and the
elderly is that it is no longer the number one
cause of death as it has been for decades.
Older adults now know more about taking care
of themselves, which improves their cardiovascular system. Cancer is now the leading
cause of death in older adults.

Age-Related Changes

Heart
- Cardiac muscle strength is diminished.
- Heart valves become thickened and more
  rigid.
- The sinoatrial node, which is responsible
  for conduction, is less efficient and
  impulses are slowed.

Blood vessels
- Arteries become less elastic.
- Capillary walls thicken and slow the
  exchange of nutrients and waste products
  between blood and tissues.
- The greater rigidity of the vascular walls
  increases both systolic and diastolic pressures.

Blood
- Blood volume is reduced owing to an age-
  related decline in total body water.

- Bone marrow activity is reduced, which
  leads to a slight drop in levels of red blood
  cells, hematocrit, and hemoglobin.
- Heart contractions may be weaker, blood
  volume decreases, and cardiac output
  drops at a rate of about 1% per year below
  the value of 5 L normally found in a younger
  person.

In summary, with normal aging, some atherosclerosis is expected, as well as decreased
cardiac output, but cardiovascular response
remains adequate if cardiac disease is not
present.

RESPIRATORY SYSTEM

Respiratory functioning shows minimal
age-related decline in healthy older adults.
The age-related changes that do affect the
respiratory system are so gradual that most
older adults compensate well for these
changes.

Age-Related Changes

Skeletal Changes
- The rib cage becomes rigid as cartilage
  calcifies.
- The thoracic spine may shorten, and osteoporosis may cause a stooped posture,
  decreasing active lung space and limiting
  thoracic movement.

Accessory Muscles
- Abdominal muscles weaken, decreasing
  both inspiratory and expiratory effort.
- The diaphragm does not appear to lose
  mass.

Intrapulmonary Changes
- Lung elastic recoil is progressively lost with
  advancing age.
- Alveoli enlarge and become thin, and
  although their number remains constant,
  the number of functioning alveoli decreases
  overall.

- The alveolus-capillary membrane thickens, reducing the surface area for gas exchange.

Functional Changes

Structural changes in the respiratory system affect the rate of air flow into and out of the lung as well as that of gas exchange at the alveolar level. Because of limited elastic recoil, residual volume increases. This means that less ventilation occurs at the bases of the lungs, and more air and secretions remain in the lungs. In addition, the shallow breathing patterns of older adults, secondary to postural changes, contribute to this reduced air flow. Decreased chest muscle strength contributes to a less effective cough response and places the older adult at greater risk of pulmonary infection. The shallow breathing pattern also affects gas exchange. Oxygen saturation is diminished. For example, the partial pressure of oxygen in alveoli (PAO_2) is about 90 mm Hg for a healthy young adult, whereas a value of 75 mm Hg at age 70 years would be acceptable. This decline may result in a decreased tolerance for exercise and the need for short rest periods during activity.

MUSCULOSKELETAL SYSTEM

Most older adults experience alterations in posture, changes in range of motion, and slowed movement. These changes account for many of the characteristics normally associated with old age.

Age-Related Changes

Bone Structure
- Loss of bone mass results in brittle, weak bones.
- The vertebral column may compress, leading to reduction in height.

Muscle Strength
- Muscle wasting occurs, and regeneration of muscle tissue slows.
- Muscles of the arms and legs become thin and flabby.
- Muscles lose flexibility and endurance with inactivity.

Joints
- Range of motion may be limited.
- Cartilage thins, so that joints may be painful, inflamed, or stiff.

Functional losses can be successfully managed with the right support devices.

Functional Changes

Loss of muscle mass is a gradual process and most older adults compensate for it well. Regular exercise has been shown to reduce bone loss and to promote increased muscle strength, as well as to improve flexibility and muscle coordination. Conversely, immobility and sedentary lifestyles lead to loss of muscle size and strength.

Loss of bone mass and bone density results in osteoporosis and porous, brittle bones that are at greater risk of fracture. This problem can be due to estrogen deficiencies and low serum calcium levels; therefore, calcium supplements and estrogens are often prescribed. In summary, changes caused by osteoporosis, lack of joint motion, and decreased muscle strength and endurance may affect the functional ability of the older adult. An effective exercise program, together with adequate diet and a healthy outlook that includes independence and an active lifestyle, can reverse or slow down musculoskeletal changes. The phrase "Use it or lose it!" directly applies to the older adult's musculoskeletal functional ability.

INTEGUMENTARY SYSTEM

Changes involving the skin probably are symbolic of the aging process more than those of any other system. The formation of wrinkles, the development of "age spots," graying of the hair, and baldness are constant reminders of growing old. In addition, no other system is so highly influenced by previous life patterns and environmental conditions, particularly exposure to the sun.

Age-Related Changes

Skin
- The skin loses elasticity, leading to wrinkles, folds, and dryness.
- The skin thins, giving less protection to underlying blood vessels.
- Subcutaneous fat diminishes.
- Melanocytes cluster, producing the skin pigmentation known as age spots.

Hair
- Decreased activity of hair follicles results in thinning of the hair.
- Decreased rate of melanin production results in loss of original color and graying.
- Women may develop hair on the chin and upper lip.

Nails
- Decreased blood flow to the nailbed may cause nails to become thick, dull, hard, and brittle, with longitudinal lines.

Sweat Glands
- Decreases in size and number occur.

Functional Changes

Intact skin is the first line of defense against bacterial invasion and minor physical trauma. Age-related skin dryness and decreased elasticity increase the risk of skin breakdown and skin tears, leading to increased potential for injury and infection. Body temperature regulation is impaired by decreased sweat production. Because of this, older adults may not exhibit diaphoresis with elevated body temperatures.

Conversely, the loss of insulation in the form of a fat layer may make older adults feel cold. They often ask for extra sweaters when younger adults are quite comfortable with the ambient temperature. Nurses need to be aware of temperature discomforts when bathing, dressing, or examining the older adult, and to respond appropriately to the older adult's concern.

Age-related changes in the integumentary system affect the essential mechanisms of body protection and temperature regulation, and also greatly influence one's perception of aging. Earlier health practices, related to nutrition, grooming, bathing, and physical activity, as well as genetic, biochemical, and environmental factors, are powerful determinants of integumentary status. The older adult who has followed a healthy lifestyle often takes pride in the moistness and softness of aging skin and reveals newfound beauty in gray hair and wise wrinkles.

GASTROINTESTINAL SYSTEM

Changes in the gastrointestinal (GI) system, although not life-threatening, often cause the greatest concern to the older adult. Indigestion, constipation, and anorexia are common GI problems that greatly affect functional status.

Age-Related Changes

Oral Cavity
- Reabsorption of bone in the jaw may loosen teeth and, thus, reduce the ability to chew.
- People with dentures must have them checked regularly to maintain a proper fit.

Esophagus
- The gag reflex weakens, causing an increased risk of food aspiration.
- Smooth muscle weakness delays emptying time.

Stomach
- Decreased gastric acid secretions may impair absorption of iron, vitamin B_{12}, and protein.

Intestines
- Peristalsis decreases.
- Weakening of the sphincter muscles leads to incompetent emptying of the bowel.

Functional Changes

The slowing of peristalsis and the loss of smooth muscle tone delay gastric emptying so that a feeling of "fullness" is present after eating only small amounts of food. In addition, delayed gastric emptying time and reduced gastric acid secretions may lead to indigestion, discomfort, and reduced appetite. Frequent small meals, rather than three large ones, may be better tolerated. Decreased peristalsis also contributes to slower transit time in the large intestine and allows more time for water reabsorption and hardening of the stool. Because of this factor, the nurse must recommend a diet adequate in fiber and fluids.

Fatigue, discomfort, activity intolerance, and sensory losses may make food preparation difficult for the older adult living at home. This problem could result in a nutritionally inadequate diet. In summary, effective GI functioning creates peace of mind for the older adult and greatly influences well-being.

GENITOURINARY SYSTEM

Changes in the genitourinary system affect the basic bodily functions of voiding and sexual performance. These issues are often difficult for the older adult to discuss. A commonly held belief holds that genitourinary problems, such as incontinence and decreased sexual response, are normal results of aging. They are not, but the belief that they are often delays the older adult from seeking treatment. Helping the older adult to maintain optimal genitourinary function is often a challenge for the nurse.

Age-Related Functions

Renal function
- Renal blood flow decreases because of decreased cardiac output and reduced glomerular filtration rate.
- Ability to concentrate urine may be impaired.

Bladder
- Loss of muscle tone and incomplete emptying may occur.
- Capacity decreases.

Micturition
- In men, increased frequency due to enlargement of the prostate is possible.
- In women, increased frequency may be caused by relaxation of the perineal muscle.

Female Reproduction
- The vulva may atrophy.
- Pubic hair may fall out.
- Vaginal secretions diminish, and vaginal walls thin and become less elastic.

Male Reproduction
- Testes decrease in size.
- Prostate may enlarge.

Functional Changes

Despite decreased renal blood flow and the loss of kidney mass, the genitourinary system continues to function normally in the absence of disease. Functional impairments result from decreased bladder capacity and include urinary frequency, nocturia, and retention of urine. These changes may eventually cause dysfunction, leading to infection, urgency, and incontinence. Although urinary incontinence is not a normal outcome of the aging process, loss of perineal muscle mass may contribute to one of the most common forms of incontinence in women, stress incontinence. This involves leakage of urine that occurs with coughing, sneezing, laughing, or lifting. Pelvic floor exercises comprise an effective strategy to strengthen muscle tone and prevent involuntary leakage. Vaginal changes may lead to painful intercourse, vaginal infections, and intense itching.

Enlargement of the prostate, which occurs in most elderly men, is most often benign. It can, however, cause urinary retention, frequency, overflow incontinence, and eventually renal damage. Therefore, older men should have regular examinations of the prostate.

Changes in voiding, particularly incontinence, and changes in sexual response may dramatically alter genitourinary function and contribute to embarrassment and general discomfort for the older adult. By demonstrating sensitivity and acceptance, the nurse can effectively intervene to improve genitourinary functional response.

NERVOUS SYSTEM

Age-related changes in the nervous system affect all body systems and involve vascular response, mobility, coordination, visual activity, and cognitive ability. Interestingly, most misconceptions about normal age-related changes involve the nervous system. For example, the misconception that mental decline or "senility" is inevitable with aging or that intellectual capacity diminishes with age. The nurse needs to teach older adults that general decline of neurological function is not an automatic response to aging and that, in the absence of disease, the older adult's neurological system functions adequately.

Age-Related Changes

Neurons
- Neurons are steadily lost in the brain and spinal cord.
- Synthesis and metabolism of neurotransmitters are diminished.
- Brain mass is lost progressively.

Movement
- The kinesthetic sense is less efficient.
- Balance may be impaired.
- Reaction time decreases.

Sleep
- Insomnia and increased night wakening may occur.
- Deep sleep (stage IV) and rapid eye movement sleep decrease.

Functional Changes

As motor neurons work less efficiently, reaction time slows and the ability to respond quickly to stimuli decreases. Research studies indicate that although response time may be prolonged, older adults are willing to give up speed for accuracy, and tend to respond more slowly but with greater precision. There appears to be little correlation between brain atrophy and cognitive loss. Older adults are generally well oriented to time, place, and person, with minimal changes in memory performance, despite decreased synthesis of neurotransmitters and diminished brain size.

Older people are particularly at risk for falls, owing to a slower reaction time in maintaining balance, and the potential for hypotensive reactions secondary to decreased blood volume. Resulting symptoms of dizziness, light-headedness, and vertigo contribute to impaired balance. Nurses should allow the older adult adequate time for position change; dangling at the bedside and standing briefly before ambulation may be indicated.

In general, older adults sleep less at night but take naps during the day, so that cumulative sleep time is usually adequate. These frequent awakenings may cause restless sleep and abrupt wakefulness that is often troubling to the older adult. Thorough sleep assessment is necessary to determine actual sleep time. Additionally, afternoon exercise and a decrease in stimulants at bedtime may be suggested by the nurse. Environmental changes, such as noise control and regulation of room temperature, may be helpful.

Common age-related changes of the nervous system, particularly slowed reaction time, affect movement, sleep, and cognition, the functions of which are vital to optimal performance of activities of daily living.

SPECIAL SENSE ORGANS

The sensory organs of sight, hearing, taste, touch, and smell facilitate communication with the environment. Loss of sensory function, particularly vision and hearing, severely alters the older adult's self-care abilities and quality of life. Age-related changes that result in loss of sensory function may be the most difficult for a person of any age to accept and cope with effectively. The nurse must be extremely sensitive to sensory changes and their impact on each person.

Age-Related Changes

Vision
- Ability to focus on close objects is diminished.
- Increased density of the lens occurs, and lipid accumulates around the iris, causing a grayish yellow ring.
- The eyes' production of tears decreases.
- The pupils decrease in size and become less responsive to light.
- Night vision decreases, and the iris loses pigment so that eye color usually becomes light blue or gray.

Hearing
- The ability to hear high-frequency tones decreases.
- The cerumen contains a greater amount of keratin so that it hardens and becomes more likely to become impacted.

Taste
- Ability to perceive bitter, salt, and sour tastes diminishes.

Touch

- Ability to feel light touch, pain, or different temperatures may decrease.

Functional Changes

Despite normal age-related changes in vision, most older adults have adequate visual function to meet self-care activities using corrective lenses. Because dark and light adaptation takes longer, simple activities, like entering or leaving a theater or going to the bathroom at night, put older people at risk for falls and injury. Yellowing of the lens makes vision for low-tone colors (violet, blue, green) difficult; use of yellow, orange, or red colors on signs or on bedroom walls increases the older adult's ability to read.

Decreased production of tears by the eye may contribute to irritation and infection; artificial tears are often prescribed. Functional hearing changes result initially in an inability to hear high-pitched tones, so that the nurse should speak in a normal tone of voice without shouting and without increasing pitch. Because it takes more sensory stimulation to trigger the taste experience, older adults may use more salt, for example, to effectively produce a salt taste on their food.

Sensory changes have a profound impact on the functional ability of older adults. The nurse must always determine whether the patient uses corrective lenses or a hearing aid and ensure that the older person has these assistive devices available at all times.

Later in this book, the reader will be able to compare abnormal physiological changes of older adults with the normal changes explained here. You, as a future gerontological nurse, should have a thorough understanding of both aspects of physiological aging.

▶ CONCLUSION

This chapter has pointed out the importance of understanding the older adult in today's society. As the number of aged individuals increases, and as more and more older adults require nursing care, you need to develop a strong knowledge base in gerontological nursing content. It is equally important to explore the myths, stereotypes, and prejudices about old age to begin the process of seeing older adults as unique individuals who have special histories and life experiences. Normal aging changes each person in a unique way. As you acquire the specific knowledge and skills to be an effective caregiver of older adults, it is hoped that you will embrace the attitude that all older adults are unique and should be encouraged to function at their full potential. With this critical understanding, we will comment again that you are the generation of nurses who will define the application of gerontological nursing. Best wishes with the task!

Elderly Navajo couple volunteers 2 days a week to deliver food for Meals on Wheels.

CASE STUDY

Ms. B., 76 years old, lives in a duplex with her 83-year-old sister. Last year, the sister had a mild stroke, leaving her with left-sided weakness. Ms. B. manages the household and coordinates her sister's care, including home health aides, physical and occupational therapy, and visits to the doctor's office.

Ms. B. describes herself as healthy. She also comments, "Okay, I had cancer of the colon 2 years ago, but I had surgery and some chemotherapy too, and now I'm okay. Oh, I sometimes get constipated but that has nothing to do with the cancer."

She states that she tires more easily these days and tries to rest every afternoon. Still, she maintains a full schedule of grocery shopping, visiting friends, cooking and cleaning, and caring for her sister's needs. She has no breathing problems, and her appetite is excellent. "I can't eat as much as I used to at each meal, but my sister and I have a snack in the afternoon and at bedtime."

She does complain about nocturnal voiding two or three times a night and has had two urinary infections this year. "Sometimes I dribble urine, and I use those pads."

Both sisters are always cold; their home is kept very warm, and they always seem to be wearing sweaters and heavy stockings. Every Sunday is beauty day at the B.'s residence, when they apply face and hand cream to dry skin, style their thinning hair, and care for their nails, which are getting thick and brittle. Both claim that they have become shorter in the past few years; Ms. B. often feels weary at night due to joint pain. She has learned to adjust her daily schedule to changes in endurance. No matter where I go, I take my time, sit down, and pace myself. I know where every bench and restaurant is in South Philadelphia.

Ms. B. has noticed that she needs to wear her glasses all the time when reading or paying bills; she invested in 100-watt light bulbs for every lamp " . . . because we both need stronger light to read by these days." She is never without her sunglasses to avoid glare; in fact, every shade is always lowered at their house during the day. Ms. B. claims she does not think as clearly lately " . . . as I used to; it takes me longer to figure things out and make decisions." But she contin-

ues to manage the household and lead an active life.

"I have my friends, my neighborhood, my home, and of course, my sister. We have been together all of our lives. We care about each other and we do pretty well, taking each day as it comes, each day expecting another good day."

Discussion

1. What age-related changes has Ms. B. experienced?
2. Would you consider Ms. B. to be a healthy older adult? Explain.

Solution

1. Ms. B. has experienced age-related changes in all the following areas:

Cardiovascular
   Decreased activity tolerance
   Fatigue with increased activity

Musculoskeletal
   Loss of muscle strength
   Height loss
   Joint pain

Integumentary
   Dry skin
   Brittle, thickened nails
   Thinning hair

Gastrointestinal
   Delayed gastric emptying leading to fullness
   Reduced GI motility

Genitourinary
   Urinary retention, which may contribute to infection
   Urgency and stress incontinence

Nervous
   Delayed reaction time

Special senses
   Diminished ability to focus on close objects
   Inability to tolerate glare
   Poor vision in reduced light

2. Ms. B. is a healthy older adult because she functions at an optimal level despite the presence of age-related changes. She feels good about her life and about her coping skills. She expects continued "good days."

STUDY QUESTIONS

Circle the correct choice(s).

1. Your client is 84 years old. What normal change in vital signs would you expect to assess?
   a. A higher than normal temperature
   b. A slower pulse
   c. A shallower breathing pattern
   d. A lower blood pressure

2. Immobility or sedentary lifestyles have what effect on the older adult?
   a. Loss of muscle size and strength
   b. Decreased serum sodium levels
   c. Loss of skin elasticity
   d. Thinning of cartilage in joints

3. Mrs. Jones, aged 86 years, complains of fullness after eating only small amounts of food. This is primarily due to which gastrointestinal change?
   a. Delayed gastric emptying time
   b. Increased gastric acid secretions
   c. Hypertonicity of gastric muscles
   d. Loss of ability to chew

4. Mrs. Smith, aged 79 years, is admitted to the hospital. Based on your understanding of normal age changes in the nervous system, what behavior might you expect Mrs. Smith to exhibit?
   a. Decreased intellectual function
   b. Forgetfulness and confusion
   c. Lack of orientation to time and place
   d. Longer response time to questions

5. Which of the following statements most accurately describes normal aging changes in the older adult?
   a. As individuals age, they become more diverse.
   b. Most older adults experience chronic illness and functional impairment.
   c. Age-related changes are similar in each older adult.
   d. Normal age changes most commonly describe decline and loss of function.

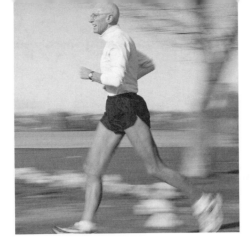

Mary Lou Long

chapter **2**

Promoting Wellness

Learning Objectives

After completing this chapter, the student will be able to:

1. Recognize aging as a normal process of living rather than a disease process.
2. Describe the role nurses play in health-promotion and disease-prevention activities for older people.
3. Describe key health-promotion and disease-prevention activities appropriate for older people.
4. Understand the importance motivation plays in the older person's ability to participate in health-promotion and disease-prevention activities.

► INTRODUCTION

One of the positive aspects of being a gerontological nurse is the variety of ways you are able to work with older people. The role of the licensed practical nurse (LPN) is critical in the care of older adults. You are the person who gives the direct care to most of the older adults who seek out health-care services. Many nurses think only of care given in a nursing home when they consider gerontological nursing, yet you have learned that only 5% of people older age 65 are at these institutions. Where are the others? What type of nursing care do they need? Many older adults need your knowledge and support in order to stay healthy. That is health promotion; something exciting and, for many nurses, something new.

The search for eternal youth has a long history. People have died in their search for the Fountain of Youth, and others have killed for what they thought would prevent them from aging. The legends surrounding the "forever young" concept are taking on a new reality and meaning for this country's aging society because people are living to be older than ever before (remember the 85+ age group and the "elite old?"). The modern version of the legend of the Fountain of Youth is embodied in the concept of health promotion. The focus is on living longer and healthier, an opportunity offered to today's society that has not existed previously.

Our society emphasizes normal age-related changes and common health problems and diseases experienced by older people. In addition, information is shared on dealing with losses related to aging, the medical treatment of chronic disease, and the financial impact of an aging society. It is our opinion that not enough attention has been given to the positive side of aging and the beneficial effects of health-promotion activities to prevent disease and to slow the effects of chronic disease. Do you think this is another form of ageism? If so, what can you do about it as a nurse?

Current health-care concepts emphasize vitality and independence for older people as a primary concern. Regardless of age, as people laugh more, walk more, eat better, relax more, and think better of themselves and their relationships, they move beyond the neutral point of good health. Many of the complaints associated with the aging process, such as joint stiffness, weight gain, fatigue, loss of bone mass, and loneliness, can be

CRITICALLY EXAMINE THE FOLLOWING:

Reread the last paragraph of the introduction. Your health would improve if you improved the management of your personal exercise, stress management, nutrition, substance abuse, relationships, and self-care. As a student in a very demanding program, you may need to examine your own health promotion critically. Make comments regarding how you can improve your health in the following areas. Be prepared to discuss them in class and relate how what you do for yourself may also assist an older adult.

1. Exercise
2. Stress management
3. Nutrition
4. Substance abuse
5. Relationships
6. Self-care

prevented or managed by basic health-promotion activities. One does not have to be free of disease to experience the benefits of health and wellness.

Most health-promotion activities focus on exercise, stress management, nutrition, and dealing with substance abuse. In addition, it is important that wellness activities for older adults include relationships and self-care.

► CHRONIC DISEASE

As an LPN giving care to older adults, you need to understand the promotion of wellness in a broad sense. This concept needs to go beyond the vision of physically well, older people living in their own homes independently. More than 80% of older adults experience at least one chronic disease condition, and as many as 50% report three chronic disease condition. Those older than 85 years old experience increased difficulty with home management activities and are more likely to depend on assistance in their living situations. Regardless of age, living arrangement, or health condition, the goal for health promotion should be to assist older adults to reach a state of optimal health—the legendary Fountain of Youth.

The most common health problems of older adults are associated with chronic disease. The most frequent of these chronic conditions include arthritis, hypertension, heart conditions, hearing impairments, and dementia. Because of these conditions, older people visit physicians more, are hospitalized more frequently, take more prescription and over-the-counter (OTC) drugs, and experience more functional problems than younger people. The focus of much of this country's medical treatment interventions is *curing* acute conditions. Chronic illnesses, the predominate Illnesses of older adults, cannot be cured but instead require management with a focus on caring.

TREATMENT STRATEGIES

Management of chronic conditions involves treating symptoms and maximizing the strengths of an older person. You need to understand the aging process and older adults in general, and then advocate and lobby for what they need. For example, for an older adult who suffers from arthritis and is in severe pain, it is important to treat the symptom of pain. If pain is minimized, the person will be better able to stay active and prevent the further disabling effects of immobility. Nurses are the key people to recognize the symptom (pain) and administer the prescribed treatment (medication). As a gerontological nurse, you must go one step further and consider the impact of the disease and its treatment on the older person's ability to perform activities of daily living (ADLs) and instrumental activities of daily living (IADL).

What could be done to prevent the onset of pain?
What will be the side effects of the pain medication?

As an LPN, you must recognize the importance of good health and its correlation with functional independence among older people; however, understanding does not always make it clear as to the kind of activities that will promote health and prevent development of

further secondary conditions that result in dependency.

▶ ILLNESS/WELLNESS AS A CONTINUUM

If you think of health as a continuum in which illness is on one end and health on the other, you will better understand the importance of health promotion. The point is that everyone wants health, and health-promotion activities are the way to achieve that goal. Physicians and nurses traditionally focus on working with patients who are on the illness end of the continuum or who have symptoms of disease or disability. As a person's health improves, traditional medicine becomes less involved in helping the person reach optimal well-being. In contrast, health-promotion efforts primarily are focused on the opposite, or wellness, side of the continuum.

In more recent years, nurses have begun to use health-promotion efforts even when dealing with people on the illness side of the continuum. For example, special exercise and nutrition programs have been designed for cardiac rehabilitation, exercise and weight-lifting programs for chair-bound persons, and weight management programs for older persons. The remainder of this chapter focuses on health-promotion activities on both the illness and wellness sides of the health continuum.

MOTIVATION

If you, as a nurse, want to be successful in promoting healthy choices in individuals in their later years, you need to understand the importance of individual motivation. Desire must be present on the part of the older adult to make a change. It is critical to explore what motivates an older person to eat right, exercise, and avoid unhealthy behaviors on an individual basis. This is true for all people, even yourself.

As a part of human behavior, motivation is the incentive or drive that causes a person to act. Incentives to take action are based on needs and desires that are both internal and external to the person. For example, an older person may have an incentive to exercise three times a week if it helps the individual experience less discomfort or immobility from arthritis. For some people, the incentive may need to be more than physical wellness. A need also may exist for a mental wellness experience, such as that derived from socialization with others while exercising, for example, in a water aerobic class or with a group doing mall walking.

The nursing challenge is to assist older adults to identify their own incentives for participation in health-promotion and disease-prevention activities. This allows the nurse to have greater insight into ways to promote health and lessens the frustration experienced from what are often incorrectly referred to as *noncompliant patients*. Compliance occurs only if the individual can personally identify a need or desire to exercise, eat correctly, reduce stress, or make other changes necessary for improved wellness. This is the motivation experienced by people in an individual way. Often, assisting to identify the motivation is one way you, the LPN, can help the older adult.

INCENTIVES

Studies have disclosed some of the reasons (incentives) for older people to participate in health-promotion behaviors. These reasons include the following:

- A belief that activities can improve fitness and health
- The enjoyment of socialization
- A belief that activities will help maintain independence
- A desire to feel good and have fun

Knowledge about why a person participates in health promotion (or the incentives for doing so) can be determined through a caring and focused interview. After personal incentives have been identified, you can reinforce them in health-promotion activities. In addition to understanding individual motivation, you will need to help individuals plan their short- and long-term goals for making health changes. The secret to success in health behavior is to assist the older adult pick personal goals with care and then learn to enjoy achieving them.

HEALTH-PROMOTION ACTIVITIES

When older adults have identified an area of health, they have an incentive to maintain or improve, the challenge is to locate a properly designed activity. Many current health-promotion activities are biased for youth and have excluded older adults by design. Four reasons underscore why the current focus on health-promotion activities is often inappropriate for older people. They are as follows:

1. The focus frequently is on life extension or on reducing the risks of premature death. For example, if a person stops smoking, reduces fat intake, and exercises, the risk of a heart attack at an early age is reduced. For elderly people who have already lived beyond the average life expectancy, life extension may not be as important as quality of life. Stopping smoking, reducing fat intake, and exercising are important at any age, but for different reasons. The focus must be on health-promotion benefits specific to an older person.
2. Emphasis is often placed on advancing "youthfulness" and preventing aging. Older people recognize that they do not fit the image of youth and have already experienced some results of aging. This does not mean self-image and appearance are not important to older people, but that the image needs to match the older person's self-perception.
3. Health-promotion programs focus on preventing chronic disease. Among older people, 50% already have three chronic diseases. When these programs focus on management of the symptoms of the disease rather than on its prevention, more older adults have a reason to participate.
4. A focus on self-responsibility for health fails to consider the limitations imposed by personal circumstances. For example, an individual who has a need and desire to walk daily for exercise may live in an unsafe neighborhood. An older adult may have a desire to eat a healthy diet but be unable to afford the proper food. The external environment may pose barriers to older people that are difficult to overcome. These problems need careful attention.

As you, the LPN, look at the key areas of health promotion for older people, your goal must be to design, plan, and provide activities that are sensitive to individual needs and responsibility. Properly designed health-promotion activities should be:

- Accessible (transportation, time of day, location)
- Enjoyable and social (mental and physical wellness)
- Reasonable (focus on the right activity for the right reason)
- Sensitive to older people's needs (hearing, vision, functional level)

Health-promotion strategies must be based on the belief that the individual is the only one who can choose a path to a healthy life. Consequently, you, the nurse, must be sure that health-promotion activities are individually designed so the pathways exist.

▶ NUTRITION

With advancing age, a person's general health is determined to a great extent by the effects of dietary patterns over the years. Staying physically and mentally active is important to all older adults. They need to understand the role proper nutrition plays in their lives, even in later years.

As bodies age, four changes occur that affect what a person needs to have optimum nutrition:

1. The body's rate of metabolism slows and no longer needs the same amount of energy and food to do the same amount of work. Older adults often comment they have not changed how they are eating and exercising, but they are now gaining weight. As people age, lean body mass decreases and body fat increases. This may result in weight gain and can lead to obesity.
2. The senses of taste and smell may be less keen. Some or all of an elderly person's teeth may need to be replaced by dental appliances. As a result, older people may find themselves eating different foods and drinking less fluid.

3. Social aspects of eating are important. As people age, they retire, families grow up and move, and spouses and friends die. This results in changes in the socialization of eating. One of the most difficult adjustments seems to be cooking for one and eating alone.
4. Environmental factors greatly influence older adult's nutritional habits. Lack of transportation to food stores and restaurants, inability to manage reading labels and shopping, and insufficient money to buy healthy food can be major barriers to eating properly.

Poor dietary habits contribute to many diseases that occur in older persons. Chronic diseases, such as heart disease and cancer, can be slowed, and for some people prevented, by avoiding obesity and decreasing the amount of fat in one's diet. Studies from the American Heart Association (2001) suggest high cholesterol levels increase the risk for atherosclerosis. The American Cancer Society found marked increases in the incidence of cancer of the uterus, gallbladder, kidney, stomach, colon, and breast associated with obesity.

Osteoporosis affects 25% of women older than 60 years of age. The loss of bone mass and bone strength as a result of this disease leads to broken hips, arms, legs, and back injuries. Osteoporosis is often referred to as a "silent" disease. Few signs or symptoms appear until a bone breaks. Adding calcium to the diet, a regular exercise regimen, avoidance of alcohol and smoking, and for women, estrogen replacement therapy are key prevention strategies.

Other chronic problems that are frequent complaints of older people include constipation, urinary incontinence, and arthritis. Nutrition plays a role in each of these conditions.

Although one-on-one teaching may be easier, group learning that incorporates an opportunity for socialization and fun is much more likely to result in positive outcomes. You, as the LPN, may want to organize a group of elderly people in the community to participate in learning nutrition principles. One of the principles that should be taught is that of the food pyramid (Fig. 2.1). This information, which is new to some people, replaced the basic four concepts that most older people have been taught.

Health-promotion activities aimed at altering a lifetime of eating habits must be reasonable, and the benefits need to be made apparent. Nurses must clearly understand what motivates the individual. In addition, they must be aware of the unique nutritional needs and problems that accompany later years.

▶ EXERCISE AND FITNESS

The 1970s saw the beginning of the fitness movement in the United States. Not until the late 1970s and early 1980s did society begin to stress the importance of fitness for older adults. Studies continue to emphasize the benefits of exercise and its importance to total health for all ages. The body's responses to exercise are fundamentally the same throughout life. Exercise stimulates the mind, maintains fitness, prevents or slows progression of some diseases, helps to establish social contacts, and generally improves the quality of life.

Fatigue and lack of energy, poor sleeping habits, and poor circulation are common reports of older adults. These problems often result in inactivity. Inactivity leads to muscle wasting and weakening of the bones. This vicious circle results in disabling conditions and functional dependency. If exercise could be packed into a pill, it would be the single most widely prescribed and beneficial medicine in the world. Chronic conditions such as heart disease, diabetes, osteoporosis, arthritis, obesity, and depression are all shown to improve or experience a slowing of progression with regular physical activity.

Physiologically, a regular exercise program can build and maintain muscle strength and endurance, and can improve the capacity of the heart, circulatory system, and lungs. The commonly heard phrase "Use it or lose it" is the overall theme for exercise and fitness in a person's later years. Exercise programs for people older than 60 years of age should emphasize a regular routine of exercise to expand and increase strength, flexibility, and endurance. This can be accomplished for individuals with a wide range of conditions, from wheelchair- or bed-bound frail elderly patients to the physically active individuals. Byproducts of a good fitness program include

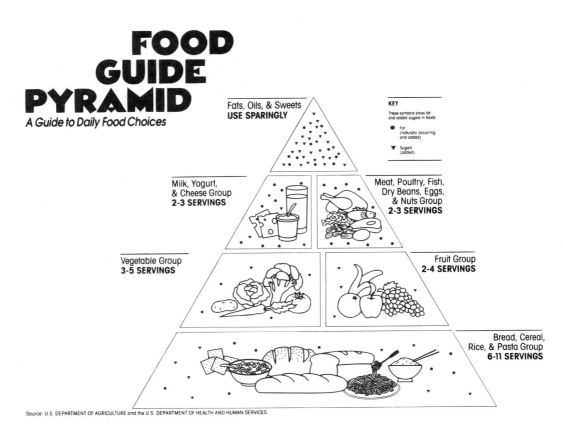

FIG. 2.1. Food guide pyramid: a guide to daily food choices. (From U.S. Department of Agriculture and U.S. Department of Health and Human Services.)

increased energy, buildup of lean body mass, and increased self-esteem.

STRENGTHENING

Strengthening exercises help build and maintain muscle condition by moving muscles against resistance. Simple strengthening exercises are needed to promote activity without tiring a person too easily. Muscle strength is also crucial to the support of joints and can help prevent problems related to arthritis. Improving muscle strength is a primary objective in slowing the progression of osteoporosis. Patients confined to bed lose bone mass very quickly. It can be restored, however, when exercise is resumed. Something as simple as doing range-of-motion exercises while holding a soup can will make a difference in strength for most older adults.

As a nurse, you must be aware of the impact a short-term illness can have on an older person. Something as commonplace as the flu can cause significant weakness and inactivity. Weak muscles lead to falls, which cause hip fractures and other injuries. If older adults are not aware of the importance of strengthening exercises, no incentive will be able to return them to the normal level of function.

Strength-building exercises are important for the patient with diabetes because the exercises help regulate glucose metabolism by increasing muscle mass. The greater the muscle mass, the greater the glycogen level in the muscles will be and the more energy in reserve for periods of exertion.

FLEXIBILITY

Flexibility exercises involve slow stretching motions. Medical and fitness experts agree that stretching is the single most important part of an exercise program designed to prevent injuries, reduce muscle tension, and maintain range of motion. As a result of the normal aging process, muscles tend to lose elasticity and tissues around the joints thicken. Flexibility exercises can delay or reverse this process by preventing muscles from becoming short and tight.

All stretching motions should be done gradually and slowly, without any sudden force or jerking motion. You should encourage a variety of stretching exercises for different parts of the body including arms, shoulders, back, chest, stomach, buttocks, thighs, and calves. All exercise routines should warm up and cool down with 5 to 15 minutes of stretching exercises. As the older person's range of motion increases, the individual will be able to reach, turn, and move in all directions with more grace and less pain.

ENDURANCE

Endurance-building or aerobic exercises improve the function of the heart, lungs, and blood vessels. A frequent report of older people is "feeling tired." Endurance-building exercises help strengthen the heart to pump blood and the lungs to exchange oxygen, and also increase the elasticity of blood vessels. These functions are a vital part of fitness and feeling good. Walking, cycling, and swimming or water aerobic exercises are excellent all-around exercises.

As stated earlier, the basic components of an exercise routine for older people include strengthening, flexibility, and endurance. In addition, attention must also be given to the simple act of breathing during exercising. Breathing is a vital part of an exercise program. As a person concentrates on the exercise, it is easy to forget to breathe. The correct breathing technique is to breathe out during vigorous effort or exertion, and breathe in as the muscles relax.

Roll breathing is also a good way to reduce tension and to induce relaxation. As a result of changes related to aging, some older people experience a general loss of elasticity of the chest muscles and some postural changes. These gradual changes often affect the way they breathe. This is especially true for frail

BOX 2.1. ROLL BREATHING

The object of roll breathing is to develop full use of the lungs. It can be practiced in any position but is best learned lying down, with the knees bent.

1. Place your left hand on your abdomen and your right hand on your chest. Notice how your hands move as you breathe in and out.

2. Practice filling your lower lungs by breathing so that your left hand goes up and down while your right hand remains still. Always inhale through your nose and exhale through your mouth.

3. When you have filled and emptied your lower lungs 8 to10 times with ease, add the second step to your breathing: Inhale first into your lower lungs as before but then continue inhaling into your upper chest. As you do so, your right hand will rise and your left hand will fall a little as your stomach is drawn in.

4. As you slowly exhale through your mouth, make a quiet, relaxing whooshing sound as first your left hand and then your right hand falls. Exhale and feel the tension leaving your body as you become more and more relaxed.

5. Practice breathing in and out in this manner for 3 to 5 minutes. Notice that the movement of your abdomen and chest is like the rolling motion of waves rising and falling in a rhythmic motion.

Roll breathing should be practiced daily for several weeks until it can be done almost anywhere, providing you with an instant relaxation tool anytime you need one. Caution: Some people get dizzy the first few times they try roll breathing. Get up slowly and with support.

Source: Reprinted with permission from Kemper, D. W., Deneen, J. E., Giuffré J. V. *Growing younger handbook* (2nd ed.). © Copyright 1992 HEALTHWISE, Incorporated, P.O. Box 1989, Boise, ID 83701. Copying of any portion of this material is not permitted without express written permission of HEALTHWISE, Incorporated.

and bed-bound elderly. The roll-breathing exercises outlined in Box 2.1 encourage deep breathing and are very helpful as a relaxation technique and a component of an exercise program.

A last comment on exercise is a caution for older adults who have not been exercising on a regular basis, who are frail, or who have cardiovascular problems. Anyone with heart problems or high blood pressure, who is overweight, or who has been told to be cautious in personal activity level should have an exercise program prescribed by a physician.

Physical fitness is one component of life that enables people to live to its fullest. As a nurse, you have a responsibility to understand and teach the importance of exercise and fitness to the elderly population.

STRESS

Stress motivates people to act, forces them to think under pressure, and challenges them to be creative, resourceful human beings. The key is to be able to strike a balance between too much stress and not enough, between positive stress (*eustress*) and stress that is harmful (*distress*).

As with all areas of health promotion, it is never too late to improve a technique. Failure to take a healthy approach to dealing with stress can greatly increase the risk of developing or worsening heart disease, cancer, and other chronic diseases.

For most older people, stress is related to three basic areas: environment, body, and mind. Environmental stressors are weather, crime, crowds, time pressures, and the demands of others. The human body can experience stress due to illness, accidents, drugs, lack of sleep, and the normal changes related to aging. Finally, the mind can create stress for people because of negative attitudes and perceptions, boredom, despair, and hopelessness.

Regularly occurring events such as trips to

the grocery store, pain from arthritis, and fear of the unknown conditions of retirement may all create stress for older people. Stress-related problems and symptoms include ulcers (stomach pain), high blood pressure (no symptoms), arthritis (joint pain, muscle tension), heart disease (chest pain, difficulty breathing), cancer (increased susceptibility), headaches (constant worry), circulatory problems (cold hands and feet), and backaches (muscle spasm and chronic pain).

One of the most important strategies for health promotion is to help older people recognize their personal reactions to stress and their bodies' physiological responses. Tools used to recognize stress are a stress log or journal of daily stressful situations, life change inventory, and stress control inventory.

After an individual has recognized personal stress and his or her personal response to it, several interventions are available to help relieve it. As a nurse, you should understand and be able to recommend appropriate stress-reducing activities. These activities may be divided into the two categories of quick relaxers and long-term stress management skills.

A quickie relaxer is something a person can do in 2 or 3 minutes to relax and counteract symptoms of distress. One of the most important, yet difficult, skills for some older people is learning simply to relax. Learning how to relax helps older people sleep better, control blood pressure, lower cholesterol, reduce headaches, relieve depression, reduce or eliminate use of drugs and alcohol, and smile more. Examples of quick relaxers include roll breathing, progressive muscle relaxation, imagining a pleasant place or situation, eye relaxation, and exercise. The importance of exercise was discussed earlier in this chapter; however, it is worth emphasizing that exercise is the most natural way to relax. For the greatest calming effect, the elderly individual can combine fitness activities with breathing and other mental relaxation techniques.

For some older people, dealing with stress requires more than a few "stress-buster" quickie techniques. If stress causes continuous physical and mental discomfort that results in illness, learning how to deal with the source of stress needs to be a major goal. This assumes that the individual understands what is causing the stress.

Using the four stress management options listed here as a teaching tool is very helpful for many people. The four basic options are:

1. Attempt symptom relief (quick techniques).
2. Accept the stressor (change perception or attitude). *Example*: Your children frequently call you at the last minute to babysit your grandchildren. You may accept the stress and decide you really do not need much time to prepare, so say yes and enjoy! Another choice is to lovingly say No!
3. Alter the stressor (change or alter the source of stress so it is no longer there). *Example*: Make the decision that you will not be able to babysit unless they let you know 1 day ahead of time.
4. Avoid the stressor (remove yourself from the stressor). *Example*: Decide you will not be a babysitter for your grandchildren. After the source of stress has been pinpointed, the older person often can decide whether to accept, alter, or avoid it.

Stress management techniques may not be familiar to many older individuals, even though stress and recognition of stress have been buzz words for some time. Teaching older people stress management can be done very successfully through either group or individual activities.

▶ LIFESTYLES

Maintaining a healthy lifestyle at any age involves more than getting fit, eating right, and coping with stress. Other challenging

Golfing, walking, and dancing provide exercise that promotes strengthening, flexibility, and endurance.

issues that people of all ages encounter are relationships, possible alcohol and drug abuse, and self-care.

RELATIONSHIPS

Human life is constantly defined and redefined by our ties to others. The term *relationship* means any significant bonding in which a person feels a strong sense of responsibility toward the physical and emotional welfare of others.

As people grow older, the reality is that all relationships eventually end. Whether through divorce or death of a spouse, child, family, friend, or pet, the loss redefines your life. An individual's ability to deal with the process of grief over the losses can result in significant personal and health changes, as well as changes in dealing with others. How strongly these changes affect the rest of one's

life depends on how well the person, and those in the personal life of an individual, cope with the loss. How people have coped with change and crisis in younger years predicts how they will deal with these same stressors later .

As years pass, life changes can become increasingly complex. Older adults must deal with changes, due to retirement, that have major impacts on home life, health, finances, and role changes. In addition, the loss of relationships may be frequent and numerous.

As a nurse, you have an opportunity to help older adults gain insight into loss and life change. Refer to Chapter 6 on End-of-Life Changes. It contains a section on the stages of grief that may be helpful to you in understanding the reactions to loss of older adults. You must assess the effect loss has on a person's ability to function with day-to-day activities. As an LPN, you must ask questions and allow the older person to share concerns. Health-promotion activities that focus on mental wellness can provide an excellent opportunity for older adults to express the concerns they face. The American Association of Retired Persons (AARP) preretirement program offers a useful notebook that helps lead discussions about the myths, fears, and reality of change as one grows older.

ALCOHOL, DRUGS, AND AGING

Abuse of alcohol and drugs among older men and women is a more serious problem than most people realize. Until recently, older problem drinkers tended to be ignored by both health professionals and the general public. The neglect occurred for several reasons:

- This country's elderly population was small, and few older individuals were identified as alcoholics.
- Chronic problem drinkers (those who had abused alcohol off and on for most of their lives) often died before old age.
- Because they often are retired or have few social contacts, older people frequently have been able to hide drinking problems.

Some families may unknowingly accept or encourage drinking in older family members. They may have the attitude that drinking should be tolerated because older people have only a limited time left to live and should be allowed to enjoy themselves. Sometimes the alcohol consumption seems to be an insignificant amount to the family, and they blame the resulting impairment on aging.

The amount, time, and place of alcohol consumption have little significance. What alcohol does to an individual's quality of life and functional ability is the critical issue that needs to be addressed. Older problem drinkers seem to be in two types. The first are chronic abusers, those who have used alcohol heavily throughout life. Approximately two thirds of older alcoholics are in this group. The second type begins excessive drinking late in life, often in response to situational factors such as retirement, lowered income, declining health, or the deaths of friends and loved ones. In these cases, alcohol is first used for temporary relief but later becomes a problem.

The physical effects of alcohol are significant for older people. Alcohol impairs mental alertness, judgment, physical coordination, and reaction time. These problems mimic and exacerbate the deleterious effects of other chronic conditions (dementia, depression, and arthritis) and increase the risks of falls and other accidents.

As people age, they appear to become less tolerant of even small amounts of alcohol, and moreover, the effect of alcohol on the body may be unusual. For example, the effects of alcohol on the cardiovascular system may mask the pain of an oncoming heart attack. Older people are the greatest consumers of prescription and OTC drugs. The combined use of alcohol and drugs increases the likelihood of a toxic or lethal affect.

Treatment efforts for older alcoholic people have not been fruitful. It is easy to overlook or accept problem drinking as a device that offers enjoyment or comfort. It is much harder to create social alternatives to the life events that lie behind alcoholism.

As a health professional, you may be tempted to rush over or omit assessment questions referring to alcohol intake. Because the nurse often plays a key role in recognizing alcohol and drug problems, you cannot afford to avoid such questions. You always should ask what the impact of this problem may be on the older person's ability to function. It becomes easy to see that the physical, mental, and social impact of drinking could contribute to alcohol dependency.

The primary health-promotion goal is helping older adults and their families recognize when alcohol is a problem. Second, straightforward information must be given to seniors regarding the effects of alcohol, especially in combination with drugs. The nurse must understand the older person's reason for drinking. Health-promotion activities that create social alternatives can be made available to the older person with an alcohol problem.

Owing to their critical importance, drug issues are covered extensively in another chapter; however, emphasis on the problem of drug dependency and abuse is important. Drug abuse depends on the relationship of the individual to the drug in question. Harmful drug relationships are frequently termed *overmedication*, *dependency*, *abuse*, *problem usage*, and *habituation*. Regardless of the reason, if an older person misuses a drug or becomes dependent on it, the effects are similar to those of problem drinking. Physical and mental impairments resulting from prescribed or OTC drugs mimic disease states and increase the risk of falls, accidents, and dependency.

One role of health promotion is to offer education and screening regarding drug use. Promoting self-responsibility is the key component. Once again, nurses must assess the impact of drug treatment on the older person's ability to complete ADLs. For example, if your patient cannot afford a prescribed drug, then it probably will not be taken as ordered. If the older adult does not understand what outcomes are expected from the drug treatment, misuse of a drug may ensue by taking it for too long or taking too much of it.

▶ SELF-CARE—TAKING CHARGE

Older adults are best qualified to keep themselves healthy and to know when they are ill. As a nurse, you need to respect and explore what the older person reports as the problem. Do not take charge and deny an older adult responsibility for personal health and health management.

Self-care, *self-help*, and *self-maintenance* are terms often used interchangeably to describe various aspects of an individual's efforts to maintain optimal health and functionality. From a nursing perspective, the focus is frequently on ADLs, the most basic self-care activities engaged in by older adults. It is not uncommon to see dependence in at least some basic ADLs for older people. Surveys show that as many as 18% of those over 65 years of age, who live in the community, are dependent in at least one ADL. In nursing homes, the prevalence is as high as 80%. In addition to ADLs, the older person needs to manage IADLs such as selecting a physician and other health-care providers, and knowing how and when to access the health-care system.

Regardless of whether the senior is attempting to overcome a functional deficit in ADLs or IADLs, the same self-care skills are needed. The art of self-care involves:

Accepting personal responsibility for your own health
Adopting healthy lifestyle habits with regard to fitness, relaxation, and nutrition
Learning how to make the changes you choose to make to do the things you want to do

Accepting personal responsibility for health behaviors applies to the "why" of the decision more than the "what." "Self-responsibility" means that the older adult does not rely solely on spouse, children, physician, or nurse to determine "what to do to be healthy." The person must be allowed to think through the options and make each decision. This does not mean a person should not seek the assistance of others, but rather that a need exists

Regardless of whether the senior is attempting to overcome a deficit in activities of daily living or make a medical decision, the person needs self-care skills.

to work in partnership with the doctor, nurse, or family (separately or together) to make the best decision.

The self-care concept emphasizes the need for encouraging individuals to take a more active role in maintaining or improving their health. Often, this process is not understood by the client, nor is it easy for older people to accomplish. Health-promotion strategies related to self-care must include helping the older adult understand how to be in charge of personal health decisions. Enabling the older person to be a wise medical consumer, and to know how and when to work and communicate as a partner with the health-care team, should be a focus of your efforts.

Your role as a health professional is twofold. First, you must offer activities to develop self-care skills: for example, one-on-one or group activities that teach how to be an informed medical consumer, or information on prevention and screening guidelines, for instance, for a mammogram or a prostate examination. Then you must ensure that the environment allows for the older adult to use the skills to make choices and assume self-responsibility. For example, if the senior wants to be a partner with the physician in a health decision, the physician should take the time to answer questions and ultimately let the treatment decision be made by the older adult. This same situation applies to nursing. For example, if the senior is expected to be involved in a self-care activity program, you, as a nurse, must be prepared to explain the benefits, procedures, and risks, and then be willing to let the senior make the decision.

▶ CONCLUSION

Until recently, older adult's needs have been ignored in the health-promotion movement. Health professionals mistakenly assumed elders had no interest in health-promotion programs. As this country has become more and more home to an aging society, these views have changed.

As a nurse, you must understand the importance of promoting wellness to all older adults, regardless of the presence or absence of disease. Attainment of a disease-free existence is not a realistic goal. Health-promotion efforts should be directed toward maintaining functional independence for older people.

Older Americans need information about how to lead healthy lifestyles. When such information and opportunity are provided, older people are willing to make the changes necessary to improve their health. Exercising regularly, maintaining a nutritious diet, managing stress effectively, taking medications safely, avoiding overuse of alcohol, and recognizing self-care as a choice are all behaviors that improve health and the quality of life. Pursuit of high-level wellness in later years is the responsibility of both the individual and society.

CASE STUDY

Mrs. C. is a 65-year-old widow who has lived alone since the death of her husband 2 years ago. She retired 1 year ago from her job of 25 years as a secretary. After retirement, she participated in a health promotion and screening clinic at the senior center. After completing a lifestyle inventory and screening, the following problems were noted in the categories of health promotion:

Nutrition: 10 lb overweight

Exercise: Does no regular exercise

Stress: Cries easily, often unable to sleep at night, complains of fatigue and generally low energy

Relationships: Misses people at work, talks about missing deceased husband

Substance abuse: Takes an OTC sleeping pill and one glass of wine before bed

Self-care: Has not seen a physician since she had a hysterectomy 10 years ago; never had a mammogram and does not perform breast self-examination; cannot recall immunization history but is sure she has not had any in the past 10 years; has never had a flu shot or pneumococcal vaccine; recently had blood pressure taken at a drug store machine, when it was 150/92.

Discussion

1. List additional assessment data that should be known in each of the categories of health promotion.
2. How might you determine Mrs. C.'s greatest concern?
3. What part does Mrs. C.'s motivation play in developing a wellness plan?
4. What conditions or disease states might develop if Mrs. C. continues with no changes in her life?
5. What might be the first priority for Mrs. C.?

Solution

1. Additional information in each category might include:

Nutrition

What are her daily eating habits? Type and amount of food and fluids? Does she eat alone?

Exercise

What is her normal daily activity level? How does this differ from her daily activity level before retirement?

Stress

What is her perception of coping with changes such as death and retirement? Any other physical complaints made, such as fatigue, headaches?

Relationships

What family or friends are important to her? In what social activities is she involved? Any hobbies?

Substance Abuse

When did she begin drinking wine every evening? When did her sleeping problems begin? Has she always taken sleeping pills?

Self-care

Does she have a primary care physician? Does she understand the importance of exercise, disease prevention? Does she know the danger of combining drugs and alcohol?

2. Asking Mrs. C. "What is your biggest worry or concern in your life at this time?" would be a beginning. Although the nurse may see many areas of concern, Mrs. C.'s own concerns are more critical.

3. If the nurse begins by focusing on what Mrs. C. considers most important, then it is easier for Mrs. C. to understand her own motivation.

4. Some potential conditions include:

Excess weight, which may lead or contribute to high blood pressure and physical limitation.

Lack of exercise, which may contribute to weight gain but also worsen arthritis and its effects on mobility.

Emotional stress, which may lead to depression.

Relationship concerns, which also may contribute to depression, isolation, and abuse of drugs and alcohol.

Combination of alcohol and OTC sleeping pills, which may lead to further sleeping problems, alcohol and drug misuse, depression, injury, and further isolation.

5. If Mrs. C. has not seen a physician for 10 years, she needs at least a baseline physical assessment. She has some significant conditions that need to be addressed such as borderline high blood pressure, sleep problems, and weight gain. In addition, she should have a basic screening related to disease prevention.

STUDY QUESTIONS

Circle the correct choice(s) to complete each statement.

1. Incentives for older persons to participate in health-promotion behaviors include:
   a. The belief that they will find the Fountain of Youth
   b. The belief that activities will help them die well
   c. The belief that activities will help keep them independent
   d. The belief that it will please their physician

2. Health-promotion programs appropriate for older people should focus on:
   a. Maintaining functional abilities
   b. Advancing youthfulness
   c. Enhancing chronic illnesses
   d. Developing dependence on others for care

3. Basic components of an exercise routine for older people are:
   a. Strengthening, endurance, and flexibility
   b. Strengthening, dieting, and power walking
   c. Strengthening, dieting, and aerobics
   d. Strengthening, aerobics, and the food pyramid

4. Age-related changes that affect nutrition include:
   a. Increase in the ability to taste
   b. Increase in body fat
   c. Increase in lean body mass
   d. Increased metabolic rate because of aging thyroid

5. Older people with a drinking problem are often ignored because:
   a. They have many social opportunities to drink.
   b. The amount of alcohol consumed may seem small.
   c. The resulting impairment may seem to be age related.
   d. So many older people do drink.

Mary Ann Anderson
Tamara Chase

chapter 3

The Management Role of the Licensed Practical/Vocational Nurse

Learning Objectives

After completing this chapter, the student will be able to:

1. Identify three management styles commonly used and determine the style that is most effective in gerontological settings.
2. Express an overall understanding of communication techniques and their use.
3. Describe two methods for managing stressful communications.
4. Describe the planning hoop and its use in setting priorities.
5. Identify three common errors made in doing employee evaluations.
6. Define Total Quality Management and explain its importance.

▶ INTRODUCTION

Administering excellent care to frail and ill individuals through the mechanism of an interdisciplinary team and, frequently, a mass of bureaucratic paperwork, requires management skills of the highest level. This is the challenge of today's licensed practical nurse (LPN): successful administration of managed care to older adults in all settings. Certain skills are critical for LPNs to master in order for you to function successfully in the management arena of health-care delivery. This chapter is designed to introduce such skills as they are used within the realm of gerontological nursing.

Some people believe that LPNs are not qualified to be managers, yet many are placed on units as charge nurses. I have worked with LPNs over my nearly 40 years of nursing and have found your colleagues to be excellent. I remember working night shift as a new graduate when an astute LPN saved the life of a surgical patient. He would have died without her critical observation and intervention. The very fact that you manage patient or resident care makes you a nurse manager. I am proud of you and what you can and will do in this wonderful profession of nursing.

▶ MANAGEMENT ROLES

The management role of the LPN is one that changes constantly, along with changes in the health-care delivery scene. It is challenging to be an LPN prepared to assume the responsibility of management. You need to recognize that the work of a licensed nurse always involves leadership skills, and the scope of responsibility frequently changes.

In some nursing homes, LPNs are directors of nursing, whereas in some hospitals, they are not allowed to administer medications. This diversity in scope of responsibility is important to understand. If a registered nurse (RN) is on the health-care team, the LPN is responsible to the RN. This is always true because of the dictates of licensure. It is possible for an RN and an LPN to have the same job description in an organization, just as it is possible for an LPN to be the director of nursing or shift supervisor. Always keep in mind that even if you and an RN have the same job description, you have different licensure; the licensure and its scope of practice are critical for you always to follow.

Look at the residents and staff in this picture. Nonverbal communication is shown clearly in each face.

The LPN should clarify, at the time of employment, the scope of responsibility and role expected to be fulfilled. Determining that the duties assigned are not in conflict with the State Nurse Practice Act also is important. As licensed nurses, all LPNs are responsible for knowing the law governing their practice. This responsibility should not be delegated to a supervisor or another nurse.

▶ MANAGEMENT STYLES

Every individual has a personal management style. This comes from the lessons learned while maturing as a person and a nurse. Nevertheless, to be a successful nurse manager, it is important to understand various management styles and master those that are most effective for you.

Three basic styles of leadership need to be understood. In addition, other leadership styles exist, and many leadership theories have been proposed. The LPN nurse manager needs to understand the basic styles and be flexible enough to incorporate other information as it becomes pertinent. The overall objective for understanding the basic styles of leadership is for the LPN to determine an effective but flexible leadership style for professional use.

AUTHORITARIAN

In the strictest sense, authoritarianism functions with a high concern for tasks done and low concern for the people who perform those tasks (Anderson, 2001). People with this leadership style work well as assembly line managers in a setting where the employees are not in a job that requires individuality, and the machinery is critical to the production of the workload. Does this description cause you to have a feeling of concern when considering an authoritarian management style for a gerontological care environment?

The authoritarian or autocratic leader tends to make all decisions in the work environment and then simply orders the employees to follow the decisions that have been made. The manager is one who has worked hard to create a power base and does not relinquish it to employees. Generally, this type of manager sees employees as irresponsible and lazy. That opinion of employees is the manager's personal justification for the control placed over them.

An authoritarian manager does not allow for creative thinking or new ideas. No opportunities are presented to try new concepts on a patient/resident care plan unless the idea is the manager's own. This type of manager is more interested in seeing that the work is done rather than that the patients are being lovingly cared for and their individual needs met. As an example of this type of management, the workload plan would require baths to be completed by 11:00 A.M. instead of treating the patients as individuals and allowing them autonomy in planning their morning care.

Situations do exist in which this type of management style is critical for success, for instance, during an emergency! If a visitor or older adult fell to the floor in cardiac arrest, this type of manager would take over, give orders, and in all likelihood, save the life of the person. However, the problem with this management style is that life is not a constant series of emergencies. This style does not allow for the creative and caring approaches that are necessary for effective gerontological nursing. Often, older persons miss out on the best possible care, and the employees miss out on opportunities to learn and grow as they implement new care practices. The managers, generally not respected or esteemed by employees, feel frustrated when their work is not valued by others.

PERMISSIVE OR LAISSEZ-FAIRE

The laissez-faire style of leadership is the exact opposite of the authoritarian style.

Essentially, this style consists of an absence of leadership (Anderson, 2001). The manager wants everyone to feel good, including himself or herself, and works hard toward that end. The basic strategy is to allow the employees to make the decisions, do the planning, set the goals, and essentially manage the organization. This manager sees employees as ambitious, responsible, intelligent, and creative. The laissez-faire manager does not require accountability from employees for their time or for the quality of work done. Initially, this may sound like an ideal management style.

It is important to examine this type of management style in relationship to organizations involved in gerontological health care. Most care given to the elderly population depends on federal approval and on complex payment systems that go through both state and federal government organizations. It is difficult to envision the federal guidelines for safety (Occupational Safety and Health Administration [OSHA]) or for nursing home licensure carried out in a permissive or laissez-faire manner. The same is true for quality assurance programs in health-care environments. Most elder-care facilities require specific attention to the paperwork that keeps an organization's doors open. It also is necessary to have layers of responsibility that ensure every person in the facility the best possible care with, again, attention to detail.

In other environments, however, laissez-faire management is very successful. A good example is a group of highly motivated, professional people, such as a group of researchers, for whom independent thinking is rewarded. Conversely, it is difficult to imagine an effective nursing home or hospital unit being managed with this style of leadership.

DEMOCRATIC OR PARTICIPATIVE

This management style has a strong valuing of the people on the team. A strong sense of a team is in existence when decisions are made through the team. The manager gathers information from the other team members and then presents it to the group. All suggestions from the group are considered before decisions are made by the group (Anderson, 2001). This is a very open system of management, yet it identifies the individuals who are responsible for the various projects being managed.

The disadvantage presented by this type of management style is that it takes a great deal of time and energy. Generally the results are positive, and the employees are very satisfied. This is a style that works well in gerontological environments because it is focused on people and includes the employee, the older adult, and the older adult's family. It is a system that considers change and improvement continuously and assigns responsibility for such ventures.

As an LPN nurse manager, you need to evaluate yourself and determine which general management style is yours. Then, consider whether it is a style that is best used in the care of older people. If it is not, you need to learn more about other management styles and with that knowledge consider making changes in yourself. You may need to find a mentor who has a management style you would like to learn more about and ask that person to assist you. This mentor could teach you, become a role model for you, and assist you in applying the management techniques you want in the real-world setting. Being a manager is a challenging facet of your professional life. Take the time to learn the skills and patterns of thought that you will need to function at your most effective level.

▶ COMMUNICATION

The most important skill for a manager, in any situation, involves communication. Nurses in gerontological care spend 85% of their time communicating with a wide variety of people who are involved in the care of older adults. This makes mastering the skills of communication essential for the successful LPN. Communication involves delivering messages that will be understood, listening to messages that may or may not be confusing, and properly interpreting messages that have been misdirected or are delivered with intense emotion, such as anger.

For the LPN, the art of communication involves various groups of people. The LPN needs to be able to communicate successfully with the older adult, the family or other members of the person's support group, and the numerous members of the interdisciplinary health-care team. Expertise in communication is demanded every day from those who manage, direct, or administer care to older people.

VERBAL COMMUNICATION

Verbal communication is the exchange of ideas and understanding that occurs through the use of spoken words and phrases. For the message to be received, the sender must use words and phrases that are appropriate for the listener. The success of all communication is measured by the question: Was the message properly received?

It should be easy to remember sitting in a class and "listening" to a lecture or presentation when you did not "receive" the message. Perhaps you were too tired to concentrate, or the instructor was boring or had inappropriate content to share. For communication to occur, being present is not enough. The critical measure is whether the listener actually understood or "received" the message.

NONVERBAL COMMUNICATION

Nonverbal communication is the ability to share messages without using words. It refers, among other things, to a person's body posture (is the person tired and slouched over, or excited and alert?), the tone and speed of the voice, the kind of clothes a person wears, and hand and facial movements. Nonverbal communication is considered to be the most honest communication a person can receive. For example, someone may say, "I'm having a great day. How are things for you?" in a cheerful-sounding way, but an examination of his appearance may indicate something different. The face is not smiling, and the posture is one of fatigue. The person's hands may be clenching and unclenching as a symptom of stress. Or take another classic example: A resident in a nursing home is asked each morning, "How are you?" and each day responds verbally, "I'm fine." The person asking the question is busy with the breakfast tray or the linen and does not look at the sad and worried face of the resident who answers with the reply that is expected, rather than with the truth.

The ability to recognize honest communication and respond to it is critical for a successful nurse manager. The nurse manager must learn to develop the refined skill of understanding nonverbal communication because it will convey valuable information about patients and employees. Nonverbal communication is an honest method of communication and will allow the LPN to follow through on problems and concerns that otherwise might not have been recognized.

COMMUNICATING WITH CLIENTS

The decision to work with the elderly population is a commitment to accept the normal physiological losses that accompany the aging process. That commitment requires knowledge of the normal changes that occur in elderly people (see Chapter 1), and the skill to work with them successfully. A tendency exists in our ageist society to negatively judge older citizens because of the normal aging processes they exhibit. Normal aging changes that might affect communication are slower speech, presbycusis (difficulty in discriminating sounds), presbyopia (difficulty seeing near objects), and overall slower movements or responses to what is being communicated. The knowledgeable LPN recognizes these as normal occurrences and responds to them with skill and compassion.

Some people are impatient and negative about the aging process. It is as if they were punishing people who had simply neglected to die young! As you know, this is ageist behavior and is unacceptable in any setting. The skills necessary for successful communication with older adults must be firmly based on respect for them as people. If that ingredient is missing, communication is unsuccessful. Consider the following strategies (not every older adult will need every strategy):

- Do not approach the person from the side because you may not be seen, and the person could be frightened by your sudden appearance. Approach only from the front. This factor is important because of the gradual loss of peripheral vision that often accompanies aging.
- Place yourself on eye level with the older person so a comfortable presence occurs during the communication process.
- Reach out and touch the person if it seems appropriate; this is often the bridge to a trusting relationship.
- It is important to speak at a normal rate and not to shout, even if the older person is having trouble hearing. Shouting does not overcome the problems of presbycusis. Speak in a normal tone and speak slower than usual, but not so slow as to insult the person.
- If the patient is having trouble hearing you, move closer and speak in a normal tone. Moving closer often allows for lip reading or the reading of facial expressions.
- Pleasantly repeat what is being said, if necessary.
- Do not be impatient or judgmental.
- Place yourself and the older adult in a setting where there is a bright light but no glaring of light.
- Use a setting without disturbing or distracting noises.
- If the older adult gets confused while speaking or responding to a question, give the person time to collect personal thoughts. Do not rush the individual.
- Repeat questions or comments in a different sentence structure if the older person is having trouble understanding what is said. Do not keep repeating the same information in the same way.
- Reflect on what the older person has said by repeating it back in a different way. For example, "Do you mean that you are lonely because your wife is in the hospital and not able to visit you here in the nursing home?"
- Listen carefully to the words used and verify what they mean.
- "Listen" carefully to the body movements and other nonverbal communication and verify what they mean.

It is critical to keep in mind that your goal is to have the message successfully received. The use of these basic, caring strategies enhances your achievement of that goal, as well as your relationship with the older adults in your care.

POINT OF INTEREST

Presbyopia and *presbycusis* are commonly used words when talking about older adults. It will complement your educational process to take the time to memorize those words and use them as you speak. Work with them and make them a natural part of your vocabulary. Make it fun!

COMMUNICATING WITH THE FAMILIES OF OLDER ADULTS

Often, the family members of older patients or residents are worried, exhausted (if there has been extensive care given at home), and experiencing feelings of guilt over the condition of their family member or the necessity of admitting their loved one to a health-care facility. Successful communication with this varied group of people is challenging because of their emotional status. The issues involved often go beyond concern over an admission to a hospital or nursing home, to such highly charged questions as the right to die, the decision whether to do an amputation, or dealing with a diagnosis such as Alzheimer's disease.

It is critical for the LPN to recognize the emotional environment of the family members before entering into any communication with them. The goal is still the same. You want the message to be received by the listener. Some communication strategies for families are:

- Listen to them before you attempt to impart information. It is essential that you evaluate the emotional environment to determine if they are able to listen to you. Often, just listening allows for you to learn critical information that you otherwise would not learn.
- Plan to spend time with the family members. They will have questions and concerns, and deserve to have them addressed.
- Family members often feel guilty over some issue with their loved one and need to have that clarified. Families need not feel guilty unless evidence of elder abuse is found.
- Find a quiet place to speak to the family. It should be a place where they can sit comfortably and be together as a group. The nurses' station is never an appropriate place for meaningful communication other than the simple sharing of facts.
- As nurse manager, the LPN needs to facilitate the sharing of information with the family. This could mean arranging an appointment with the social worker or assisting a family member to reach the physician.
- The older adult's family is as important as the older person. Generally, strong personal

The interdisciplinary team conference is a place where the licensed practical nurse needs to assume the role of advocate for the older person as well as to teach and explain nursing concepts to the other team members.

relationships that are interdependent exist. Always treat the family members with the high level of respect and concern that you use with the older adult.

INTERDISCIPLINARY TEAM COMMUNICATION

It is unrealistic to give quality care to older adults without the support of an interdisciplinary team (IDT). Generally, the care given to older people in all settings is based on the interdisciplinary approach. It is critical that the nurse manager be an active and contributing part of this team. Generally, the nurse is with the patients 24 hours a day, or if the older person is a home patient, the nurse generally sees the individual more frequently than other members of the team. This constant attendance of the nurse to the patient provides a vast amount of personal and pertinent information. Therefore, it is essential that the nurse manager be active in contributing to the knowledge base and planning of the IDT.

Again, concern arises over how to share information the nurse has gathered about the older person. It needs to be shared with skill so that the message is received. This process is different in a group setting than it is with an individual patient or family members. The group consists of professionals who have specialized knowledge regarding the older person. Unfortunately, rarely is there sufficient time to discuss the patients in a thorough and relaxed manner. Often, a time crunch exists in

IDT planning that establishes a unique atmosphere for communication. The following are strategies for communicating with an IDT:

- Come prepared! There is no time to waste in these meetings, whether in groups or one-on-one.
- Plan ahead and have priority concerns in your mind or on a piece of paper.
- Remember that this is not a team of nurses, and they may not understand a nursing concept that is very familiar to you. Because nursing is its own specialty, you may be asked to justify your requests or concerns or to teach the team about a nursing concept.

In most situations, the nurse has the role of patient/resident advocate. This occurs naturally because of the amount of time nursing personnel spend with patients compared with that spent by other disciplines. This time allows for personal information and concerns to be communicated. It is critical that the patient advocacy role be accepted by the nurse, so that the patient is protected from the system and its potentially depersonalizing effects.

▶ ADDITIONAL COMMUNICATION SKILLS

Very specific skills are necessary for successful communication, and each of these skills can be used appropriately in all settings. Such skills are necessary to clarify communication errors, or potential errors, and are commonly necessary in difficult situations. They are important for every LPN to add to the communication skills checklist, and their importance can be compared with that of being expert at cardiopulmonary resuscitation (CPR). You may not use the skills very often, but when they are necessary, you need to know how to use them.

ASSERTIVE COMMUNICATION SKILLS

The normal physiological reaction to being attacked physically or verbally is "fight or flight." This reaction occurs without thinking about it; it is normal physiology. When a situation occurs in which you are being attacked verbally or feel threatened by what is being said or done, the normal response is to fight back (an argument) or to take flight (avoidance). In the framework of assertive communication, these two normal responses are more formally identified as: *aggressive*—fight, or *passive*—flight. The third concept that belongs on a continuum between these two is *assertive*—dealing with the problem.

Ideally you will use assertive behavior when someone has violated the rights of an individual either verbally or physically. Assertive behavior is the most effective response to that violation. The major rule regarding the concept of assertive communication is simply that the assertive response *must not* violate the rights of the person who just infringed on your rights. What does that look like? An argument is the best example. Someone comes to the nurses' station and criticizes you in an angry, loud manner. Of course, there are residents or patients, visitors, and coworkers in the area listening to this *aggressive* communication. It is embarrassing and humiliating to be the victim of a communication delivered in such an inappropriate way. The normal physiological response is to either run away, perhaps crying (*passive*), or to scream back (*aggressive*). Screaming back or starting an argument is a violation of the other person's rights. It does not matter if he or she deserves it, it is still wrong. The *passive* behavior or running away does not violate the other person's rights, but it does prevent a resolution of the problem.

Assertive communication requires that the person being violated not respond in a normal physiological fashion to the situation. Instead, it is necessary to resist the normal response and use the skills of communication to promote problem solving. Assertive communication often follows this response format:

- "I *feel*"—Tell the other person how the aggressive attack made you feel. Perhaps you feel frustrated, devalued, angry, or frightened. Many other options are available for you to describe how you feel about what has been said.
- "*When you*"—Describe for the person the behavior that has caused you to feel the way you do. It could be when you raise your voice at me, talk about private concerns in public, demand things from me that I cannot do, or criticize me in front of others. Again, many other statements could be used here. The statements used must not be personal statements that attack the other person.
- "*We should*"—Together determine a solution

to the problem. This is difficult to do because it is not one of the two normal and usual responses. Use it anyway. Take a deep breath and simply ask what can the two of you do to prevent this from happening again. Be open minded and expect that there will be more hostility because of the discomfort that comes to the aggressive person with your unusual approach. It is hoped that the two of you can resolve the problem. If not, you still have done a good thing. Another skill that may help you in this type of situation is active listening.

ACTIVE LISTENING

Another communication skill that complements assertive behavior is that of *active listening*. Most people respond to aggressive and negative remarks with defensive communication. While the aggressor is making comments, the person being attacked generally is mentally preparing the defense to the aggressor's attack. These are the defensive comments that often provoke an argument. They follow the script of "It is not my fault, now let me tell you why!"

Active listening requires that the person being verbally attacked listen to what is being said. Because of the natural inclination to prepare a defense, this is a challenging thing to do. Just listen and, while listening, try to determine the cause of the problem beyond the apparent anger.

The person who is out of control must be removed to a private setting, such as an office or the clean holding area. This prevents that individual from self-embarrassment in front of others, and it places you in an environment with fewer distractions.

After the angry person has finished saying all the aggressive things there are to say, he or she will take a deep breath and stop talking. This is where the person uneducated in communication skills presents their defense. But you, the nurse manager, need skills beyond the ordinary person. Active listening is one of those skills. The deep breath is the signal to use the information you learned, while listening, to clarify the problem and negotiate a solution.

Comments like "You seem so frustrated with . . ." or "It is unlike you to be so upset." "How can I help?" are effective ones to use. They are not what the aggressive person expects to hear and generally prevent the person from losing control again. They are helpful comments that show caring and problem-solving skills. These are hallmark behaviors for nurse managers. The next move is for the two people involved to sit down and rationally look at the problem and work on a solution. The whole process begins with the nurse being able to stop "self-defending" and focus on listening.

The format for active listening is:

- Remove the conversation to a private setting.
- Listen.
- Do not prepare a defense.

- Listen for the deep breath that means the person has finished speaking.
- Show support for the other person's feelings.
- Negotiate how to resolve the problem.

Some LPNs reading this text may feel concern over being responsible for assertive communication and active listening skills. They are two of many possible communication skills that could have been discussed in this book. They are listed for a very specific purpose. LPNs, in management roles, have very challenging positions that may place them in serious situations that must be managed rather than ignored. Some people will say, "But I am just an LPN!" and feel that their role does not involve managing and solving problems of this nature. However, it is important to recognize that, if you are a nurse manager, you have an obligation to develop the skills necessary for managing these acute and potentially destructive problems.

▶ THE PLANNING HOOP

Every day, decisions must be made regarding the workload of the LPN and others that affect the scope of LPN practice. These are decisions that should be made with careful thought and planning rather than casually and without attention to detail. The decision that may be required of you could be as simple as who will get first bath as you give morning care; but even this decision may have serious implications for the patients or residents who are receiving your care. Other decisions that will be required of the LPN nurse manager could be counseling an employee whose behavior is unacceptable, making care assignments, confronting a doctor or therapist with an alternate plan of care for a resident, or managing daily staffing. None of these tasks, and the many others that are required of a nurse manager, are easy or simple. They require the highest level of skill and attention to manage the process of making such decisions effectively.

To set priorities and make excellent decisions, the LPN nurse manager must understand the importance of planning, which is an intelligent process of thinking based on facts and information, rather than on emotion and wishes. An example is the holiday schedule. Staff members want Christmas Day off to be with their families. You, the manager, want

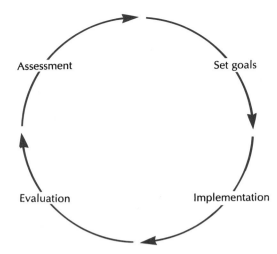

FIG. 3. 1. The planning hoop. The effective nurse manager must learn that planning is critical to getting the total workload done effectively.

everyone on your staff to be happy, but you have a clear picture as to what would happen if you granted everyone's wishes for Christmas Day! Instead, you need to intelligently make a rotation plan for the holidays, or perhaps draw names out of a hat, assign requests according to seniority, or determine some other way for the Christmas Day shift to be adequately staffed.

Planning is a process that never ends. It can be thought of as a hoop with notches where you stop and enter another phase of the planning process; then you continue going around the hoop over and over again. It is unrealistic to develop a plan and think that it will never change. It may be perfect for the moment, a week, or even an entire year; but the complexity of health care and the individuality of clients and staff require that your excellent plan be continuously re-evaluated. The planning (Fig. 3.1) hoop begins with an assessment.

ASSESSMENT

What is the problem or potential problem that concerns you? You know how to do a physical assessment. This is a similar process. Look at the problem from "head to toe" and assess what really is wrong. If it is a staffing problem in a nursing home, look at the mix of licensed and unlicensed personnel. Is it right for the needs of the residents?

Is the problem a lack of knowledge? If it is,

you need to assess where the lack is, who needs to know the information, and how to most effectively teach it. Do not be distracted by other issues as you do your assessment. Keep focused on the problem you are trying to resolve and learn all you can about it. Otherwise, it would be similar to trying to assess two residents at the same time. One does not get a clear picture of the problem unless a very focused effort is made. The next step in the planning hoop is to set goals.

GOAL SETTING

Now that you have a complete set of data regarding the problem, you have enough information to set goals. This, again, is very similar to the nursing process. Instead of writing a care plan, you are preparing a plan to resolve a management problem. Make the goals reasonable and achievable. As we saw, not everyone can have Christmas Day off. If the problem is an unbalanced mix of licensed and unlicensed personnel, your goal could be to correct the mix through attrition and selective hiring within the next 6 months. If the problem is knowledge, your goal would be to have 100% of your staff attend a class on the information needed by a specific date. The goals should be meaningful and demonstrate your most careful and organized thinking.

IMPLEMENTATION

This is the test of good planning. Was your assessment done accurately and are your goals realistic? Perhaps the actual implementation requires you to not hire an RN or LPN when they apply because your staff has too great a proportion of licensed personnel. Or implementation may mean you need to find the budget money to pay the staff to attend the education program you determined they needed. In addition, you need a plan for getting everyone to attend. This could involve bonus money or other rewards, and in all likelihood, it would mean presenting the education program several times. Implementation is the actual performance of your plan.

EVALUATION

Did your plan work? Was Christmas Day successfully staffed and did the staff feel that the staffing decisions were made with fair-

ness? Within 6 months, was your staff mix at the level at which you needed it to be? How effective was your education program? Did it bring about the change you wanted? Such questions initiate the process of evaluation. A nurse manager cannot just do something and consider the problem solved. Instead, a careful evaluation must be performed so the cycle of the planning hoop can begin again. That is right; once you have evaluated your plan, you need to do another assessment and begin the circle again!

Many people do not spend a great deal of time planning solutions to the unit's problems. The profession of nursing is filled with "doing types" of people. One of the critical skills of being a manager is to learn to quit "just doing" and begin planning "to do." It is a challenge to take the time necessary to plan because planning does not enter into the conventional description of a "good nurse."

When a person is planning, that person is sitting somewhere quietly thinking. The profession of nursing generally does not see that as productive because beds need to be made, and there are baths and treatments to be given. With those unfinished care issues, how can a real nurse take the time to just sit and think? A real nurse manager soon learns that doing the thinking or planning is critical to getting the total workload done effectively. So, fight the urge to be busy when planning is needed. Teach the staff that the time you spend planning is critical to the overall picture of care for patients and job satisfaction for them. Be courageous enough to use the planning hoop to resolve problems and prevent new ones. Because if you do not, you will become a victim of crisis management!

CRISIS MANAGEMENT

A crisis manager is a person who does not take the time to plan. This manager waits until the week before Christmas to resolve the problem of the staffing crisis. A great deal of hysteria, excess energy, and distress are involved in solving problems when they occur rather than in foreseeing them and taking the time to plan a solution for the problem. The phrase "All I do is run around and put out fires!" is indicative of the crisis manager. It is not effective management and can be prevented by the implementation of the planning hoop into your management style. Look to the future and anticipate problems. Then, devise a plan for solving them before a crisis happens.

Some situations still will become a crisis for even the best manager. Accept that, solve the problem, design a plan so it will not be a crisis the next time, and move on to the next situation.

▶ PRIORITY SETTING

Every LPN has learned how to prioritize the work of giving patient or resident care. Traditionally, the sickest patient receives the nurse's attention first and the least seriously ill person waits until last. This concept assumes that each patient is assessed and observed frequently, rather than being ignored until her or his turn comes to receive care.

Priority setting in management situations has a similar format. The priority of each management problem is determined after the assessment of the situation has been completed. The method for determining priority problems generally is based on determining what is essential for the organization or the person at the time. Staffing for Christmas Day is essential, as is giving pain medications in a timely manner.

The nurse manager needs to think of the entire organization when determining priorities. They often are divided into two categories: (1) concerns that relate to patient or resident care, and (2) concerns that relate to the process of running the business of the institution.

Each category should be considered separately, although a great deal of overlap of concerns occurs in implementing problem solutions. Each concern needs to be listed as a *need* or a *want*. Obviously, needs should be met before wants. It is helpful to use this method for categorizing your management concerns before prioritizing them.

▶ MANAGING PERSONNEL

As a nurse manager, you will be involved in, if not responsible for, the hiring and evaluating of employees. This is a critical aspect of your job and one that requires the highest level of professional skill and performance. This work cannot be done by intuition or "best guess." All personnel decisions directly affect the lives of the employees of the institution. These people deserve as much care and attention as the patients.

The hiring process is where the employee begins a career with your organization or, if not employed, will leave with an impression that will be taken out to the community. It should be your desire to have that impression be a good one. Many legal issues are involved in the hiring process. Be sure to clarify them with your personnel manager or administrator. Laws exist that involve the advertisement of a job and how the interview is conducted, and federal rules identify questions that cannot be asked in an interview because of concern over discrimination. Be alert to these rules and follow them.

The philosophy of interviewing someone for employment is to find someone who fits with the philosophy and image of your institution. The applicant needs the licensure or certification that the job description demands and the experience to perform the job at a satisfactory level. The interview also allows the nurse manager to determine the shift availability and whether the potential employee is available for part-time or full-time work. Moreover, an effort should be made to learn the specific interests of the applicant so plans can be made to use any special skills and knowledge the person possesses. The screening process of the personnel department presumably will eliminate anyone unqualified for the job. It is not necessary for unqualified people to be interviewed.

INTERVIEW

The purpose of the interview is to exchange information. Be prepared to give positive information about your facility to all applicants whether they are to be employed or not. Remember, you want applicants to say favorable things about your organization even if they are not selected for the job. During the interview, the nurse manager is expected to determine the applicant's:

- Dependability
- Skill level
- Willingness to assume the responsibilities of the job
- Willingness and ability to work with others
- Interest in the job
- Adaptability
- Consistency of goals with available opportunities

• Conformity of manner and appearance to job requirements

The interview has definite purposes and should be carried out in a professional manner. It is not the place for social chit-chat; however, some warm and friendly comments at the beginning of the interview should put the applicant at ease so the interview can be emotionally comfortable.

The greatest predictor of the applicant's future success is past performance. Is this someone who has worked with the older adults previously and enjoyed it? Has the applicant sought additional educational experiences that will enhance work in your type of setting? Was this person a desirable employee at the last place of employment or, if a new graduate, a good student? These critical pieces of information should be noted on the application and verified in the interview.

It is your responsibility, as the nurse manager, to set the tone for honesty in the interview. Be specific and direct in your comments. It is helpful to have an interview guide available to use for every interview. This guide is a written document that contains questions, directions, and pertinent information to be shared with the applicant. The presence of an interview guide ensures you, the applicant, and the institution that the same process is being used in every interview. It avoids gathering of prejudicial information and provides consistency in the interview process.

Questions on the interview guide should cover subjects such as which shifts the applicant is willing to work, whether part-time or full-time work is desired, and feelings about working with older people. It also could contain a brief case study or scenario about a gerontologically focused situation that requires a response from the applicant. The presence of two or three such questions gives you additional information about the potential employee. All applicants must be asked the same questions to avoid discrimination or the appearance of discrimination in choosing future employees. You also need to carefully review the Title VII Civil Rights Act before conducting any interviewing. This federal law prohibits discrimination in any personnel decision on the basis of race, color, sex, age, religion, or national origin. A comfortable format for an interview is presented below:

• Use an opening to establish rapport, and put the applicant at ease.
• Share the interview procedure with the applicant.
• Discuss the applicant's interests in being employed at your facility.
• Obtain an educational history.
• Discuss future plans of the applicant, for example, upward mobility, future education.
• Share case studies and situations and discuss them.
• Inform the applicant about the organization.
• Allow time for the applicant to ask questions and get answers.
• Close by clarifying how to reach the applicant after the interview, informing the person when the decision will be made, and thanking the applicant for considering your organization for employment.

EMPLOYEE EVALUATION

After the nurse manager has made a decision to hire an applicant, a very focused effort must be made to give that person a thorough and extensive orientation to the job, its standards, and its expectations. The quality of personnel hired and retained in the organization determines the success of the organization. The quality of the orientation directly determines the overall success for both the organization and the employee.

After the employee has had the opportunity to work with other qualified employees and to establish an effective working routine, a new employee can be allowed to work independently. A resource person should always be available, in some way, to the new employee for the first 3 months of employment. This provision indicates that a sincere effort is being made to ensure success for both the organization and the employee.

Each organization has an established process for evaluating employees. The first evaluation may come at 3 months, 6 months, or 12 months. Earlier and more frequent evaluations take more of the manager's time but also provide regular feedback for the employee. Overall, it is generally time well spent. Your organization also should have an established written form for evaluating employees. Again, this process should be consistent for all employees to avoid discrimination.

For all employing organizations, a performance appraisal may be based on the five basic realistic assumptions outlined below:

1. The appraisal will help an employee improve the management of the workload.
2. Employee appraisal is a difficult process, but a skill that can be mastered with hard work.
3. Few people like the current form (a perfect one simply does not exist!).
4. The appraisal will be made by the employee's supervisor.
5. Information must be gathered on a day-to-day basis.

The challenge to the nurse manager is that the performance appraisal must accurately reflect the person's actual job performance. It cannot contain prejudicial information, hearsay, or undocumented information. It is designed to be helpful to the employee and, by assisting the employee to improve, it will be helpful to the organization.

Traditionally, potential evaluation problems can contribute to a less than accurate evaluation. The first one is *leniency error*. This occurs when a supervisor wants everyone to be buddies or be the manager's best friend. It results when the manager "looks the other way" or gives an employee the "benefit of the doubt" rather than finding out what really happened.

A competent nurse manager cannot afford to be "best friends" with employees. The manager needs to be the manager. It is critical to success for the manager to be an honest and fair person who does not lose the ability to be objective. The leniency error does not help an employee improve, and it does not contribute to the overall functioning of the organization.

The *recency error* is an indication of a manager who has forgotten the basic assumptions of evaluation, and who has not kept records of employee performance over the year. Because of the lack of written record, the manager then evaluates only on what is remembered most recently. All employees know when their annual review is scheduled and often find it easy to "look good" during the time just before their evaluation. Again, this type of evaluation process enhances neither the performance of the employee nor that of the organization.

The *halo error* is allowing one trait to influence the entire evaluation. It could be either a strongly positive trait or a strongly negative one. Either way, it clouds the objective evaluation of an employee if only the halo behavior is remembered. Evaluations need to be fair and comprehensive regarding the employee's behavior and skills.

The evaluation process is critical to the growth and stability of the organization. Evaluation standards cannot be successful if they are ambiguous. The process of rewarding a strong employee and counseling a poor employee must be valid. This happens only if the manager maintains a professional and consistent attitude toward the evaluation process.

Negative or probationary evaluations are very difficult for all managers to give. Use the same process you would use for a positive evaluation. Make it fair and comprehensive, and share the information you have in a professional manner. For all terminations, the process of counseling the employee must be carefully documented over time. This is an act of fairness toward the employee and a protection against litigation for the institution.

The licensed practical nurse is often responsible for making the care assignments to nursing assistants.

MAKING CARE ASSIGNMENTS FOR OLDER ADULTS

One of the day-to-day management skills used by LPNs is that of making care assignments for older adults. The skill of making effective assignments is critical to any clinical area. The goal of making successful care assignments is to match the worker with the older person in a manner that allows for the best nursing care to be administered and received. As the manager, you also need to focus on an assignment that affords the highest level of employee satisfaction. This requires sensitivity, awareness of the skills and attitudes of others, and the ability to form a plan and to follow through on it. Several aspects of making care assignments should be examined.

When making care assignments, you must consider the personal skills of each person you are managing. You have learned how to assess older adults, now your question might be "How do I accurately assess a nursing assistant's skills?" Dr. Patricia Benner, who developed the nursing theory *From Novice to Expert* describes a specific way to identify clinical skills. Benner's theory focuses on intensive care, registered nurses, and their clinical expertise along the five points of:

- Novice
- Advanced Beginner
- Competent
- Proficient
- Expert

Dr. Benner's theory was designed for RNs. However, national research is currently being done to determine if the five points of clinical expertise will identify the clinical skills of certified nursing assistant (CNAs).

As a nurse manager, it is important for you to understand the five points of clinical expertise and how you can use them to identify skill levels for CNAs and other personnel who work under your direction. The five points are:

1. *Novice*—CNAs performing at this level have no prior experience with certain situations. They will not understand the detailed information regarding what is happening. They simply do not have the experience to understand what is going on in the situation. For example, a CNA may have several years of employment as a CNA but may not have any experience working on an Alzheimer's unit. As a nurse manager, you should be aware of such a lack of skill and may want to assign a novice CNA to work several shifts with a CNA who is experienced caring for people with Alzheimer's disease.

2. *Advanced Beginner*—CNAs functioning at this level can demonstrate limited acceptable performance. Advanced beginners generally have had multiple clinical experiences, independently or with a mentor, so they have a general understanding of the clinical situation. Advanced beginners perform tasks using behavior that follows instructions only rather than appropriate behavior for a specific situation.

   You, as the nurse manager, may ask a CNA to assist a resident into the shower. When the CNA enters the room, the resident is found confused and combative. Rather than gauging the situation and deciding that this may not be the best time to give this resident a shower, the CNA does everything possible to complete the task of giving the shower. The focus is on the task, not the aspects of the specific situation, nor the needs of the older person.

3. *Competent*—The competent CNA has an increased level of skill and ability. The knowledge is based on following the posi-

tive role-modeling of other CNAs as well as dealing with a variety of situations where clinical skills were learned. However, the competent CNA still focuses on organizing the assigned tasks. The competent CNA makes sure the time is managed well in an effort to complete the tasks on the list, instead of basing work decisions on the older person's needs.

As a nurse manager, it is critical that you make sure that the resident's needs are actually being met by the CNA in a timely manner. Otherwise, those you manage may give care based on a schedule and a list, rather than the needs of older adults.

4. *Proficient*—The proficient CNA is much more comfortable with clinical skills, and has the ability to deal with different situations as they arise. The proficient CNA engages more with the older adult and family instead of focusing on required tasks. The focus of the CNAs nursing care is on the needs of the older person, rather than a list. An advantage to working with proficient CNAs is their ability to reprioritize the workload based on resident/patient needs. As a nurse manager, you may delegate several things to the proficient CNA who will then decide in what order they should be completed.

5. *Expert*—The expert CNA has experienced many different situations, and has learned from the experiences. These experiences assist the CNA in making decisions based more on intuition (referred to by Benner as intuitive knowing) than timetables and rules. The expert CNA knows the older adult's patterns of behavior and is able to anticipate the unexpected. This complexity of skill and thinking assists the CNA to make decisions based on the "big picture" or the holistic needs of the person receiving care.

As an example, the expert CNA walks into a room where an older adult is behaving differently, and spends time with the person trying to identify the problem. The expert CNA will take vital signs and ask questions so there are data to report to the licensed nurse. The expert CNA will know what to do for this patient.

Are you able to identify where your CNAs fit in Benner's five points of clinical expertise? Do you have a new CNA who is still working at the novice level? If so, that person should be assigned to older adults who only require basic skills that were learned in the CNA class. The novice CNA also should be assigned to an expert CNA who can assist with care when needed, as well as serve as a positive role model. Novice CNAs should not be assigned to give care to challenging clients. They could be assigned to work with another CNA who has the challenging resident, and in that way, have experiences that eventually will lead the CNA to the level of expert without hurting an older person in the learning process.

Do you also have a CNA who has worked at the facility for several years, is very familiar with the residents, and has excellent clinical skills? That is the CNA who should be assigned to the most challenging older adults so they, the older adults, can benefit from the CNA's skills and knowledge. This may not always be the sickest person on the unit. The assignment could be to the latest admission in which the older person and the family are having a difficult time adjusting to the transitional stress of the admission.

It is important when developing staffing patterns that a team should not consist of a novice CNA and a novice-licensed nurse. A better staffing pattern would be an expert CNA with a novice nurse or expert nurse with a novice CNA. The mix of novice and the levels of expertise that lead to expert are important to acknowledge and use as you manage care.

Once you, as the nurse manager, have identified the "expertise" levels of each nursing assistant, you should praise each one for their special skills and allow them to use them. Assist employees to develop skills related to their interests and abilities, and recognize them for the skills they develop. Assign staff older adults who will benefit from their skill and knowledge. This enhances both quality of care and employee self-esteem. This, in turn, enhances the entire organization.

When working with older adults, it is generally more effective to assign the same employee to an older person for several days in succession. This allows the caregiver to learn the personal needs and nuances of the persons receiving care, and address them successfully. When a "new" person is assigned to an older person each day, it puts a demand on the older adult to need to explain again that he cannot hear out of his right ear, or that he wants two cups of coffee on his breakfast tray, or that it is his right knee that does not work very well. Generally, a comfortable camaraderie and sense of teamwork develops between the caregiver and the care receiver that enhances the work of healing when they are allowed to work together over time.

Sometimes a difficult or demanding older person requires more energy and patience than most employees can provide day after day. When this occurs, the nurse manager should rotate the assignment in a direct effort to avoid burnout of the employees.

Another consideration for making assignments is that of physical demands. Often when caring for older adult or chronically ill persons, a heavy physical demand is made in turning, positioning, and assisting the older person to ambulate. When the nurse manager makes the assignment, the physical, muscular work of the care should be considered in order not to overwork a particular employee. Another consideration is the geographic placement of the rooms. It is unnecessary to make assignments that require an employee to travel to both ends of the hall or in other diverse patterns. Make a strong effort to group the room numbers assigned to avoid unnecessary walking. Most workdays are tiring enough.

DELEGATION

As the LPN manager, you need to know what is involved in delegating to CNAs and unlicensed assistive personnel (UAP). The goal is to delegate tasks while maintaining quality patient and resident care. Your first step is to familiarize yourself with the Nurse Practice Act for the state where you work. This document defines the roles and responsibilities of a licensed nurse. You need to determine if your Nurse Practice Act allows for delegation, and if so, are there any limitations as to what you can delegate to a CNA or UAP. Your next step is to become familiar with the policy and procedures for your facility as well as the written job descriptions. Any job you assign must be within the employee's job description. Once you have identified a task that can be delegated, you want to use sound delegation approaches. You also will want to keep in mind how delegating this task will affect the safety of the older adult. Has the older person been accurately assessed and are there any safety issues that need to be addressed? The

National Council of State Boards of Nursing (NCSBN) has developed guidelines to help nurses ensure safe and proper delegation. The NCSBN has developed the "Five Rights of Delegation," which provides a checklist nurses can use to when making delegation decisions. The Five Rights of Delegation are:

1. The right task
2. The right circumstances
3. The right person
4. The right direction
5. The right supervision

In general, CNAs and UAPs can do tasks that assist older adults with basic needs and activities of daily living. They cannot assess, plan, or evaluate any aspects of patient care. If an older person is taking Lanoxin for his heart, the nurse can delegate to the CNA the task of taking an apical pulse and notifying the nurse what the heart rate is once the pulse is taken. The CNA cannot decide if the older adult can have medication based on the pulse the CNA took. In addition, the nurse will make the decision as to when the pulse should be checked again. It is very important, when working with CNAs and UAPs, that the nurse give clear instructions as to what time the task should be completed and whether they need to report back to you directly once they have completed the task. It is wise to encourage CNAs and UAPs to take notes as you are giving them the information regarding the delegated assignment. When delegating a task to a CNA or UAP, you must remember that you still are responsible for the older adult's care. If you delegate a task to a novice CNA or UAP, and the task should have been delegated to an expert CNA or UAP; or if you do not give proper supervision, you may be held responsible for the outcome of the care. If, however, you delegate to the appropriate person and provide appropriate supervision, the CNA or UAP may be liable for his or her own actions.

As a manager, you should always be willing to delegate certain projects. As organizational needs arise, you may be assigned a project that will not allow you to complete your regular workload. This is a good time to delegate routine work that can be done by someone else.

In your role as an LPN, you will find it necessary to do effective delegation. Does that mean that you delegate the projects that you do not want to do? Does delegating make you a lazy person? The answer to both of these questions is "No." Delegation of routine tasks to someone else frees the manager to work on more complicated unit needs. Because delegation is critical to effective management, you want to make sure you are doing it as efficiently as possible. When delegating to anyone, your responsibility as the manager is to identify if they have the basic skills or education necessary to complete the assignment. You also should make sure they have the time to complete the assignment by the deadline without requiring them to put aside their regular job responsibilities. Delegating to someone who is interested in the assignment, and who will have to live with the outcomes of the assignment is a good choice.

Once the individual is identified, you should give the person clear and direct instructions on what is to be done including why they are doing the assignment. How the person completes the assignment should be an individual choice. This is the really hard part. Once you delegate a responsibility in the manner described earlier, just leave it and allow the person to do the work. You can "check in," determine whether the person needs something, or just observe so you can step in if there is a critical situation. Giving the employee autonomy in deciding how to complete the assignment is a positive factor for the employee and the key to successful delegation. It also is important that you do not oversupervise the employee. If you are going to watch and participate in every step of the project, then you may want to ask yourself why you chose to delegate it.

Definite time lines for completion of any delegated project should be discussed, and the manager should check in periodically to ensure that the deadline will be met. Monitoring the assignment periodically allows for questions and discussion regarding the project as the work is being done. Being available for interaction is an important concept. You always should be available to assist the employee if he or she is having difficulty. Taking the delegated project back would be a last-resort behavior because it makes the employee feel like a failure and "demotivates" rather than motivates. When the project is complete, you must evaluate the performance, giving both praise and additional information to the employee. This lets the person know what was done well and what may be done

differently next time they are assigned a similar assignment. Delegation is an effective way to assist someone to move from novice to expert because of the opportunity to develop new skills and have new experiences.

PROVIDING TRAINING FOR YOUR EMPLOYEES

This chapter has discussed management concepts needed to supervise employees. Now the question is, "What is the nurse manager's role in providing continuing education to the staff?" What can the nurse manager do to move CNAs from novice care providers to expert care providers? Health care changes on a regular basis, and we, as licensed professionals are all trying to keep up with the changes. It is important for unlicensed health-care providers to keep up with health-care changes as well. As a nurse manager, you need to assist with this endeavor. There are several areas of education that need to be addressed. The first is the orientation process for new employees. It is suggested that orientation programs for new CNAs should extend to at least 3 months. An orientation program should match, one on one, a new or novice CNA with a veteran or expert CNA. The program should provide the new CNA the information needed to function as an effective member of the nursing team at the end of the orientation period. The orientation information should include the policies and procedures for the facility, information about the daily operation and schedules for the facility, and most important, detailed information about the older adults and the specific skills needed to give excellent nursing care.

The expert CNA who is willing to be a role-model and mentor the new employee should be a valued employee who consistently demonstrates expert clinical skills and care behaviors. This is a CNA who demonstrates willingness to orient the new employees as well. It is appropriate to demonstrate valuing of employees who participate in the orientation program through some type of a reward.

The novice CNAs must have continuity of instruction throughout the orientation. If the facility has five units, the CNA should spend equal amounts of time on each unit. The time spent should be consecutive days so the CNA can become acquainted with the staff and procedures on one unit before moving to the next. This also provides consistency of care for the older adults who are getting to know the new employee.

At the end of the orientation period, the new employee should be evaluated. It is at this time the nurse manager must decide if the employee is acceptable for the facility. If you are not satisfied with the employee's performance, a plan of action should be developed to assist the employee in meeting the requirements necessary for successful employment. This also may be the time when the nurse manager may make the difficult decision to release the employee.

Once a nurse manager hires an employee an effort should be made to increase and maintain the skills of the employee. There are various ways to accomplish this goal. Mentorship programs match individuals together when one person has the required skills and the other needs to learn them. These programs generally last for a longer period of time than orientation, and in most cases, are less formal. A CNA who is interested in becoming an LPN may be matched with an LPN who is interested in helping the CNA be prepared for nursing school. Or you may have an employee who works well with people with Alzheimer's disease and their families. This individual could work as a mentor for other employees who would like to posses the same skills.

Some facilities are using clinical ladder models to increase employee skills. Different levels of knowledge are identified as well as ways to obtain and document the skills. When an employee meets the requirements of one level or "rung" of the ladder, there often is a promotion. When employees have met the requirements for an advanced level, they often are recognized with a ceremony and a monetary award, an increase in pay, or a set one-time dollar amount. Facilities have found that clinical ladders can assist with employee retention as well as improve employee morale. The benefit to the facility is better patient care. The improvement in care is a result of the facility seeking to prepare its own expert CNAs, LPNs, and RNs.

▶ MANAGING THE QUALITY OF CARE

The process of managing and evaluating the quality of health care is not new. Florence Nightingale (1859) urged that all nursing care be carefully evaluated. Because of her innovative nursing care practices and her ability to measure and evaluate nursing care, she was able to measure changes in the health of patients. At one hospital during the Crimean War, she measured a decrease in patient mortality of 50% down to 20% after her nursing-care ideas were instituted. Different outside organizations measure the quality of care given in hospitals and nursing homes. The Joint Commission on Accreditation of Hospitals (JCAH) was founded in 1952 to evaluate health-care services. Two nursing organizations followed this trend in the late 1950s. The American Nurses Association developed and published standards of care for the various nursing specialties and the National League of Nursing published standards that the public could expect from nursing education. Quality health care is the right of persons who enter the health-care system. The organizations just listed provide outside evaluation of the organization. Other methods for making self-evaluation that involve the LPN also exist.

TOTAL QUALITY MANAGEMENT

Total quality management (TQM) is a management philosophy that emphasizes a commitment of excellence throughout the entire health-care organization. The principles are widely used throughout many business organizations in addition to health care. The overall purpose of TQM is to improve quality of service and ensure customer satisfaction.

The four major characteristics of TQM are (1) customer/client focus, (2) total organizational involvement, (3) use of quality tools and statistics for measurement, and (4) identification of key processes for improvement. The LPN is involved in all four aspects of the TQM process.

Most nurses naturally believe that their focus is the customer or client. This is the overall theme of TQM and calls for all personnel in each department to focus on the needs of the client. An example would be a smoother admission process, given that process is often an area that provokes customer complaints. Another example is the housekeeper responding to the patient. This could be simply friendly visiting or putting aside the housekeeper's usual work to go get a nurse for a patient.

The customer focus of TQM is most effective

when all employees in a hospital or nursing home respond to the challenge to focus on the needs of the patient. This philosophy eliminates the idea of "That is not my job!" Instead, everyone works toward the overall goal of satisfied customers. This may make it necessary for a nurse to assist the housekeeper in making beds because of the large number of admissions and discharges done in one shift. Or a physician may need to transport a patient from the emergency room to the unit; respiratory therapists may assist patients to the toilet; the unit secretary may need to transport patients who are being discharged to their car. The point is that everyone is committed to the idea of customer satisfaction and is willing to fulfill whatever role might be necessary and safe to meet that commitment.

The use of high-quality tools and statistics to measure the level of care that is being given is an important consideration. An organization cannot determine whether the quality of care is being improved unless accurate measurement takes place. This generally is not the responsibility of the LPN, but an upper management or administrative assignment.

The LPN may need to complete forms or make reports that contribute to overall measurement of the work being done, but such an assignment will be made by someone else in the system to you, as the LPN.

The fourth component of TQM is identification of key processes for improvement. All activities in an organization can be described in terms of people working together. The term identification of key processes refers to the efficiency or effectiveness of the work people or teams do together. One example is the PDCA cycle. This is the Plan, Do, Check, and Act cycle. It very simply defines the process a group or team should be following as they do their work.

▶ CONCLUSION

Many skills are needed by the nurse manager, but this is just a chapter, not a management textbook. The case study at the end of the chapter will give you practice in considering management issues. Finally, it is important for you to find a mentor to assist you with the real world of management.

CASE STUDY

It is 7:35 A.M. and you are the nurse in charge of a 25-bed skilled nursing facility (SNF) unit at the nursing home where you work. The night nurse went home early because she was ill, and you have just discovered that only half of the 6:00 A.M. medications have been distributed. You have a new LPN orienting with you, but she is a recent graduate, and you are not yet sure of her skill level.

You have an 8:00 A.M. meeting with the social worker and a family who is struggling with the decision of whether to allow their mother to die or to place her on stronger life-support mechanisms. The final concern you have is making up the payroll. It is your responsibility to have the paperwork completed on the payroll by 9:00 A.M. If the payroll forms are not in the personnel office, a 3-day delay will occur in paying the employees on your unit. It is the week before Christmas.

As you are struggling to set priorities for the morning, Dr. N. comes onto the unit in a rage and begins talking to you in a raised voice and with an angry nonverbal appearance. This is a physician who is known as a bully with both nurses and families, yet you have learned by working with him that he really does care for his residents. You stop everything you are doing to listen to him degrade you with his unprofessional manner. The halls are full of residents and employees who are watching this situation. As the charge nurse, you are responsible for all activities on the unit.

Please make a priority list with an explanation for the ranking of each item. Then, in narrative form, describe how you would implement the priority list you have made. Good luck!

Discussion

PRIORITY LIST

1.
EXPLANATION:
2.
EXPLANATION:
3.
EXPLANATION:
4.
EXPLANATION:

Solution

1. The medications must be distributed.

EXPLANATION: The medications are already an hour and a half late. This could have very serious physiological consequences for the frail elderly residents on the unit. This is a critical need.

2. The physician must be managed.

EXPLANATION: He is preventing me from resolving the other problems on the unit, and some of them are critical. In addition, he is very disruptive to the people (including residents) on the unit.

3. The meeting with the social worker and the resident's family.

EXPLANATION: This is a very emotional situation for this family, and it is unethical and unkind to ask them to wait or come back at a more convenient time. An issue of this importance cannot be delayed once people are ready to deal with it. It is listed third because the meeting could go ahead without me since the social worker will be there.

4. The payroll forms need to be completed.

EXPLANATION: It is unfair not to have the employees paid in a timely manner. Yet people are always more important than paperwork. This could wait because paperwork does not bleed, die, or have feelings.

NARRATIVE EXPLANATION OF THIS LIST

I would ignore the physician and his screaming; in the meantime I would call an experienced nurse on another unit. I would quickly explain to her the medication errors and the availability of only my newly hired LPN for assistance. My request would be for her to come to my floor and work with the new LPN to pass the medications that were missed. I am asking her for 30 minutes of her time in an emergency situation. I would not turn this assignment over to the new LPN because I am unsure of her skill level. This is a critical situation that demands immediate correction by someone with a very high skill level.

Because I know the physician really cares about his residents, I would resist the desire to humor him; instead, I would let him know that I had a resident emergency and could see him about his problem after 10:30 A.M. This is not a good example of problem solving with him, but it is an excellent example of setting priorities. He might still be angry with me, but I would be keeping my residents in the best health possible with my decisive action. My hope would be that his natural caring for residents would prevail, and he would cooperate in this situation.

I would notify the social worker that I would be at the meeting, but that I might be late. And finally, I would call the personnel office and explain to them that a crisis involving the residents occurred and that the paperwork would be delivered to them by noon. If that did not allow for the employees on the unit to be paid in a timely manner, I would request that an employee from their office come to the floor and do the necessary paperwork.

I would not give lengthy explanations to any of these people. Instead, I would count on my professional reputation to underlie the urgency of the situation. After the day was under control and all of the problems resolved, I would very conscientiously go to each person involved and thank him or her for their cooperation and give the explanation each person deserves. I would call the night nurse and let him or her know of the situation, and ask the nurse to come in within 24 hours to complete the medication error forms. I already would have made the necessary phone calls to the physicians informing them of the medication errors.

STUDY QUESTIONS

Circle the correct choice(s) to complete each statement.

1. Every LPN must practice within the definition of the State Nurse Practice Act. The best way for an LPN to determine whether the current job description is within the current Nurse Practice Act is to:
   a. Ask the supervisor.
   b. Discuss it with the personnel office during the hiring interview.
   c. Read the Nurse Practice Act.
   d. Ask another LPN.

2. The authoritarian style of leadership is the most effective to use in gerontological settings because:
   a. The work gets done in a timely manner.
   b. Geriatric settings have many emergencies to manage.
   c. Authoritarian leaders are very person focused.
   d. Authoritarian leadership is not strongly compatible with elder-care settings.

3. The most honest form of communication is:
   a. Nonverbal communication

   b. Verbal communications with facial movements
   c. Sitting quietly and listening
   d. The written word

4. Assertive communication is:
   a. Inappropriate for an LPN to use
   b. A meaningful way to share angry feelings
   c. A learned behavior that allows for effective communication
   d. A normal physiological response to stressful communication

5. The purpose of an employee interview is to:
   a. Learn the prejudices of the applicant before employment
   b. Exchange information
   c. Fill the employment quota of minorities
   d. Make new friends

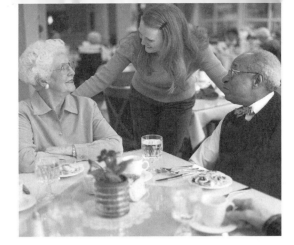

Kathleen R. Culliton

chapter 4

The Use of the Nursing Process and Nursing Diagnosis in the Care of Older Adults

Learning Objectives

After completing this chapter, the student will be able to:

1. Describe the nursing process as a problem-solving technique in the context of the older adult's assessment, plan of care, nursing interventions, and nursing documentation.
2. Identify the use of the nursing process minimum data set (MDS) and resident assessment protocols (RAPs) in developing nursing care plans for residents in nursing facilities.
3. Use the nursing process to develop a care plan for the presented case study.

▶ INTRODUCTION

Licensed practical nurses (LPNs) work in a variety of care settings. Each setting may require the practical nurse to function in a different capacity, yet each practice area expects you be involved with the assessment, planning, implementation, and evaluation of older adults and the care they receive.

▶ ENVIRONMENTS OF CARE

HOME CARE

A relatively new practice area for LPNs is working in home care. Practical nurses in home care work under the direction of a registered nurse. They provide nursing care such as changing dressings, monitoring blood glucose levels, administering medications, and assessing the status of chronic disease processes in the older adult's home.

HOSPITAL CARE

LPNs work in a variety of capacities with the acutely ill older person who is hospitalized. Often, they are paired with a registered nurse to form a care team in providing nursing care. Other care delivery models may require the LPN to have specific tasks on the unit, such as treatments or passing medications for all of the patients on the unit.

LONG-TERM CARE FACILITIES

The LPN may be employed in many types of long-term care facilities. Skilled nursing facilities and nursing facilities were previously thought of as nursing homes. They generally provide a high level of nursing intervention. Assisted living facilities provide care to older persons who may need assistance with activities of daily living (ADLs) but who do not require complex, skilled intervention (Eliopolous, 2001). Continuing care retirement communities have several levels of care including those offered in a skilled nursing facility, assisted living, and independent living apartments. Wellness clinics are frequently provided for independent apartment living residents. LPNs could be employed in any one of these long-term care settings.

In the long-term care environment, the practical nurse collects admission data,

provides input to the plan of care, carries out the nursing interventions that are outlined in the plan of care, and evaluates the effectiveness of these interventions in meeting the goals of the older adult's care plan. Often the LPN confers with the interdisciplinary health care team (IDT) to share observations and clarify the plan of care. Very often, the LPN in these settings is responsible for working with nursing assistants to be sure the plan of care is carried out. Practical nurses even call physicians to clarify orders and to report changes in the resident's health status. The practice of LPNs in nursing facilities is the practice model referred to for this chapter.

▶ THE NURSING PROCESS

An LPN walks into a resident's room and finds the person with a supper tray in place. The resident is unable to talk and is turning blue. The nurse thinks that the resident is choking. Quickly, the nurse moves the meal tray out of the way and uses a two-handed thrust under the resident's diaphragm to attempt to dislodge the food that is obstructing the airway. After the nurse does the abdominal thrusts, the resident is assessed for respiratory movements. If the person is breathing again, the nurse takes a deep breath, cuts the resident's meat into smaller pieces, and observes the resident eating the rest of the meal. If the resident is not breathing, the nurse may attempt another abdominal thrust or reposition the resident so another abdominal thrust can be done from behind.

This short scenario is an example of the nursing process (Fig. 4.1). When the LPN entered the room and saw the older person with hands clenched on throat and turning blue, the nurse was collecting data. In a split second, the nurse identified the resident's problem as choking. The nurse's next thought was to set a goal for this resident's care: The resident will expel the food that is causing the choking. With the goal of expelling the lodged food, the nurse designs the plan from nursing knowledge and immediately implements abdominal thrusts. After the nursing intervention, the nurse evaluates the situation to determine whether the resident has expelled the food. If the resident has not, the nurse must rethink and redesign the plan and immediately implement the revised nursing actions.

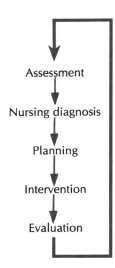

FIG. 4.1. Nursing process model. The circular nature of this model demonstrates that the process is ongoing.

The nursing process is a problem-solving model that describes what nurses do. It identifies the way nurses approach patient care and recognizes the ongoing and changeable nature of the care that nurses provide, care that is based on the individual needs of the patient.

Nurses are faced with many patient or resident care problems every day. The nursing process provides a structure for nurses to plan and give high-quality, individualized care.

ASSESSMENT

The first step in the nursing process is to collect all the information the nurse will need to clearly identify the older person's strengths, and current and potential problems. Usually, the assessment starts with the call or written summary from the agency or department that is transferring the older adult to your nursing care area. The information that it is important to receive before the actual transfer of the person includes:

- Name, age, insurance identification numbers
- Medical diagnoses, advanced directives, disease prognosis
- Family support
- Need for equipment (Does the person need special equipment, such as a special bed, oxygen, intravenous [IV] setup, or feeding pump?)

- Functional ability (How does the person transfer, ambulate, move in bed, bathe, toilet, and eat?)
- Medications (Which prescription and over-the-counter medication does the person take?)
- Cognitive ability (Is the client oriented? How is the person's memory?)
- Special needs (Is the person depressed, at risk for skin breakdown or other health risks?)

This information is very important for the preparation of the older person's bed and room, and makes the transfer to your care as smooth as possible.

Once the older person is transferred, the nurse makes a focused assessment that culminates in a comprehensive assessment. The admission assessment includes observations, physical examination, review of laboratory values, interview of the older adult and his or her family, and a nursing history.

In 1987, the federal government enacted legislation that set minimum standards for the assessment and care planning processes in nursing facilities certified for Medicare reimbursement. This legislation is known as the Omnibus Budget Reconciliation Act of 1987 (OBRA 1987). This was followed by OBRA 1990, which clarified some of the questioned areas of OBRA 1987. The minimum data set (MDS) and resident assessment protocols (RAPs) were a part of the legislation that had been implemented across the country in nursing facilities that accept Medicare and Medicaid funding as reimbursement for the care they provide. The MDS and the RAPs are two components of the mandated assessment process entitled the Resident Assessment Instrument (RAI).

The MDS provides an outline of the most essential information that must be collected about every resident admitted to a nursing facility. Nursing observations, physical assessment, health history, and interview of the older adult and the family, and completion of the RAPs added to the MDS make a comprehensive assessment. (An example of a comprehensive assessment is included in the case study at the end of this chapter and in the Appendix at the end of the book.)

What does a nurse do with all the information that has been collected during assessment? The MDS refers care providers to a list of problem areas that must be addressed in the plan of care. Each of these problem areas also has an RAP that lists areas that require further assessment and consideration before designing the plan of care (Box 4.1)

Frequently, the RAPs are not actually incorporated into the assessment process. These protocols, however, extend the assessment from the minimum information of the MDS and offer a more thorough review of the problem area identified by the MDS.

THE NURSING DIAGNOSIS

Developing the nursing diagnosis is a primary responsibility of the registered nurse. It involves the use of diagnostic reasoning to reflect the older person's strengths, problems, and potential problems. The registered nurse considers the assessment data and organizes them to decide whether they meet criteria for a specific nursing diagnosis. The North American Nursing Diagnosis Association (NANDA) has identified diagnoses that are widely accepted and understood by multiple disciplines and are viewed as the national standards for nursing diagnoses. The NANDA diagnoses are not specific to older people, but they are useful in providing consistent expression of nursing diagnoses for all disciplines and in all settings. An example of a NANDA diagnosis is: *Comfort altered, Pain, related to: degenerative joint disease.*

In the long-term care setting, nurses often prefer to use nursing diagnoses that incorporate the MDS language and format.

An example of an MDS-related nursing diagnosis is: Potential for joint pain due to degenerative joint disease. Common nursing diagnoses for older adults include:

- Self Care Deficit
- Physical Mobility, impaired
- Nutrition, altered: less than body requirements
- Injury, high risk for
- Urinary Elimination, altered
- Constipation
- Thought Process, altered
- Skin Integrity, impaired: high risk for

It is the responsibility of the registered nurse to ensure that nursing diagnoses address the comprehensive assessment. The nursing diagnosis is an important part of the nursing process and addresses the potential and actual problems of the older adult.

NURSING DIAGNOSIS AND MEDICAL DIAGNOSIS

There are two basic ways to communicate the nature of an older adult's health problems.

One way is by medical diagnoses and the other is by nursing diagnoses. Medical diagnoses are made by a physician and describe a disease or a disease process. Diseases are diagnosed by identifying a specific group of signs and symptoms. For example, diabetes mellitus is diagnosed when a person has elevated fasting blood sugar levels, weight loss, thirst, and a large urine output. A person who has an area of dead brain tissue on magnetic resonance imaging (MRI) and computerized tomography (CT) scan, along with speech and swallowing difficulty and left-sided paralysis, would be diagnosed with a cerebrovascular accident (CVA). Both of these medical diagnoses are common for older adults and communicate information to the nurse about what physical or psychological processes are happening to the person.

The major problem with planning care based only on medical diagnoses is that they do not describe the individual problems of the older adult or the impact the disease has on the person's day-to-day life. Nursing diagnoses, on the other hand, are specific to the individual older person's nursing care needs and frequently relate to the areas in which the older person has difficulty functioning.

For example, an obese person who is newly diagnosed with diabetes mellitus may have the following nursing diagnoses:

- Nutrition, altered: more than body requirements and Knowledge Deficit related to poor dietary practices
  A long-term diabetes patient may be experiencing problems with a heel ulcer that will not heal. In this case, the nursing diagnosis would be:
- Skin Integrity, altered
  Both of these people have the same medical diagnoses but different health-care needs, as shown in their nursing diagnoses.

PLANNING

After organizing the assessment data and noting the nursing diagnoses identified by the registered nurse, the practical nurse, working with the older adult, the family, and the health-care team, begins the planning part of the nursing process. The planning portion of the nursing process includes setting priorities, identifying goals and outcomes of care, and designing and documenting interventions.

Setting Priorities

The nurse reviews the nursing diagnoses and places them in priority order. Remember the example at the beginning of this section? Removing the lodged food so the resident could breathe would be a higher priority than putting on the resident's shoes!

One of the most popular models used to assist the nurse in setting priorities is Abraham Maslow's hierarchy of needs. This framework gives life-sustaining needs the highest priority. These needs are followed by safety and security needs, love and belonging needs, self-esteem needs, and self-actualization needs.

Because the nursing process is focused on the older person as an individual, it also is necessary to consider the priorities of the resident. Often, a resident will state that the highest priority is to go home. The resident may refuse treatments, medications, and activities that will maintain personal health because no one is assisting in the patient's discharge. Although discharge may not be realistic (at this time), you, as the nurse, will probably be more successful in providing nursing care if the plan of care addresses discharge to home as a high priority.

This is an example of how the nutrition nursing diagnosis can be considered:

- Nutrition, altered: less than body requirements
  Resident refuses to eat and drink.
  Discuss with the resident what is usually eaten at home and how it is prepared.
  Review how the person's current health status would affect the ability to buy food, prepare it, and eat at home.

Discuss strategies and plans for ensuring that the resident is able to eat after returning home.

Include the resident's food preferences in meals.

GOAL SETTING OR IDENTIFYING OUTCOMES

After identifying the priorities for the resident's care, the nurse identifies goals or outcomes for each of the nursing diagnoses. Setting goals is something that most of us do all of the time. Sometimes our personal goal may be to clock out on time or to survive a busy day. The goals that are part of the planning process, however, describe the specific resident outcomes and identify the goals that direct nursing care. To direct care and describe outcomes, goals must be:

- *Measurable*—measurable outcomes need to be identified. "Eating 100% of a meal" can be measured, whereas it is difficult to measure "appetite will improve."
- *Realistic*—the goal must fit in with the resident's abilities. "The resident will recall the correct date and time" is probably an unrealistic goal for a resident with Alzheimer's disease.
- *Specific*—the goal should identify certain behaviors or conditions to aid in their attainment and evaluation. "The resident will feel better" is not specific. It could be better worded as, "The resident will state that he has less nausea."
- *Timely*—a time frame needs to be established for the attainment of each goal. "The resident will walk 100 feet" does not specify a time frame for achievement of this goal. Adding "by the end of December" provides a time frame.
- *Attainable*—the goal should be written in such a way as to communicate a motivating factor to the resident and the nursing care staff. For an older adult with left hemiplegia, a goal such as "The resident will be independent in self-care by the end of the

When setting goals, carefully consider a holistic approach to meet them. Does this older woman walk better when her family is present? Does she eat better when she has lunch with her granddaughter? Holistic considerations are essential to meaningful goals and their achievement.

year" may be a strong motivator to work harder at the occupational and physical therapy sessions.

In nursing facilities, the documentation regulations under OBRA 1987 and OBRA 1990 require that the status of goal attainment be systematically addressed. These documentation requirements are the monthly summaries (a comprehensive review of outcomes every 30 days) and the quarterly reviews (comprehensive interdisciplinary review of the resident's plan of care every 90 days) (Box 4.2). With new admissions or specific insurance carriers, the nurse may be required to conduct monthly comprehensive assessments of the outcome of care. This provides a 30- or 90-day time framework in which goals can be designed. It also helps the nurse to think about what is realistic in that specific time frame. For a resident who is rehabilitating after having a hip replacement, "Ambulate independently" may be a realistic goal in 6 months. "Stand and walk 10 steps with a walker" may be a more realistic goal for 30 days. The following are examples of goals:

BOX 4.2. ASSESSMENTS NEEDED FOR EACH NURSING HOME RESIDENT

COMPREHENSIVE ADMISSION ASSESSMENT including
RESIDENT ASSESSMENT INSTRUMENT (RAI)

1. Minimum data set (MDS)
2. Resident assessment protocols
3. Ongoing nursing assessment

ANNUAL REASSESSMENT including RAI
SIGNIFICANT CHANGE IN STATUS ASSESSMENT including RAI
QUARTERLY ASSESSMENT including part of MDS

- The resident will eat more than 75% of each meal for the next 30 days.
- The resident will toilet independently when reminded to go to the bathroom for the next 90 days.
- The resident will attend one activity daily for the next 90 days.
- The resident will have no signs and symptoms of a urinary tract infection for the next 90 days.
- The resident's supplemental oxygen needs will be decreased to 1 L in the next 30 days.

Look back at these goals. What do you notice about them? Each goal identifies something that the resident will or will not do, or will or will not experience. The resident's behavior is the major focus of goals as outcomes. Nursing care is not part of the goal. Bathe the resident is a nursing intervention, not an outcome or a goal. Nursing standards also are not part of the goal statements. "Administer all medications within 30 minutes of their ordered time" is a nursing standard, not a resident goal.

Designing and Documenting the Plan of Care

Once the goals or outcomes of care are identified, the practical nurse, along with the other members of the IDT, begin to plan the activities that will help the older person reach the goals. The planning phase involves discussion and pen-and-paper activity. Discussing and documenting the plan of care allows input from all members of the team to be communicated to all staff members who are providing care for that resident. Standards of nursing practice and federal regulations require that

each resident have a written, comprehensive, and interdisciplinary plan of care. The plan of care includes the problem or potential prob-

CRITICALLY EXAMINE THE FOLLOWING:

Identify the correctly stated resident-based outcomes or goals in the following list. When the outcomes or goals are not properly expressed, explain what is wrong.

1. The resident will walk more in the next 90 days.
2. The nurse will toilet the resident every 2 hours for the next 30 days.
3. The resident will have no areas of skin breakdown in the next 90 days.
4. The resident's nutrition will improve.
5. The resident will drink 1500 mL a day for the next 90 days.

The correct answers and rationales follow.

1. This goal is not measurable. It would be better stated as follows: "the resident will walk 100 ft in the next 90 days."
2. This is a nursing intervention rather than a goal. It would be better stated as follows: "the resident will void when toileted by the nursing staff every 2 hours for the next 90 days."
3. This is a realistic, specific, and attainable goal. The outcome of care can be measured.
4. This is a noble goal, but it is not specific or measurable. It would be better stated as follows: "the resident will gain 2 lbs in the next 30 days."
5. This is a realistic, specific, and attainable goal. The outcome of care can be measured.

lem to be identified, the actions or interventions to be taken to address the problem, the person or discipline responsible for each action, and the goals to be achieved. An example of interventions in an interdisciplinary plan of care follows:

• Document percentage of food eaten at each meal—nursing
• Feed resident and assess swallowing ability—speech therapy
• Review dietary preferences—dietary services
• Promote feeding of self—restorative nursing

The focus of this chapter is on developing interdisciplinary plans of care using the nursing process. As you can see, all disciplines caring for the resident need to be represented in an actual plan of care. This is an important criterion for planning interventions: planned interventions must complement the interventions of other therapies. For example, it would be confusing for the resident to be ambulated with a walker by physical therapy and encouraged to walk with two canes by the nursing staff.

It is critical that members of all disciplines discuss and develop the components of the interdisciplinary plan of care so that confusion among the staff does not occur. Residents who are asked to perform one way in physical therapy and another way on the nursing unit can become confused as to how they should perform. A coordinated approach between physical therapy and nursing helps residents improve quickly and maintain function longer. A coordinated approach among all disciplines enhances the effectiveness of the care given to the resident and minimizes duplication of efforts.

Nursing interventions also must consider the safety of the resident. "Administering a diuretic and a sleeping pill at bedtime" is an unsafe nursing action. The resident may fall while going to the bathroom at night if still groggy from the sleeping pill. Transferring a resident who is able to stand only with the assistance of just one staff member, may place that resident at risk of falling.

Selected nursing interventions should help to attain the identified goal. If a resident's goal is to "lose 1 lb a week," giving "dietary supplements between meals and at bedtime" would not assist in achieving this weight loss. When the resident's goal is "will ambulate 100 ft by the end of the month," a nursing intervention must state that the nursing staff will assist the resident to ambulate.

Nursing interventions also must be realistic for the resident, staff, resources, and equipment. A reality in the workplace is that there often is not extra time for staff to talk to the residents. Therefore, providing 30 minutes of one-on-one time discussing pain every shift is an unrealistic intervention. Stating that each staff member "will ask the resident about hip pain whenever he or she interacts with the resident" is a more realistic intervention.

To be successful and effective, nursing interventions must be developed with input from the certified nursing assistants (CNAs). CNAs are important members of the interdisciplinary team. Nursing assistants spend more time with clients in nursing facilities, assisted living facilities, retirement communities, and sometimes in the client's home than any other member of the IDT. They can offer important specific information for the assessment of the client. Because CNAs are so familiar with the daily routine and functioning of the clients, they can offer pertinent, realistic suggestions for individualized interventions to deal with specific problems. They also are frequently the first people to notice subtle changes in residents' conditions that may indicate onset of a new problem or success or failure of an intervention. A care plan meeting, including representatives of all disciplines, is generally held to discuss assessment information and develop the interdisciplinary plan of care. The CNA, who works with the resident to be discussed, must be invited to this meeting and arrangements made to facilitate the CNA's attendance. The time away from the unit for the CNA is minimal compared with the value of the CNAs input into the care planning process.

Successful nursing interventions require the resident's input and should be important to the resident. A resident may not want to "lift weights to strengthen and increase flexibility of his arms" but may be very willing to "comb his hair and wash his face." "Encourage the resident to drink 1000 mL of water" may not work as well as "encourage the resident to drink 1000 mL of fruit juice and water."

Nursing interventions also must include continuing assessment and monitoring of disease processes and effects of medications and treatments. If a resident has an IV, the IV site must be "assessed every shift for signs of infiltration, irritation, and infection." If a resident is receiving therapy with digoxin (Lanoxin), the "apical pulse must be taken and recorded before each dose." Residents with congestive heart failure (CHF) should be "assessed for edema and dyspnea."

Remember that the plan of care is part of the resident's permanent record. It needs to be routinely reviewed and updated as the resident's health status improves or declines. The monthly and quarterly review times provide an excellent opportunity to revise the care plan to ensure that the resident is receiving appropriate nursing care.

IMPLEMENTATION

Implementation is the part of the nursing process that nurses do best. Being at the bedside of the resident providing care is one of the most rewarding aspects of being a nurse. Implementation means actually putting the plan of care into action. Along with providing the nursing care that has been outlined in the resident's nursing care plan, the LPN continues to collect data that can be used to update and revise the plan of care.

Many interventions from the plan of care are assigned to CNAs. This is another strong reason for having CNAs attend the care plan development meeting. If the CNAs have an opportunity to provide input into the plan of care, and they are present when it is discussed and developed, they will be more likely to carry out the interventions than if they are merely told what to do or handed a care plan to read.

Every visit with the resident is an opportunity to reassess your nursing diagnoses and their implementation.

Because nursing assistants on all shifts cannot attend the care plan meeting, a major challenge for the practical nurse is communicating the plan of care back to all CNAs. A variety of communication techniques can be used. Some facilities provide nursing assistants with written assignments that list all of the interventions for each resident. Many facilities place the plan of care in a book and make it available to the staff. Very often, however, the book is rarely consulted. Meeting regularly with nursing assistants to discuss the plan of care, giving each CNA written assignments with information on the plan of care, and using primary CNAs who care for the same residents each day, will ensure the implementation of the plan of care and make it a working document rather than a useless piece of paper completed only to comply with regulations.

Another difficult aspect of implementation is that it also must be documented. Charting is an important part of implementing the plan of care. Documentation of interventions requires not only recording that the intervention was done, but also the resident's responses to the intervention. An entry such as the following provides no information about the resident's response to the treatment:

12/16/93 1420 Wet to dry saline packing to coccyx ulcer

A better picture is given in the following chart:

12/16/93 1420 Wet to dry saline packing to coccyx pressure ulcer. Ulcer is 3 × 2 cm and 1.5 cm deep. Ulcer margins are pink, and there is granulation tissue evident. Small amount of yellow serous drainage on old packing. Resident complained of pain when old packing was removed and new packing inserted. Two small (6-mm) scabs on left buttocks from tape irritation. No redness or drainage noted.

Every visit with the resident is an opportunity to reassess your nursing diagnoses and their implementation. A simple model that can be used to document the nursing process with nursing interventions and resident responses is presented below:

Assessment What the nurse observed and assessed
Objective measurements (blood pressure, laboratory values)
What the resident did (response to nursing intervention)

What the resident said

Action What the nurse did (nursing interventions): treatments, turning the resident, giving a medication, increasing the oxygen flow rate, hanging a tube feeding, inserting a catheter

Plan What the nurse plans to do: call the doctor, call the family, reassess with the next treatment, refer resident to social services

The assessment-action-plan charting format is simple, yet it sets up a framework for documenting the nursing process in a narrative format.

CNAs also may be involved in documentation and may provide information for the practical nurse's documentation. Flow sheets that include interventions from the plan of care and activities from the resident's day can be completed by nursing assistants. Flow sheets can be used to document such interventions as ADLs, walking programs, bowel and bladder training programs, and dietary intake and feeding programs. Results and trends from the flow sheets can be incorporated into the LPNs regular progress charting.

EVALUATION

Evaluation is the final step in the nursing process. The main purpose of evaluation is to decide If the resident has met the identified goals and to assess the outcomes of the nursing care provided. Remember how, in the discussion of implementation, the importance of assessing the resident and documenting the resident's responses to care was emphasized? The chart and resident assessments are reviewed as part of evaluation.

When goals have been stated in measurable terms, the LPN should be able to review all of the data and decide whether the goal has been met, has been partially met, or remains unmet. This is a straightforward look at the

resident's response to the nursing interventions. The evaluation of goal achievement needs to be documented in a monthly summary, quarterly review, or the nursing notes.

Evaluation also requires that the nurse review the nursing process. This helps to keep the plan of care up to date and reflects changes in the resident's health status. It also is an opportunity to decide which nursing interventions were ineffective (Box 4.3).

The reassessment of the resident and the plan of care in evaluation really addresses the dynamic strength of the nursing process. Although it follows specific, organized steps, no step excludes collecting more data. This is done by assessing the resident, updating goals and interventions, and conducting an ongoing evaluation of the outcome of the care that is provided. Nurses seem to use the nursing process even when they do not identify it as such. Here are some examples.

Mary Jones always was incontinent during the 1:00 A.M. rounds. The nursing staff decided to toilet her at 12:30 A.M.

In this example, the nursing staff assessed incontinence as a problem. Their unstated goal was, "the resident will not be incontinent at 1:00 A.M. rounds." Their intervention was to toilet the resident 30 minutes before she was usually incontinent. After toileting the resident at 12:30 A.M., the resident would be checked for urinary incontinence at 1 A.M. If she was not incontinent, the goal would be achieved and the staff would continue to toilet the resident at 12:30 A.M. to maintain that outcome. If the resident was toileted at 12:30 A.M. and she still was incontinent at 1:00 A.M., the staff may decide to toilet the resident at midnight. The care plan and charting examples provided in Figure 4.2 demonstrate the use of evaluation.

As this example shows, evaluation is ongoing and takes place daily, not just at the mandatory reassessment intervals. Thus, evaluation does not take place only when the quarterly assessment is due. Would you continue to carry out an intervention that was not working for 3 months until the quarterly review was due? Many people help you evaluate the plan of care each day. Residents give you information by their behavior and by telling you if an intervention is helping or not. Families tell you about changes they notice. Nursing assistants frequently note subtle changes in residents and may alter interventions to accommodate the change in the residents.

Making daily changes in the actual care given is common. Translating these changes into the written plan of care is less common. For the sake of communication and consistency among all staff, it is very important to be sure that the written plan of care is updated to reflect the actual care you want to be given.

▶ COMPUTERS AND THE NURSING PROCESS

More and more nursing facilities throughout the country are installing computers to help nursing staff complete the MDS assessment and care plans. The practical nurse may be asked to enter MDS data directly on the computer or to complete the written form while another nurse enters the assessment data on the computer for all residents. Many different kinds of software are available that can be used by nurses to complete the MDS, RAPs, and care plans. Each software program is somewhat different, and generally no one program will do everything that you want it to do.

If you have never worked on a computer before, you may be fearful of using it for your assessment and care plans. Completing the MDS and the care plan on the computer, however, has many benefits that warrant overcoming your fears. One of the most time-consuming portions of the MDS is computing the triggers, that is, identifying the potential problem areas that need to be further assessed through the RAPs. Most MDS software packages compute the triggers in a matter of seconds. Completing the interdisciplinary care plan on the computer saves the nurse from a great deal of handwriting and lends itself to regular updating without further lengthy handwriting. Some software packages will print out nursing assistant forms that include all the interventions from the plan of care assigned to the nursing assistant. These forms can be used as assignment sheets that communicate the plan of care to the CNA.

▶ CONCLUSION

As an LPN, you have major responsibilities for delivering meaningful nursing care to residents in long-term care facilities. Your responsibilities include the management of care given by nursing assistants, working with the IDT, completing documents required by the federal government, and delivering excellent care to the frail and vulnerable people in your care. It is essential that you understand and become highly skilled in the content of this chapter. Best wishes as you proceed to meet that objective.

Nursing Diagnosis Problems Addressed	Goals Outcomes of Care	Nursing Interventions	Evaluation
Physical Mobility, impaired related to musculoskeletal impairment as manifested by inability to transfer and ambulate without assistance	Resident will increase ambulation with walker in PT to independent use with minimal supervision in 90 days	■ Assess and document: Orthostatic BPs (lying/sitting/ standing) ROM and strength of legs and arms Walking ability with walker and amount of assistance needed ■ Have walker in resident's reach at all times and use for all transfers and walking in room ■ Physical therapy for quad-strengthening exercises and ambulation with walker ■ Put on jogging pants for daily physical therapy	

FIG. 4.2. Sample care plan.

DOCUMENTATION

October 11, 1994, 1:45 p.m.: Resident is transferred from bed to wheelchair with assistance of one. Uses walker to steady himself when standing. Ambulates with hold-on assistance from physical therapist using a walker. Ambulated two steps withou hold-on assistance before becoming unsteady. Orthostatic BPs lying—138/82, sitting—110/80, standing—106/76, complained of being light-headed when he sat up. Dizziness passed in 5 minutes. Instructed to move slowly from lying-sitting-standing positions and not to move to another position until any dizziness or light-headedness passes. Will review medications and fluid intake for possible causes of orthostatic hypotension.

CASE STUDY

RESIDENT ADMISSION

December 1, 1997, 1 P.M.: Mr. B., 82-year-old white widowed male, is admitted to Room 112 of Quality Care Health Facility from Mercy Hospital via ambulance accompanied by daughter-in-law. Admitted with diagnosis of fractured left wrist, multiple hematomas and abrasions, Alzheimer's disease, diabetes mellitus, and a history of CHF. Dr. Ben Johnston notified of admission and verified orders. Dietary notified of 2 g sodium/no concentrated sweets diet. Medication orders faxed to the pharmacy:

furosemide (Lasix) 40 mg q.d. for CHF and COPD
digoxin (Lanoxin) 0.125 mg q.d. for CHF
potassium chloride (K-tabs) 2 tabs q.d. for CHF
glipizide (Glucotrol) 5 mg q. A.M. for diabetes
oxazepam (Serax) 20 mg q.h.s. for insomnia
haloperidol (Haldol) 1 mg b.i.d. for agitation
ducosate (Dulcolax) sodium suppository q.d. prn constipation
acetaminophen (Tylenol) gr 10 q.4h. p.r.n. pain
hydrocolloid gel (DuoDerm) to open area on coccyx change q.o.d.
mupirocin (Bactroban) to abrasions b.i.d.
nystatin (Mycostatin) ointment to perineal rash b.i.d. 3 to 10 days
Ace wrap and splint to left wrist at all times return to clinic in 2 weeks

Son has durable power of attorney for both financial and health-care decisions, and has signed the advanced directive form for "Do Not Resuscitate." Resident has a living will, and his wishes are known to his family.

Daughter-in-law reports that he has no known allergies, wears bifocals and reads large-print Reader's Digest occasionally, has upper and lower dentures, does not use a hearing aid, and has minimal difficulty hearing unless in a noisy room. Uses a cane to ambulate. Height—5' 9"; weight—124 lb.

Mr. B. is alert and oriented to self and daughter-in-law but states that it is 1936, that the season is winter, the month is September, and that he is in Denver. Since his wife died 6 months ago, he has been living with his son and his family. His daughter-in-law has been his principal caregiver. Caring for Mr. B. has been quite stressful at times. He does not strike out but repeatedly asks the same questions over and over, even when the question has been answered. His daughter-in-law took a leave of absence from her job because Mr. B. could no longer stay in the house alone without becoming very anxious. He would call friends on the phone repeatedly and ask for his deceased wife. He would often go for walks and get lost.

Mr. B. was admitted to Mercy Hospital after he had fallen on an uneven sidewalk four blocks from home and suffered a concussion, multiple facial hematomas, abrasions on his right arm and shoulder, a fractured left wrist, and a large hematoma on his left hip. His daughter-in-law had been in the basement folding laundry when Mr. B. left the house. The family is expressing much guilt over the decision to place Mr. B. in a long-term care facility, but they admit that he would be safer there.

Mr. B is able to walk with his cane but favors the left hip when he stands and is very unsteady. He forgets where he is and cries out for help. He is able to dress himself but must have supervision to remind him of what he is doing. Mr. B. is able to feed himself but has not been eating and has lost a significant amount of weight in the past 3 months. Mr. B. has been generally continent of his bladder and bowel except while in the hospital, where he was incontinent of both.

Mr. B. was an accountant before he retired, and he would often spend hours with a paper and pencil "doing the books." He has always enjoyed classical music and was quite an accomplished pianist. He had season tickets to the ballet and the opera, and would go often before his wife died 6 months ago.

CHF = congestive heart failure; COPD = chronic obstructive coronary disease, b.i.d. = twice daily; p.r.n. = as needed; q. A.M. = every morning; q.o.d. = every other day; q.4h. = every 4 hours; q.h.s. = before bedtime, every hour of sleep.

Physical Assessment

General Appearance	Thin white male
Head and Neck	White hair. Scalp dry with multiple areas of white dry flaking. Face symmetrical, two 5-cm hematomas on left cheek and jaw. Two-centimeter hematoma on left forehead, skin also is dry. Eyes are clear with no drainage, conjunctivae pink, pupils are equal at 5 mm and react briskly to light, consensual, and accommodative. No drainage from nose; patient is able to breathe through both nostrils. No drainage from ears. Did not appropriately respond when asked in a whisper to raise his arm. Oral mucous membranes are pink and dry. No denture irritation noted. No saliva pooling noted between gum and cheek. Tongue pink with no coating; remains at midline when extended from mouth. Throat dry with no pharyngeal drainage or redness noted: no cervical lymph nodes palpable: no thyroid nodules or enlargement palpated.
Chest	Symmetrical chest movements. Breath sounds clear throughout except for expiratory crackle in base of left lower lobe that cleared with cough. Apical pulse—78 and regular. No extra heart sounds noted. Back has multiple waxy, light brown to medium brown, 2 to 3 cm flat raised lesions. Moderate kyphosis of spine.
Abdomen and Buttocks	Large (8 × 12 cm) hematoma over left hip and left lower abdominal area. Hard stool in rectum. Active bowel sounds in all quadrants. Abdomen soft. No masses palpable. A 2 × 1.5 cm stage 2 pressure ulcer over coccyx that is oozing serous drainage. Three small fluid-filled vesicles in gluteal fold of right buttocks.
Genitourinary	Normal male genitalia. Urinary meatus reddened.
	Urine dark amber and foul smelling. Fiery red rash noted on inner aspects of both upper thighs and scrotum.
Extremities	Full range of motion (ROM) of shoulders, elbows, right wrist, and fingers. Left wrist is splinted with a rigid plastic splint and wrapped with an Ace bandage that he is constantly unwrapping. Radial and brachial pulses strong and equal bilaterally. Healing abrasions noted over lateral aspect of left upper arm and left shoulder. Limited ROM of both hips with complaints of pain with movement of left hip. Full ROM of both knees and ankles. Femoral and popliteal pulses strong and equal bilaterally. Left pedal pulse weak and 1+ pitting edema noted in left ankle. Right pedal pulse strong and right ankle edematous with no pitting noted. Homans' sign not present bilaterally, and no complaints of calf tenderness to palpation. One-centimeter eschar noted along medial nail of the left great toe. No drainage noted, but there is slight redness around the eschar.

December 6, 2:00 P.M.: Mr. B. was found in another resident's room pulling clothes out of the closet. This is a daily occurrence. Mr. B. cannot explain why he is in the other resident's room and does not know the way back to his room. He yells at his roommate to get out and yells randomly at other residents in the facility. When he is in his room, he cries for help but does not have any requests or needs when the staff members answer. He went 3 days without having a bowel movement and was incontinent of stool in the hallway 30 minutes after being given a suppository. Mr. B. attends activities when asked to go, but he often leaves the activity early. He naps for 1 to 2 hours in the afternoon and is awake frequently at night, where he has to be reminded to stay in bed. He was found one night stuck between the side rails and incontinent of urine.

The MDS for Mr. B. is shown in Figure 4.3.

MINIMUM DATA SET (MDS) — *VERSION 2.0*
FOR NURSING HOME RESIDENT ASSESSMENT AND CARE SCREENING
BASIC ASSESSMENT TRACKING FORM

SECTION AA. IDENTIFICATION INFORMATION		GENERAL INSTRUCTIONS

GENERAL INSTRUCTIONS

Complete this information for submission with all full and quarterly assessments (Admission, Annual, Significant Change, State or Medicare required assessments, or Quarterly Reviews, etc.).

1. RESIDENT NAME ✱
George T. Blair
a. (First)   b. (Middle Initial)   c. (Last)   d. (Jr./Sr.)

2. GENDER ✱
1. Male   2. Female | 1 |

3. BIRTHDATE ✱
| 1 0 | – | 1 5 | – | 1 9 1 5 |
Month   Day   Year

4. RACE/ETHNICITY ✱
1. American Indian/Alaskan Native
2. Asian/Pacific Islander
3. Black, not of Hispanic origin
4. Hispanic
5. White, not of Hispanic origin | 5 |

5. SOCIAL SECURITY AND MEDICARE NUMBERS ✱ [C in 1st box if non Med. no.]
a. Social Security Number
| 0 0 5 | – | 0 6 | – | 7 8 0 0 |
b. Medicare number (or comparable railroad insurance number)
| 0 0 5 0 6 7 8 0 0 A |

6. FACILITY PROVIDER NO. ✱
a. State No.
| |
b. Federal No. | 5 4 0 9 |

7. MEDICAID NO. ["+" if pending, "N" if not a Medicaid ✱ recipient]
| N |

8. REASONS FOR ASSESSMENT
[Note—Other codes do not apply to this form]
a. Primary reason for assessment
1. Admission assessment (required by day 14)
2. Annual assessment
3. Significant change in status assessment
4. Significant correction of prior assessment
5. Quarterly review assessment
0. *NONE OF ABOVE* | 1 |

b. *Special codes for use with supplemental assessment types in Case Mix demonstration states or other states where required*
1. *5 day assessment*
2. *30 day assessment*
3. *60 day assessment*
4. *Quarterly assessment using full MDS form*
5. *Readmission/return assessment*
6. *Other state required assessment*

9. SIGNATURES OF PERSONS COMPLETING THESE ITEMS:
a. Signatures A. Jones, R.N.   Title   12/2/2002   Date

b.   Date

✱ = Key items for computerized resident tracking
▨ = When box blank, must enter number or letter
| a. | = When letter in box, check if condition applies

Code "NA" if information unavailable or unknown.

TRIGGER LEGEND

1 - Delirium
2 - Cognitive Loss/Dementia
3 - Visual Function
4 - Communication
5A - ADL-Rehabilitation
5B - ADL-Maintenance
6 - Urinary Incontinence and Indwelling Catheter
7 - Psychosocial Well-Being
8 - Mood State
9 - Behavioral Symptoms
10A - Activities (Revise)
10B - Activities (Review)
11 - Falls
12 - Nutritional Status
13 - Feeding Tubes
14 - Dehydration/Fluid Maintenance
15 - Dental Care
16 - Pressure Ulcers
17 - Psychotropic Drug Use
17* - For this to trigger, O4a, b, or c must = 1-7
18 - Physical Restraints

Form 1728HH   © 1995 Briggs Corporation, Des Moines, IA 50306   (800) 247-2343   PRINTED IN U.S.A.
R196   Copyright limited to addition of trigger system.

1 of 8

FIG. 4.3. Sample minimum data set.

MINIMUM DATA SET (MDS) — *VERSION 2.0*
FOR NURSING HOME RESIDENT ASSESSMENT AND CARE SCREENING
BACKGROUND (FACE SHEET) INFORMATION AT ADMISSION

SECTION AB. DEMOGRAPHIC INFORMATION

1.	DATE OF ENTRY	Date the stay began. Note — Does not include readmission if record was closed at time of temporary discharge to hospital, etc. In such cases, use prior admission date.

$$\boxed{1\ 2} - \boxed{0\ 1} - \boxed{1\ 9\ 9\ 7}$$
Month — Day — Year

2.	ADMITTED FROM (AT ENTRY)	1. Private home/apt. with no home health services 2. Private home/apt. with home health services 3. Board and care/assisted living/group home 4. Nursing home 5. Acute care hospital 6. Psychiatric hospital, MR/DD facility 7. Rehabilitation hospital 8. Other	**1**
3.	LIVED ALONE (PRIOR TO ENTRY)	0. No 1. Yes 2. In other facility	**0**
4.	ZIP CODE OF PRIOR PRIMARY RESIDENCE		**84403**
5.	RESIDEN-TIAL HISTORY 5 YEARS PRIOR TO ENTRY	*(Check all settings resident lived in during 5 years prior to date of entry given in item AB1 above.)* Prior stay at this nursing home — a. Stay in other nursing home — b. Other residential facility — board and care home, assisted living, group home — c. MH/psychiatric setting — d. MR/DD setting — e. *NONE OF ABOVE* — f. ✓
6.	LIFETIME OCCUPA-TION(S) *(Put "/" between two occupations)*	accountant
7.	EDUCATION *(Highest level completed)*	1. No schooling 5. Technical or trade school 2. 8th grade/less 6. Some college 3. 9-11 grades 7. Bachelor's degree 4. High school 8. Graduate degree	**7**
8.	LANGUAGE	*(Code for correct response)* a. Primary Language 0. English 1. Spanish 2. French 3. Other	**0**
		b. If other, specify	
9.	MENTAL HEALTH HISTORY	Does resident's RECORD indicate any history of mental retardation, mental illness, or developmental disability problem? 0. No 1. Yes	**0**
10.	CONDITIONS RELATED TO MR/DD STATUS	*(Check all conditions that are related to MR/DD status that were manifested before age 22, and are likely to continue indefinitely)* Not applicable — no MR/DD (Skip to AB11) — a. MR/DD with organic condition Down's syndrome — b. Autism — c. Epilepsy — d. Other organic condition related to MR/DD — e. MR/DD with no organic condition — f.
11.	DATE BACK-GROUND INFORMA-TION COMPLETED	

$$\boxed{1\ 2} - \boxed{0\ 2} - \boxed{1\ 9\ 9\ 7}$$
Month — Day — Year

▨ = When box blank, must enter number or letter

a.☐ = When letter in box, check if condition applies

Code "NA" if information unavailable or unknown.

SECTION AC. CUSTOMARY ROUTINE

1.	CUSTOMARY ROUTINE	*(Check all that apply. If all information UNKNOWN, check last box only)*

(In year prior to DATE OF ENTRY to this nursing home, or year last in community if now being admitted from another nursing home)

CYCLE OF DAILY EVENTS	
Stays up late at night (e.g., after 9 pm)	a.
Naps regularly during day (at least 1 hour)	b.
Goes out 1+ days a week	c.
Stays busy with hobbies, reading, or fixed daily routine	d.
Spends most of time alone or watching TV	e.
Moves independently indoors (with appliances, if used)	f. ✓
Use of tobacco products at least daily	g.
NONE OF ABOVE	h.
EATING PATTERNS	
Distinct food preferences	i.
Eats between meals all or most days	j.
Use of alcoholic beverage(s) at least weekly	k.
NONE OF ABOVE	l. ✓
ADL PATTERNS	
In bedclothes much of day	m.
Wakens to toilet all or most nights	n. ✓
Has irregular bowel movement pattern	o.
Showers for bathing	p.
Bathing in PM	q.
NONE OF ABOVE	r.
INVOLVEMENT PATTERNS	
Daily contact with relatives/close friends	s. ✓
Usually attends church, temple, synagogue (etc.)	t.
Finds strength in faith	u.
Daily animal companion/presence	v.
Involved in group activities	w.
NONE OF ABOVE	x.
UNKNOWN — Resident/family unable to provide information	y.

END

SECTION AD. FACE SHEET SIGNATURES

SIGNATURES OF PERSONS COMPLETING FACE SHEET:

A. Jones, R.N.		12/2/2002
a. Signature of RN Assessment Coordinator		Date
b. Signatures Title Sections		Date
c.		Date
d.		Date
e.		Date
f.		Date
g.		Date

NOTE: Normally, the MDS Face Sheet is completed once, when an individual first enters the facility. However, the face sheet is also required if the person is reentering this facility after a discharge where return had not previously been expected. It is **not** completed following temporary discharges to hospitals or after therapeutic leaves/home visits.

Form 1728HH © 1995 Briggs Corporation, Des Moines, IA 50306 (800) 247-2343 PRINTED IN U.S.A.
Copyright limited to addition of trigger system.

2 of 8

MDS 2.0   10/18/94N

Resident __George Blair__   Numeric Identifier __784393__

MINIMUM DATA SET (MDS) — *VERSION 2.0*
FOR NURSING HOME RESIDENT ASSESSMENT AND CARE SCREENING
FULL ASSESSMENT FORM
(Status in last 7 days, unless other time frame indicated)

SECTION A. IDENTIFICATION AND BACKGROUND INFORMATION

1. RESIDENT NAME
George T. Blair
a. (First)　b. (Middle Initial)　c. (Last)　d. (Jr./Sr.)

2. ROOM NUMBER `112`

3. ASSESSMENT REFERENCE DATE
a. Last day of MDS observation period
`12` – `14` – `2002`
Month　Day　Year
b. Original (0) or corrected copy of form (enter number of correction) `0`

4a. DATE OF REENTRY Date of reentry from most recent temporary discharge to a hospital in last 90 days) (or since last assessment or admission if less than 90 days)
____ – ____ – ____
Month　Day　Year

5. MARITAL STATUS
1. Never married 3. Widowed 5. Divorced
2. Married 4. Separated
`3`

6. MEDICAL RECORD NO. `784393`

7. CURRENT PAYMENT SOURCES FOR N.H. STAY
(Billing Office to indicate; check all that apply in last 30 days)
Medicaid per diem `a.`
Medicare per diem `b.✓`
Medicare ancillary part A `c.`
Medicare ancillary part B `d.`
CHAMPUS per diem `e.`
VA per diem `f.`
Self or family pays for full per diem `g.`
Medicaid resident liability or Medicare co-payment `h.`
Private insurance per diem (including co-payment) `i.`
Other per diem `j.`

8. REASONS FOR ASSESSMENT
[Note—If this is a discharge or reentry assessment, only a limited subset of MDS items need be completed]
a. Primary reason for assessment
1. Admission assessment (required by day 14)
2. Annual assessment
3. Significant change in status assessment
4. Significant correction of prior assessment
5. Quarterly review assessment
6. Discharged—return not anticipated
7. Discharged—return anticipated
8. Discharged prior to completing initial assessment
9. Reentry
0. NONE OF ABOVE
`1`
b. Special codes for use with supplemental assessment types in Case Mix demonstration states or other states where required
1. 5 day assessment
2. 30 day assessment
3. 60 day assessment
4. Quarterly assessment using full MDS form
5. Readmission/return assessment
6. Other state required assessment

9. RESPONSIBILITY/ LEGAL GUARDIAN
(Check all that apply)
Legal guardian `a.`
Other legal oversight `b.`
Durable power of attorney/health care `c.`
Durable power of attorney/ financial `d.`
Family member responsible `e.`
Patient responsible for self `f.`
NONE OF ABOVE `g.`

10. ADVANCED DIRECTIVES
(For those items with supporting documentation in the medical record, check all that apply)
Living will `a.✓`
Do not resuscitate `b.✓`
Do not hospitalize `c.`
Organ donation `d.`
Autopsy request `e.`
Feeding restrictions `f.`
Medication restrictions `g.`
Other treatment restrictions `h.`
NONE OF ABOVE `i.`

SECTION B. COGNITIVE PATTERNS

1. COMATOSE (Persistent vegetative state/no discernible consciousness)
0. No 1. Yes (If yes, skip to Section G)
`0`

2. MEMORY (Recall of what was learned or known)
a. Short-term memory OK—seems/appears to recall after 5 minutes
0. Memory OK 1. Memory problem 2
`1`
b. Long-term memory OK—seems/appears to recall long past
0. Memory OK 1. Memory problem 2
`1`

☐ = When box blank, must enter number or letter.
`a.` = When letter in box, check if condition applies
Code "NA" if information unavailable or unknown.

Form 1728HH © 1995 Briggs Corporation, Des Moines, IA 50306 (800) 247-2343 PRINTED IN U.S.A.
Copyright limited to addition of trigger system.

---

3. MEMORY/ RECALL ABILITY
(Check all that resident was normally able to recall during last 7 days)
Current season `a.`
Location of own room `b.`
Staff names/faces `c.`
That he/she is in a nursing home `d.`
NONE OF ABOVE are recalled `e.✓`

4. COGNITIVE SKILLS FOR DAILY DECISION-MAKING
(Made decisions regarding tasks of daily life)
0. INDEPENDENT—decisions consistent/reasonable
1. MODIFIED INDEPENDENCE—some difficulty in new situations only 2
2. MODERATELY IMPAIRED—decisions poor; cues/ supervision required 2
3. SEVERELY IMPAIRED—never/rarely made decisions 2, 5B
`3`

5. INDICATORS OF DELIRIUM— PERIODIC DISORDERED THINKING/ AWARENESS
(Code for behavior in the last 7 days.) [Note: Accurate assessment requires conversations with staff and family who have direct knowledge of resident's behavior over this time.]
0. Behavior not present
1. Behavior present, not of recent onset
2. Behavior present, over last 7 days appears different from resident's usual functioning (e.g., new onset or worsening)
a. EASILY DISTRACTED—(e.g., difficulty paying attention; gets sidetracked) 2 = 1, 17* `1`
b. PERIODS OF ALTERED PERCEPTION OR AWARENESS OF SURROUNDINGS—(e.g., moves lips or talks to someone not present; believes he/she is somewhere else; confuses night and day) 2 = 1, 17* `1`
c. EPISODES OF DISORGANIZED SPEECH—(e.g., speech is incoherent, nonsensical, irrelevant, or rambling from subject to subject; loses train of thought) 2 = 1, 17* `0`
d. PERIODS OF RESTLESSNESS—(e.g., fidgeting or picking at skin, clothing, napkins, etc.; frequent position changes; repetitive physical movements or calling out) 2 = 1, 17* `0`
e. PERIODS OF LETHARGY—(e.g., sluggishness; staring into space; difficult to arouse; little body movement) 2 = 1, 17* `0`
f. MENTAL FUNCTION VARIES OVER THE COURSE OF THE DAY—(e.g., sometimes better, sometimes worse; behaviors sometimes present, sometimes not) 2 = 1, 17* `0`

6. CHANGE IN COGNITIVE STATUS
Resident's cognitive status, skills, or abilities have changed as compared to status of 90 days ago (or since last assessment if less than 90 days)
0. No change 1. Improved 2. Deteriorated 1, 17* `0`

SECTION C. COMMUNICATION/HEARING PATTERNS

1. HEARING (With hearing appliance, if used)
0. HEARS ADEQUATELY—normal talk, TV, phone
1. MINIMAL DIFFICULTY when not in quiet setting 4
2. HEARS IN SPECIAL SITUATIONS ONLY—speaker has to adjust tonal quality and speak distinctly 4
3. HIGHLY IMPAIRED/absence of useful hearing 4
`1`

2. COMMUNICATION DEVICES/ TECHNIQUES
(Check all that apply during last 7 days)
Hearing aid, present and used `a.`
Hearing aid, present and not used regularly `b.`
Other receptive comm. techniques used (e.g., lip reading) `c.`
NONE OF ABOVE `d.`

3. MODES OF EXPRESSION
(Check all used by resident to make needs known)
Speech `a.`
Writing messages to express or clarify needs `b.`
American sign language or Braille `c.`
Signs/gestures/sounds `d.`
Communication board `e.`
Other `f.`
NONE OF ABOVE `g.`

4. MAKING SELF UNDERSTOOD
(Expressing information content—however able)
0. UNDERSTOOD
1. USUALLY UNDERSTOOD—difficulty finding words or finishing thoughts 4
2. SOMETIMES UNDERSTOOD—ability is limited to making concrete requests 4
3. RARELY/NEVER UNDERSTOOD 4
`1`

5. SPEECH CLARITY
(Code for speech in the last 7 days)
0. CLEAR SPEECH—distinct, intelligible words
1. UNCLEAR SPEECH—slurred, mumbled words
2. NO SPEECH—absence of spoken words
`0`

6. ABILITY TO UNDERSTAND OTHERS
(Understanding verbal information content—however able)
0. UNDERSTANDS
1. USUALLY UNDERSTANDS—may miss some part/ intent of message 2, 4
2. SOMETIMES UNDERSTANDS—responds adequately to simple, direct communication 2, 4
3. RARELY/NEVER UNDERSTANDS 2, 4
`2`

7. CHANGE IN COMMUNICATION/ HEARING
Resident's ability to express, understand, or hear information has changed as compared to status of 90 days ago (or since last assessment if less than 90 days)
0. No change 1. Improved 2. Deteriorated 17*
`0`

3 of 8

MDS 2.0 10/18/94N

70　FOUNDATIONS OF CARE FOR THE OLDER ADULT

Resident __George Blair__   Numeric Identifier __784393__

5.	**CHANGE IN BEHAVIORAL SYMPTOMS**	Resident's behavior status has changed as compared to **status of 90 days ago** (or since last assessment if less than 90 days) 0. No change 1. Improved 2. Deteriorated **1, 17*** **2**

SECTION D. VISION PATTERNS

1.	**VISION**	*(Ability to see in adequate light and with glasses if used)* 0. *ADEQUATE*—sees fine detail, including regular print in newspapers/books 1. *IMPAIRED*—sees large print, but not regular print in newspapers/books **3** 2. *MODERATELY IMPAIRED*—limited vision; not able to see newspaper headlines, but can identify objects **3** 3. *HIGHLY IMPAIRED*—object identification in question, but eyes appear to follow objects **3** 4. *SEVERELY IMPAIRED*—no vision or sees only light, colors, or shapes; eyes do not appear to follow objects	**1**
2.	**VISUAL LIMITATIONS/ DIFFICULTIES**	Side vision problems—decreased peripheral vision (e.g., leaves food on one side of tray, difficulty traveling, bumps into people and objects, misjudges placement of chair when seating self) **3**	a.
		Experiences any of following: sees halos or rings around lights; sees flashes of light; sees "curtains" over eyes	b.
		NONE OF ABOVE	c. ✔
3.	**VISUAL APPLIANCES**	Glasses; contact lenses; magnifying glass 0. No 1. Yes	**1**

SECTION E. MOOD AND BEHAVIOR PATTERNS

1.	**INDICATORS OF DEPRESSION, ANXIETY, SAD MOOD**	*(Code for indicators observed in last 30 days, irrespective of the assumed cause)* 0. Indicator not exhibited in last 30 days 1. Indicator of this type exhibited up to five days a week 2. Indicator of this type exhibited daily or almost daily (6, 7 days a week)	

VERBAL EXPRESSIONS OF DISTRESS

a. Resident made negative statements—e.g., "Nothing matters; Would rather be dead; What's the use; Regrets having lived so long; Let me die" 1 or 2 = **8**	**0**	h. Repetitive health complaints—e.g., persistently seeks medical attention, obsessive concern with body functions 1 or 2 = **8**	**0**
b. Repetitive questions—e.g., "Where do I go; What do I do?" 1 or 2 = **8**	**2**	i. Repetitive anxious complaints/concerns (non-health related)—e.g., persistently seeks attention/reassurance regarding schedules, meals, laundry/clothing, relationship issues 1 or 2 = **8**	**0**
c. Repetitive verbalizations—e.g., calling out for help ("God help me") 1 or 2 = **8**	**0**	**SLEEP-CYCLE ISSUES** j. Unpleasant mood in morning 1 or 2 = **8**	**0**
d. Persistent anger with self or others—e.g., easily annoyed, anger at placement in nursing home; anger at care received 1 or 2 = **8**	**1**	k. Insomnia/change in usual sleep pattern 1 or 2 = **8**	**0**
e. Self deprecation—e.g., "I am nothing; I am of no use to anyone" 1 or 2 = **8**	**0**	**SAD, APATHETIC, ANXIOUS APPEARANCE** l. Sad, pained, worried facial expressions—e.g., furrowed brows 1 or 2 = **8**	**0**
f. Expressions of what appear to be unrealistic fears—e.g., fear of being abandoned, left alone, being with others 1 or 2 = **8**	**0**	m. Crying, tearfulness 1 or 2 = **8** n. Repetitive physical movements—e.g., pacing, hand wringing, restlessness, fidgeting, picking 1 or 2 = **8, 17***	**0** **0**
g. Recurrent statements that something terrible is about to happen—e.g., believes he or she is about to die, have a heart attack		**LOSS OF INTEREST** o. Withdrawal from activities of interest—e.g., no interest in longstanding activities or being with family/ friends 1 or 2 = **7, 8**	**0**
		p. Reduced social interaction 1 or 2 = **8**	**0**

2.	**MOOD PERSISTENCE**	One or more indicators of depressed, sad or anxious mood were not easily altered by attempts to "cheer up", console, or reassure the resident over last 7 days 0. No mood indicators 1. Indicators present, easily altered **8** 2. Indicators present, not easily altered **8**	**2**
3.	**CHANGE IN MOOD**	Resident's mood status has changed as compared to status of 90 days ago (or since last assessment if **less than 90 days**) 0. No change 1. Improved 2. Deteriorated **1, 17***	**2**
4.	**BEHAVIORAL SYMPTOMS**	*(A) Behavioral symptom frequency in last 7 days* 0. Behavior not exhibited in last 7 days 1. Behavior of this type occurred 1 to 3 days in last 7 days 2. Behavior of this type occurred 4 to 6 days, but less than daily 3. Behavior of this type occurred daily *(B) Behavioral symptom alterability in last 7 days* 0. Behavior not present OR behavior was easily altered 1. Behavior was not easily altered	(A) (B)

a. WANDERING (moved with no rational purpose, seemingly oblivious to needs or safety) A = 1, 2, or 3 = **9, 11**	**3**	**2**
b. VERBALLY ABUSIVE BEHAVIORAL SYMPTOMS (others were threatened, screamed at, cursed at) A = 1, 2, or 3 = **9**	**3**	**2**
c. PHYSICALLY ABUSIVE BEHAVIORAL SYMPTOMS (others were hit, shoved, scratched, sexually abused) A = 1, 2, or 3 = **9**	**0**	**0**
d. SOCIALLY INAPPROPRIATE/DISRUPTIVE BEHAVIORAL SYMPTOMS (made disruptive sounds, noisiness, screaming, self-abusive acts, sexual behavior or disrobing in public, smeared/threw food/feces, hoarding, rummaged through others' belongings) A = 1, 2, or 3 = **9**	**3**	**2**
e. RESISTS CARE (resisted taking medications/injections, ADL assistance, or eating) A = 1, 2, or 3 = **9**	**0**	**0**

SECTION F. PSYCHOSOCIAL WELL-BEING

1.	**SENSE OF INITIATIVE/ INVOLVEMENT**	At ease interacting with others	a.
		At ease doing planned or structured activities	b.
		At ease doing self-initiated activities	c.
		Establishes own goals **7**	d.
		Pursues involvement in life of facility (e.g., makes/keeps friends; involved in group activities; responds positively to new activities; assists at religious services)	e.
		Accepts invitations into most group activities	f. ✔
		NONE OF ABOVE	g.
2.	**UNSETTLED RELATIONSHIPS**	Covert/open conflict with or repeated criticism of staff **7**	a.
		Unhappy with roommate **7**	b. ✔
		Unhappy with residents other than roommate **7**	c. ✔
		Openly expresses conflict/anger with family/friends **7**	d.
		Absence of personal contact with family/friends	e.
		Recent loss of close family member/friend	f. ✔
		Does not adjust easily to change in routines	g.
		NONE OF ABOVE	h.
3.	**PAST ROLES**	Strong identification with past roles and life status **7**	a. ✔
		Expresses sadness/anger/empty feeling over lost roles/status	b.
		Resident perceives that daily routine (customary routine, activities) is very different from prior pattern in the community **7**	c.
		NONE OF ABOVE	d.

SECTION G. PHYSICAL FUNCTIONING AND STRUCTURAL PROBLEMS

1.	(A)	**ADL SELF-PERFORMANCE—(Code for resident's PERFORMANCE OVER ALL SHIFTS during last 7 days—Not including setup)** 0. *INDEPENDENT*—No help or oversight—OR—Help/oversight provided only 1 or 2 times during last 7 days 1. *SUPERVISION*—Oversight, encouragement or cueing provided 3 or more times during last 7 days—OR—Supervision (3 or more times) plus physical assistance provided only 1 or 2 times during last 7 days 2. *LIMITED ASSISTANCE*—Resident highly involved in activity; received physical help in guided maneuvering of limbs or other nonweight bearing assistance 3 or more times—OR—More help provided only 1 or 2 times during last 7 days 3. *EXTENSIVE ASSISTANCE*—While resident performed part of activity, over last 7-day period, help of following type(s) provided 3 or more times: —Weight-bearing support —Full staff performance during part (but not all) of last 7 days 4. *TOTAL DEPENDENCE*—Full staff performance of activity during entire 7 days 8. *ACTIVITY DID NOT OCCUR* during entire 7 days

(B)	**ADL SUPPORT PROVIDED—(Code for MOST SUPPORT PROVIDED OVER ALL SHIFTS during last 7 days; code regardless of resident's self-performance classification)** 0. No setup or physical help from staff 1. Setup help only 2. One person physical assist 3. Two+ persons physical assist 8. ADL activity itself did not occur during entire 7 days

			(A) SELF-PERF	(B) SUPPORT
a.	BED MOBILITY	How resident moves to and from lying position, turns side to side, and positions body while in bed A = 1 - **5A** ; A = 2, 3, or 4 = **5A, 16** ; A = 8 - **16**	0	0
b.	TRANSFER	How resident moves between surfaces—to/from: bed, chair, wheelchair, standing position (EXCLUDE to/from bath/toilet) A = 1, 2, 3, or 4 = **5A**	0	0
c.	WALK IN ROOM	How resident walks between locations in his/her room A = 1, 2, 3, or 4 = **5A**	2	2
d.	WALK IN CORRIDOR	How resident walks in corridor on unit A = 1, 2, 3, or 4 = **5A**	2	2
e.	LOCOMOTION ON UNIT	How resident moves between locations in his/her room and adjacent corridor on same floor. If in wheelchair, self-sufficiency once in chair A = 1, 2, 3, or 4 = **5A**	2	2
f.	LOCOMOTION OFF UNIT	How resident moves to and returns from off unit locations (e.g., areas set aside for dining, activities, or treatments). If facility has only one floor, how resident moves to and from distant areas on the floor. If in wheelchair, self-sufficiency once in chair A = 1, 2, 3, or 4 = **5A**	2	2
g.	DRESSING	How resident puts on, fastens, and takes off all items of street clothing, including donning/removing prosthesis A = 1, 2, 3, or 4 = **5A**	3	2
h.	EATING	How resident eats and drinks (regardless of skill). Includes intake of nourishment by other means (e.g., tube feeding, total parenteral nutrition) A = 1, 2, 3, or 4 = **5A**	1	1
i.	TOILET USE	How resident uses the toilet room (or commode, bedpan, urinal); transfers on/off toilet, cleanses, changes pad, manages ostomy or catheter, adjusts clothes A = 1, 2, 3, or 4 = **5A**	2	1
j.	PERSONAL HYGIENE	How resident maintains personal hygiene, including combing hair, brushing teeth, shaving, applying makeup, washing/drying face, hands, and perineum (EXCLUDE baths and showers) A = 1, 2, 3, or 4 = **5A**	2	2

Form 1728HH   © 1995 Briggs Corporation, Des Moines, IA 50306 (800) 247-2343 PRINTED IN U.S.A. Copyright limited to addition of trigger system.

MDS 2.0   10/18/94N

Resident __George Blair__   Numeric Identifier __784393__

2.	BATHING	How resident takes full-body bath/shower, sponge bath, and transfers in/out of tub/shower (EXCLUDE washing of back and hair). **Code for most dependent in self-performance and support.** A = 1, 2, 3 or 4 = **5A**		
		(A) BATHING SELF-PERFORMANCE codes appear below.	**(A)**	**(B)**
		0. Independent—No help provided		
		1. Supervision—Oversight help only		
		2. Physical help limited to transfer only	3	2
		3. Physical help in part of bathing activity		
		4. Total dependence		
		8. Activity itself did not occur entire 7 days		
		(Bathing support codes are as defined in Item 1, code B above)		

3.	TEST FOR BALANCE (See training manual)	*(Code for ability during test in the last 7 days)* 0. Maintained position as required in test 1. Unsteady, but able to rebalance self without physical support 2. Partial physical support during test; or stands (sits) but does not follow directions for test 3. Not able to attempt test without physical help		
		a. Balance while standing		2
		b. Balance while sitting—position, trunk control 1, 2, or 3 = **17***		1

4.	FUNCTIONAL LIMITATION IN RANGE OF MOTION (see training manual)	*(Code for limitations during last 7 days that interfered with daily functions or placed resident at risk of injury)*		
		(A) RANGE OF MOTION 0. No limitation 1. Limitation on one side 2. Limitation on both sides	**(B) VOLUNTARY MOVEMENT** 0. No loss 1. Partial loss 2. Full loss	**(A)**	**(B)**

			(A)	(B)
	a. Neck		0	0
	b. Arm—Including shoulder or elbow		0	0
	c. Hand—Including wrist or fingers		1	2
	d. Leg—Including hip or knee		2	1
	e. Foot—Including ankle or toes		0	0
	f. Other limitation or loss		0	0

5.	MODES OF LOCOMOTION	*(Check all that apply during last 7 days)*		
		Cane/walker/crutch a. ✔	Wheelchair primary mode of locomotion d.	
		Wheeled self b.		
		Other person wheeled c.	NONE OF ABOVE e.	

6.	MODES OF TRANSFER	*(Check all that apply during last 7 days)*		
		Bedfast all or most of time **16** a.	Lifted mechanically d.	
		Bed rails used for bed mobility or transfer b. ✔	Transfer aid (e.g., slide board, trapeze, cane, walker, brace) e.	
		Lifted manually c.	NONE OF ABOVE f.	

7.	TASK SEGMEN-TATION	Some or all of ADL activities were broken into subtasks during **last 7 days** so that resident could perform them 0. No 1. Yes	1

8.	ADL FUNCTIONAL REHABILITA-TION POTENTIAL	Resident believes he/she is capable of increased independence in at least some ADLs **5A**	a.
		Direct care staff believe resident is capable of increased independence in at least some ADLs **5A**	b. ✔
		Resident able to perform tasks/activity but is very slow	c.
		Difference in ADL Self-Performance or ADL Support, comparing mornings to evenings	d.
		NONE OF ABOVE	e.

9.	CHANGE IN ADL FUNCTION	Resident's ADL self-performance status has changed as compared to status of **90 days ago** (or since last assessment if less than 90 days) 0. No change 1. Improved 2. Deteriorated	0

SECTION H. CONTINENCE IN LAST 14 DAYS

1.	CONTINENCE SELF-CONTROL CATEGORIES *(Code for resident's PERFORMANCE OVER ALL SHIFTS)*
	0. **CONTINENT**—Complete control (includes use of indwelling urinary catheter or ostomy device that does not leak urine or stool)
	1. **USUALLY CONTINENT**—BLADDER, incontinent episodes once a week or less; BOWEL, less than weekly
	2. **OCCASIONALLY INCONTINENT**—BLADDER, 2 or more times a week but not daily; BOWEL, once a week
	3. **FREQUENTLY INCONTINENT**—BLADDER, tended to be incontinent daily, but some control present (e.g., on day shift); BOWEL, 2-3 times a week
	4. **INCONTINENT**—Had inadequate control. BLADDER, multiple daily episodes; BOWEL, all (or almost all) of the time

a.	BOWEL CONTI-NENCE	Control of bowel movement, with appliance or bowel continence programs, if employed 1, 2, 3 or 4 = **16**	3
b.	BLADDER CONTI-NENCE	Control of urinary bladder function (if dribbles, volume insufficient to soak through underpants), with appliances (e.g., foley) or continence programs, if employed 2, 3 or 4 = **6**	3

2.	BOWEL ELIMIN-ATION PATTERN	Bowel elimination pattern regular—at least one movement every three days a.	Diarrhea c.	
		Constipation **17*** b.	Fecal impaction **17*** d.	
			NONE OF ABOVE e. ✔	

3.	APPLIANCES AND PROGRAMS	Any scheduled toileting plan a. ✔	Did not use toilet room/commode/urinal f.
		Bladder retraining program b.	Pads/briefs used **6** g.
		External (condom) catheter **6** c.	Enemas/irrigation h.
		Indwelling catheter **6** d.	Ostomy present i.
		Intermittent catheter **6** e.	NONE OF ABOVE j.

4.	CHANGE IN URINARY CONTI-NENCE	Resident's urinary continence has changed as compared to status of **90 days ago** (or since last assessment if less than 90 days) 0. No change 1. Improved 2. Deteriorated	2

SECTION I. DISEASE DIAGNOSES

Check only **those diseases that have a relationship** to current ADL status, cognitive status, mood and behavior status, medical treatments, nursing monitoring, or risk of death. (Do not list inactive diagnoses.)

1.	DISEASES	*(If none apply, CHECK the NONE OF ABOVE box)*	
		ENDOCRINE/METABOLIC/NUTRITIONAL	Hemiplegia/Hemiparesis v.
		Diabetes mellitus a. ✔	Multiple sclerosis w.
		Hyperthyroidism b.	Paraplegia x.
		Hypothyroidism c.	Parkinson's disease y.
		HEART/CIRCULATION	Quadriplegia z.
		Arteriosclerotic heart disease (ASHD) d.	Seizure disorder aa.
		Cardiac dysrhythmias e.	Transient ischemic attack (TIA) bb.
		Congestive heart failure f. ✔	Traumatic brain injury cc.
		Deep vein thrombosis g.	**PSYCHIATRIC/MOOD**
		Hypertension h.	Anxiety disorder dd.
		Hypotension **17*** i.	Depression **17*** ee.
		Peripheral vascular disease **16** j.	Manic depression (bipolar disease) ff.
		Other cardiovascular disease k.	Schizophrenia gg.
		MUSCULOSKELETAL	**PULMONARY**
		Arthritis l.	Asthma hh.
		Hip fracture m.	Emphysema/COPD ii.
		Missing limb (e.g., amputation) n.	**SENSORY**
		Osteoporosis o.	Cataracts **3** jj.
		Pathological bone fracture p.	Diabetic retinopathy kk.
		NEUROLOGICAL	Glaucoma **3** ll.
		Alzheimer's disease q.	Macular degeneration mm.
		Aphasia r.	**OTHER**
		Cerebral palsy s.	Allergies nn.
		Cerebrovascular accident (stroke) t.	Anemia oo.
		Dementia other than Alzheimer's disease u.	Cancer pp.
			Renal failure qq.
			NONE OF ABOVE rr.

2.	INFECTIONS	*(If none apply, CHECK the NONE OF ABOVE box)*	
		Antibiotic resistant infection (e.g., Methicillin resistant staph) a.	Septicemia g.
			Sexually transmitted diseases h.
		Clostridium difficile (c. diff.) b.	Tuberculosis i.
		Conjunctivitis c.	Urinary tract infection in last 30 days **14** j.
		HIV infection d.	Viral hepatitis k.
		Pneumonia e.	Wound infection l.
		Respiratory infection f.	NONE OF ABOVE m. ✔

3.	OTHER CURRENT OR MORE DETAILED DIAGNOSES AND ICD-9 CODES	Dehydration 276.5 = **14**		
		a. Fx L wrist	814.00
		b. Hematomas	924.8
		c. Abrasions	919.0
		d.	
		e.	

SECTION J. HEALTH CONDITIONS

1.	PROBLEM CONDITIONS	*(Check all problems present in last 7 days unless other time frame is indicated)*	
		INDICATORS OF FLUID STATUS	Dizziness/Vertigo **11, 17*** f.
		Weight gain or loss of 3 or more pounds within a 7 day period **14** a.	Edema g. ✔
		Inability to lie flat due to shortness of breath b.	Fever **14** h.
			Hallucinations **17*** i.
		Dehydrated; output exceeds input **14** c.	Internal bleeding j.
		Insufficient fluid; did NOT consume all/almost all liquids provided during last 3 days **14** d. ✔	Recurrent lung aspirations in last 90 days **17*** k.
			Shortness of breath l.
		OTHER	Syncope (fainting) **17*** m.
		Delusions e.	Unsteady gait **17*** n. ✔
			Vomiting o.
			NONE OF ABOVE p.

Form 1728HH © 1995 Briggs Corporation, Des Moines, IA 50306 (800) 247-2343 PRINTED IN U.S.A.
Copyright limited to addition of trigger system.

5 of 8

MDS 2.0   10/18/94N

Resident __George Blair__   Numeric Identifier __784393__

2.	PAIN SYMPTOMS	*(Code the **highest level of pain** present in **the last 7 days**)*		
		a. FREQUENCY with which resident complains or shows evidence of pain	**b. INTENSITY** of pain 1. Mild pain 2. Moderate pain 3. Times when pain is horrible or excruciating	
		0. No pain *(skip to J4)* 1. Pain less than daily 2. Pain daily	**2**	**2**

3.	PAIN SITE	*(If pain present, **check all sites** that apply in **last 7 days**)*			
		Back pain	a.	Incisional pain	f.
		Bone pain	b.	Joint pain (other than hip)	g. ✔
		Chest pain while doing usual activities	c.	Soft tissue pain (e.g., lesion, muscle)	h.
		Headache	d.	Stomach pain	i.
		Hip pain	e. ✔	Other	j.

4.	ACCIDENTS	*(Check all that apply)*			
		Fell in past 30 days 11, 17*	a.	Hip fracture in last 180 days 17*	c.
		Fell in past 31-180 days 11, 17*	b.	Other fracture in last 180 days	d. ✔
				NONE OF ABOVE	e.

5.	STABILITY OF CONDITIONS	Conditions/diseases make resident's cognitive, ADL, mood or behavior patterns unstable—(fluctuating, precarious, or deteriorating)	a.
		Resident experiencing an acute episode or a flare-up of a recurrent or chronic problem	b.
		End-stage disease, 6 or fewer months to live	c.
		NONE OF ABOVE	d. ✔

SECTION K. ORAL/NUTRITIONAL STATUS

1.	ORAL PROBLEMS	Chewing problem	a.
		Swallowing problem 17*	b.
		Mouth pain 15	c.
		NONE OF ABOVE	d. ✔

2.	HEIGHT AND WEIGHT	Record *(a.)* height in inches and *(b.)* weight in pounds. Base weight on most recent measure in **last 30 days**; measure weight consistently in accord with standard facility practice—e.g., in a.m. after voiding, before meal, with shoes off, and in nightclothes.		
		a. HT (in.) **6 9**	b. WT (lb.) **1 2 4**	

3.	WEIGHT CHANGE	a. Weight loss—5% or more in **last 30 days**; or 10% or more in **last 180 days** 0. No 1. Yes 12	**1**
		b. Weight gain—5% or more in **last 30 days**; or 10% or more in **last 180 days** 0. No 1. Yes	**0**

4.	NUTRI- TIONAL PROBLEMS	Complains about the taste of many foods 12	a.	Leaves 25% or more of food uneaten at most meals 12	c. ✔
		Regular or repetitive complaints of hunger	b.	NONE OF ABOVE	d.

5.	NUTRI- TIONAL APPROACH- ES	*(Check all that apply in last 7 days)*			
		Parenteral/IV 12, 14	a.	Dietary supplement between meals	f.
		Feeding tube 13, 14	b.	Plate guard, stabilized built-up utensil, etc.	g.
		Mechanically altered diet 12	c.	On a planned weight change program	h.
		Syringe (oral feeding) 12	d.	NONE OF ABOVE	i. ✔
		Therapeutic diet 12	e.		

6.	PARENTERAL OR ENTERAL INTAKE	*(Skip to Section L if neither 5a nor 5b is checked)*	
		a. Code the proportion of **total calories** the resident received through parenteral or tube feedings in the **last 7 days** 0. None 3. 51% to 75% 1. 1% to 25% 4. 76% to 100% 2. 26% to 50%	**0**
		b. Code the average fluid intake per day by IV or tube in **last 7 days** 0. None 3. 1001 to 1500 cc/day 1. 1 to 500 cc/day 4. 1501 to 2000 cc/day 2. 501 to 1000 cc/day 5. 2001 or more cc/day	**0**

SECTION L. ORAL/DENTAL STATUS

1.	ORAL STATUS AND DISEASE PREVEN- TION	Debris (soft, easily movable substances) present in mouth prior to going to bed at night 15	a.
		Has dentures or removable bridge	b. ✔
		Some/all natural teeth lost—does not have or does not use dentures (or partial plates) 15	c.
		Broken, loose, or carious teeth 15	d.
		Inflamed gums (gingiva); swollen or bleeding gums; oral abscesses; ulcers or rashes 15	e.
		Daily cleaning of teeth/dentures or daily mouth care—by resident or staff Not ✓ = 15	f. ✔
		NONE OF ABOVE	g.

SECTION M. SKIN CONDITION

1.	ULCERS (Due to any cause)	*(Record the number of ulcers at each ulcer stage—regardless of cause. If none present at a stage, record "0" (zero). Code all that apply during **last 7 days**. Code 9 = 9 or more.) [**Requires full body exam.**]*	Number at Stage
		a. **Stage 1.** A persistent area of skin redness (without a break in the skin) that does not disappear when pressure is relieved.	**0**
		b. **Stage 2.** A partial thickness loss of skin layers that presents clinically as an abrasion, blister, or shallow crater.	**1**
		c. **Stage 3.** A full thickness of skin is lost, exposing the subcutaneous tissues—presents as a deep crater with or without undermining adjacent tissue.	**0**
		d. **Stage 4.** A full thickness of skin and subcutaneous tissue is lost, exposing muscle or bone.	**0**

2.	TYPE OF ULCER	*(For each type of ulcer, **code for the highest stage** in the **last 7 days** using scale in item M1—i.e., 0=none; stages 1, 2, 3, 4)*	
		a. Pressure ulcer—any lesion caused by pressure resulting in damage of underlying tissue 1 = 16; 2, 3, or 4 = 12, 16	**2**
		b. Stasis ulcer—open lesion caused by poor circulation in the lower extremities	**0**

3.	HISTORY OF RESOLVED ULCERS	Resident had an ulcer that was resolved or cured in **LAST 90 DAYS** 0. No 1. Yes 16	**0**

4.	OTHER SKIN PROBLEMS OR LESIONS PRESENT	*(Check all that apply during **last 7 days**)*	
		Abrasions, bruises	a. ✔
		Burns (second or third degree)	b.
		Open lesions other than ulcers, rashes, cuts (e.g., cancer lesions)	c. ✔
		Rashes—e.g., intertrigo, eczema, drug rash, heat rash, herpes zoster	d.
		Skin desensitized to pain or pressure 16	e.
		Skin tears or cuts (other than surgery)	f.
		Surgical wounds	g.
		NONE OF ABOVE	h.

5.	SKIN TREAT- MENTS	*(Check all that apply during **last 7 days**)*	
		Pressure relieving device(s) for chair	a.
		Pressure relieving device(s) for bed	b.
		Turning/repositioning program	c.
		Nutrition or hydration intervention to manage skin problems	d.
		Ulcer care	e. ✔
		Surgical wound care	f.
		Application of dressings (with or without topical medications) other than to feet	g. ✔
		Application of ointments/medications (other than to feet)	h. ✔
		Other preventative or protective skin care (other than to feet)	i.
		NONE OF ABOVE	j.

6.	FOOT PROBLEMS AND CARE	*(Check all that apply during **last 7 days**)*	
		Resident has one or more foot problems—e.g., corns, calluses, bunions, hammer toes, overlapping toes, pain, structural problems	a.
		Infection of the foot—e.g., cellulitis, purulent drainage	b.
		Open lesions on the foot	c.
		Nails/calluses trimmed during **last 90 days**	d.
		Received preventative or protective foot care (e.g., used special shoes, inserts, pads, toe separators)	e.
		Application of dressings (with or without topical medications)	f.
		NONE OF ABOVE	g. ✔

SECTION N. ACTIVITY PURSUIT PATTERNS

1.	TIME AWAKE	*(Check appropriate time periods over **last 7 days**)* Resident awake all or most of the time (i.e., naps no more than one hour per time period) in:		
	10B only if BOTH N1a = ✓ and N2 = 0	Morning 10B	a. ✔	Evening c.
		Afternoon	b.	NONE OF ABOVE

(IF RESIDENT IS COMATOSE, SKIP TO SECTION O)

2.	AVERAGE TIME INVOLVED IN ACTIVITIES	*(When awake and not receiving treatments or ADL care)* 0. Most—more than 2/3 of time 10B 1. Some—from 1/3 to 2/3 of time 2. Little—less than 1/3 of time 10A 3. None 10A	**1**

3.	PREFERRED ACTIVITY SETTINGS	*(Check all settings in which activities are preferred)*			
		Own room	a.		
		Day/activity room	b.	Outside facility	d.
		Inside NH/off unit	c.	NONE OF ABOVE	e.

4.	GENERAL ACTIVITY PREFER- ENCES (Adapted to resident's current abilities)	*(Check all PREFERENCES whether or not activity is currently available to resident)*			
		Cards/other games	a.	Trips/shopping	g.
		Crafts/arts	b.	Walking/wheeling outdoors	h.
		Exercise/sports	c.	Watching TV	i.
		Music	d. ✔	Gardening or plants	j.
		Reading/writing	e.	Talking or conversing	k.
		Spiritual/religious activities	f.	Helping others	l.
				NONE OF ABOVE	m.

Form 1728HH © 1995 Briggs Corporation, Des Moines, IA 50306 (800) 247-2343 PRINTED IN U.S.A.
Copyright limited to addition of trigger system.

6 of 8

MDS 2.0 10/18/94N

Resident __George Blair__   Numeric Identifier __784393__

5.	PREFERS CHANGE IN DAILY ROUTINE	Code for resident preferences in daily routines 0. No change 1. Slight change 2. Major change	
		a. Type of activities in which resident is currently involved 1 or 2 = **10A**	0
		b. Extent of resident involvement in activity 1 or 2 = **10A**	0

SECTION O. MEDICATIONS

1.	NUMBER OF MEDICATIONS	(Record the number of different medications used in the last 7 days; enter "0" if none used)	10
2.	NEW MEDICA-TIONS	(Resident currently receiving medications that were initiated during the last 90 days) 0. No 1. Yes	1
3.	INJECTIONS	(Record the number of DAYS injections of any type received during the last 7 days; enter "0" if none used)	0
4.	DAYS RECEIVED THE FOLLOWING MEDICATION	(Record the number of DAYS during last 7 days; enter "0" if not used. Note—enter "1" for long acting meds used less than weekly) (NOTE: For **17** to actually be triggered, O4a, b, or c MUST = 1-7 AND at least one additional item marked **17*** must be indicated. See sections B, C, E, G, H, I, J, and K.)	

a. Antipsychotic 1-7 = **17**	7	d. Hypnotic	7
b. Antianxiety 1-7 = **11, 17**	2	e. Diuretic 1-7 = **14**	7
c. Antidepressant 1-7 = **11, 17**			

SECTION P. SPECIAL TREATMENTS AND PROCEDURES

1.	SPECIAL TREAT-MENTS, PROCE-DURES, AND PROGRAMS	a. SPECIAL CARE—Check treatments or programs received during the last 14 days

TREATMENTS			PROGRAMS	
Chemotherapy	a.	Ventilator or respirator		l.
Dialysis	b.	Alcohol/drug treatment program	m.	
IV medication	c.	Alzheimer's/dementia special care unit	n.	
Intake/output	d.	Hospice care	o.	
Monitoring acute medical condition	e.	Pediatric unit	p.	
Ostomy care	f.	Respite care	q.	
Oxygen therapy	g.	Training in skills required to return to the community (e.g., taking medications, house work, shopping, transportation, ADLs)	r.	
Radiation	h.			
Suctioning	i.			
Tracheostomy care	j.			
Transfusions	k.	NONE OF ABOVE	s.	✓

b. THERAPIES—Record the number of days and total minutes each of the following therapies was administered (for at least 15 minutes a day) in the last 7 calendar days (Enter 0 if none or less than 15 min. daily) [Note—count only post admission therapies]
(A) = # of days administered for **15** minutes or more
(B) = total # of **minutes** provided in last 7 days

	DAYS (A)	MINUTES (B)
a. Speech-language pathology and audiology services	0	
b. Occupational therapy	0	
c. Physical therapy	0	
d. Respiratory therapy	0	
e. Psychological therapy (by any licensed mental health professional)	0	

2.	INTERVEN-TION PROGRAMS FOR MOOD, BEHAVIOR, COGNITIVE LOSS	(Check all interventions or strategies used in last 7 days—no matter where received)	
		Special behavior symptom evaluation program	a.
		Evaluation by a licensed mental health specialist in last 90 days	b.
		Group therapy	c.
		Resident-specific deliberate changes in the environment to address mood/behavior patterns—e.g., providing bureau in which to rummage	d.
		Reorientation—e.g., cueing	e.
		NONE OF ABOVE	f. ✓

3.	NURSING REHABILI-TATION/ RESTOR-ATIVE CARE	Record the NUMBER OF DAYS each of the following rehabilitation or restorative techniques or practices was provided to the resident for more than or equal to 15 minutes per day in the last 7 days (Enter 0 if none or less than 15 min. daily.)	

a. Range of motion (passive)	0	f. Walking	
b. Range of motion (active)	0	g. Dressing or grooming	0
c. Splint or brace assistance	0	h. Eating or swallowing	0
TRAINING AND SKILL PRACTICE IN:		i. Amputation/prosthesis care	0
		j. Communication	
d. Bed mobility	0	k. Other	0
e. Transfer	0		

4.	DEVICES AND RESTRAINTS	(Use the following codes for last 7 days:) 0. Not used 1. Used less than daily 2. Used daily	
		Bed rails	
		a. —Full bed rails on all open sides of bed	2
		b. —Other types of side rails used (e.g., half rail, one side)	0
		c. Trunk restraint 1 = 11, 18. 2 = 11, 16, 18	0
		d. Limb restraint 1 or 2 = 18	0
		e. Chair prevents rising 1 or 2 = 18	0

5.	HOSPITAL STAY(S)	Record number of times resident was admitted to hospital with an overnight stay in last 90 days (or since last assessment if less than 90 days). (Enter 0 if no hospital admissions)	1
6.	EMERGENCY ROOM (ER) VISIT(S)	Record number of times resident visited ER without an overnight stay in last 90 days (or since last assessment if less than 90 days). (Enter 0 if no ER visits)	0
7.	PHYSICIAN VISITS	In the LAST 14 DAYS (or since admission if less than 14 days in facility) how many days has the physician (or authorized assistant or practitioner) examined the resident? (Enter 0 if none)	0
8.	PHYSICIAN ORDERS	In the LAST 14 DAYS (or since admission if less than 14 days in facility) how many days has the physician (or authorized assistant or practitioner) changed the resident's orders? Do not include order renewals without change. (Enter 0 if none)	0
9.	ABNORMAL LAB VALUES	Has the resident had any abnormal lab values during the last 90 days (or since admission)? 0. No 1. Yes	1

SECTION Q. DISCHARGE POTENTIAL AND OVERALL STATUS

1.	DISCHARGE POTENTIAL	a. Resident expresses/indicates preference to return to the community 0. No 1. Yes	0
		b. Resident has a support person who is positive toward discharge 0. No 1. Yes	0
		c. Stay projected to be of a short duration—discharge projected within 90 days (do not include expected discharge due to death) 0. No 2. Within 31-90 days 1. Within 30 days 3. Discharge status uncertain	0
2.	OVERALL CHANGE IN CARE NEEDS	Resident's overall self sufficiency has changed significantly as compared to status of 90 days ago (or since last assessment if less than 90 days) 0. No change 1. Improved—receives fewer supports, needs less restrictive level of care 2. Deteriorated—receives more support	2

SECTION R. ASSESSMENT INFORMATION

1.	PARTICI-PATION IN ASSESSMENT	a. Resident: 0. No 1. Yes	0
		b. Family: 0. No 1. Yes 2. No family	1
		c. Significant other: 0. No 1. Yes 2. None	0

2. SIGNATURES OF PERSONS COMPLETING THE ASSESSMENT:

a. A. Jones, R.N. (O,P,Q,R)
   Signature of RN Assessment Coordinator (sign on above line)

b. Date RN Assessment Coordinator signed as complete

Month	Day	Year
1 2	1 4	2 0 0 2

	Other Signatures	Title	Sections	
c.	J. Spencer, LPN	(A,B,C,D,J,K,L)	12/12/97	
d.	M. Moeller, LPN	(G,H,I,M)	12/14/02	Date
e.	J. Miller, TRT	(N)	12/14/02	Date
f.	A. Schmidt, MSW	(E,F)	12/10/02	Date
g.				Date
h.				Date

TRIGGER LEGEND

1 - Delirium	5B - ADL-Maintenance	10A - Activities (Revise)	14 - Dehydration/Fluid Maintenance
2 - Cognitive Loss/Dementia	6B - Urinary Incontinence and Indwelling Catheter	10B - Activities (Review)	15 - Dental Care
3 - Visual Function	7 - Psychosocial Well-Being	11 - Falls	16 - Pressure Ulcers
4 - Communication	8 - Mood State	12 - Nutritional Status	17 - Psychotropic Drug Use
5A - ADL-Rehabilitation	9 - Behavioral Symptoms	13 - Feeding Tubes	17* - For this trigger, O4a, b, or c must = 1-7
			18 - Physical Restraints

Form 1728HH © 1995 Briggs Corporation, Des Moines, IA 50306 (800) 247-2343 PRINTED IN U.S.A.
Copyright limited to addition of trigger system.

7 of 8

MDS 2.0   10/18/94N

| Resident's Name: George T. Blair | | Medical Record No.: 784393 | | |

1. Check if RAP is triggered.
2. For each triggered RAP, use the RAP guidelines to identify areas needing further assessment. Document relevant assessment information regarding the resident's status.
   - Describe:
     —Nature of the condition (may include presence or lack of objective data and subjective complaints).
     —Complications and risk factors that affect your decision to proceed to care planning.
     —Factors that must be considered in developing individualized care plan interventions.
     —Need for referrals/further evaluation by appropriate health professionals.
   - Documentation should support your decision-making regarding whether to proceed with a care plan for a triggered RAP and the type(s) of care plan interventions that are appropriate for a particular resident.
   - Documentation may appear anywhere in the clinical record (e.g., progress notes, consults, flowsheets, etc.).
3. Indicate under the Location of RAP Assessment Documentation column where information related to the RAP assessment can be found.
4. For each triggered RAP, indicate whether a new care plan, care plan revision, or continuation of current care plan is necessary to address the problem(s) identified in your assessment. The Care Planning Decision column must be completed within 7 days of completing the RAI (MDS and RAPs).

A. RAP Problem Area	(a) Check if Triggered	Location and Date of RAP Assessment Documentation	(b) Care Planning Decision—check if addressed in care plan
1. DELIRIUM	✓	Mood + behavior problems \ Admit notes \ Nsg notes	✓
2. COGNITIVE LOSS	✓	Poor STM + LTM \ Nsg. notes	✓
3. VISUAL FUNCTION	✓	Wears glasses \ Admit note	✓
4. COMMUNICATION	✓	Difficulty making needs \ Nsg. Known + following instruc \ notes	✓
5. ADL FUNCTIONAL/ REHABILITATION POTENTIAL	✓	Assist c ADL's \ Nsg. notes	✓
6. URINARY INCONTINENCE AND INDWELLING CATHETER	✓	Incont. of urine \ Admit note \ Nsg. note	✓
7. PSYCHOSOCIAL WELL-BEING	✓	Verbally abusive \ Nsg. note	✓
8. MOOD STATE	✓	Expressions of distress \ Nsg. note	✓
9. BEHAVIORAL SYMPTOMS	✓	Wandering + inapprop. behavior \ Nsg. notes	✓
10. ACTIVITIES			
11. FALLS	✓	Fell in last 2 wks \ Admit note	✓
12. NUTRITIONAL STATUS	✓	Wgt. loss, spec. diet \ Admit note \ Nsg note	
13. FEEDING TUBES			
14. DEHYDRATION/FLUID MAINTENANCE	✓	Constipation \ Nsg. note	✓
15. ORAL/DENTAL CARE			
16. PRESSURE ULCERS	✓	Coccyx pressure ulcer \ Admit note	✓
17. PSYCHOTROPIC DRUG USE	✓	Haldol bid + \ Admit note Oxazepam HS \ Nsg note	✓
18. PHYSICAL RESTRAINTS			

B. A. Jones, R.N.
1. Signature of RN Coordinator for RAP Assessment Process

2. | 1 | 2 | – | 1 | 4 | – | 2 | 0 | 0 | 2 |
   Month   Day   Year

A. Jones, R.N.
3. Signature of Person Completing Care Planning Decision

4. | 1 | 2 | – | 1 | 4 | – | 2 | 0 | 0 | 2 |
   Month   Day   Year

Form 1728HH © 1995 Briggs Corporation, Des Moines, IA 50306 (800) 247-2343 PRINTED IN U.S.A.
Copyright limited to addition of trigger system.   8 of 8

MDS 2.0 10/18/94N

RESIDENT ASSESSMENT PROTOCOL TRIGGER LEGEND FOR REVISED RAPS (FOR MDS VERSION 2.0)

Resident _____ Numeric Identifier _____

Key:
- ● = One item required to trigger
- ❷ = Two items required to trigger
- ★ = One of these three items (O4a, O4b, O4c), plus at least one other item (●) required to trigger
- ●★ = Psychotropic Drug Use triggered only when at least one of the three items (O4a, O4b, O4c) identified by ★ also apply
- ⓐ = When both ADL triggers present, maintenance takes precedence

Proceed to RAP Review once triggered

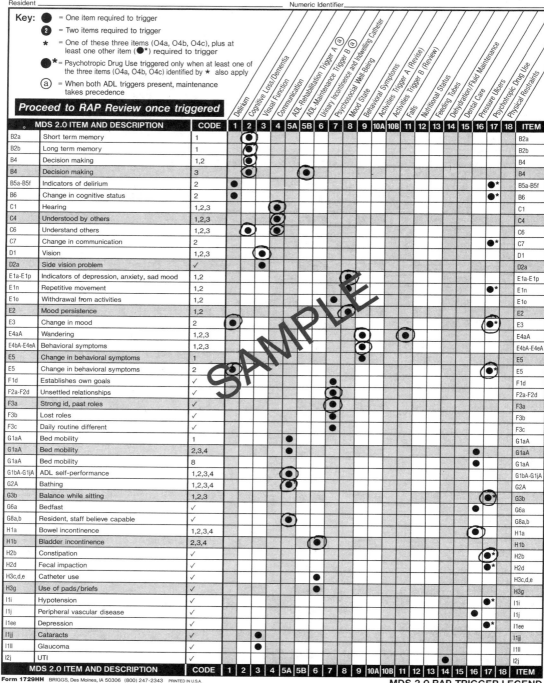

MDS 2.0 ITEM AND DESCRIPTION		CODE	1 Delirium	2 Cognitive Loss/Dementia	3 Visual Function	4 Communication	5A ADL-Rehabilitation Trigger A ⓐ	5B ADL-Maintenance Trigger B ⓐ	6 Urinary Incontinence and Indwelling Catheter	7 Psychosocial Well-Being	8 Mood State	9 Behavioral Symptoms	10A Activities Trigger A (Revise)	10B Activities Trigger B (Review)	11 Falls	12 Nutritional Status	13 Feeding Tubes	14 Dehydration/Fluid Maintenance	15 Dental Care	16 Pressure Ulcers	17 Psychotropic Drug Use	18 Physical Restraints	ITEM
B2a	Short term memory	1		●																			B2a
B2b	Long term memory	1		●																			B2b
B4	Decision making	1,2		●																			B4
B4	Decision making	3		●			●																B4
B5a-B5f	Indicators of delirium	2	●																		●★		B5a-B5f
B6	Change in cognitive status	2	●																		●★		B6
C1	Hearing	1,2,3				●																	C1
C4	Understood by others	1,2,3				●																	C4
C6	Understand others	1,2,3		●		●																	C6
C7	Change in communication	2				●															●★		C7
D1	Vision	1,2,3			●																		D1
D2a	Side vision problem	✓			●																		D2a
E1a-E1p	Indicators of depression, anxiety, sad mood	1,2									●												E1a-E1p
E1n	Repetitive movement	1,2																			●★		E1n
E1o	Withdrawal from activities	1,2									●												E1o
E2	Mood persistence	1,2									●												E2
E3	Change in mood	2	●								●										●★		E3
E4aA	Wandering	1,2,3										●		●									E4aA
E4bA-E4eA	Behavioral symptoms	1,2,3										●											E4bA-E4eA
E5	Change in behavioral symptoms	1										●											E5
E5	Change in behavioral symptoms	2										●									●★		E5
F1d	Establishes own goals	✓							●														F1d
F2a-F2d	Unsettled relationships	✓							●														F2a-F2d
F3a	Strong id, past roles	✓							●														F3a
F3b	Lost roles	✓							●														F3b
F3c	Daily routine different	✓							●														F3c
G1aA	Bed mobility	1					●																G1aA
G1aA	Bed mobility	2,3,4					●													●			G1aA
G1aA	Bed mobility	8																		●			G1aA
G1bA-G1jA	ADL self-performance	1,2,3,4					●																G1bA-G1jA
G2A	Bathing	1,2,3,4					●																G2A
G3b	Balance while sitting	1,2,3													●					●★		G3b
G6a	Bedfast	✓																		●			G6a
G8a,b	Resident, staff believe capable	✓					●																G8a,b
H1a	Bowel incontinence	1,2,3,4																		●			H1a
H1b	Bladder incontinence	2,3,4							●														H1b
H2b	Constipation	✓																		●★			H2b
H2d	Fecal impaction	✓																			●★		H2d
H3c,d,e	Catheter use	✓							●														H3c,d,e
H3g	Use of pads/briefs	✓							●														H3g
I1i	Hypotension	✓																			●★		I1i
I1j	Peripheral vascular disease	✓																		●			I1j
I1ee	Depression	✓																			●★		I1ee
I1jj	Cataracts	✓		●																			I1jj
I1ll	Glaucoma	✓		●																			I1ll
I2j	UTI	✓														●							I2j
MDS 2.0 ITEM AND DESCRIPTION		CODE	1	2	3	4	5A	5B	6	7	8	9	10A	10B	11	12	13	14	15	16	17	18	ITEM

Form 1729HH BRIGGS, Des Moines, IA 50306 (800) 247-2343 PRINTED IN U.S.A.
R396

MDS 2.0 RAP TRIGGER LEGEND
MDS 2.0 10/18/94N

Key:
- ● = One item required to trigger
- ② = Two items required to trigger
- ★ = One of these three items (O4a, O4b, O4c), plus at least one other item (●*) required to trigger
- ●* = Psychotropic Drug Use triggered only when at least one of the three items (O4a, O4b, O4c) identified by ★ also apply
- ⓐ = When both ADL triggers present, maintenance takes precedence

Proceed to RAP Review once triggered

Column legend (1–18):
1 Delirium · 2 Cognitive Loss/Dementia · 3 Visual Function · 4 Communication · 5A ADL-Rehabilitation Trigger A ⓐ · 5B ADL-Maintenance Trigger B ⓐ · 6 Urinary Incontinence and Indwelling Catheter · 7 Psychosocial Well-Being · 8 Mood State · 9 Behavioral Symptoms · 10A Activities Trigger A (Revise) · 10B Activities Trigger B (Review) · 11 Falls · 12 Nutritional Status · 13 Feeding Tubes · 14 Dehydration/Fluid Maintenance · 15 Dental Care · 16 Pressure Ulcers · 17 Psychotropic Drug Use · 18 Physical Restraints

MDS 2.0 ITEM	DESCRIPTION	CODE	1	2	3	4	5A	5B	6	7	8	9	10A	10B	11	12	13	14	15	16	17	18
I3	Dehydration diagnosis	276.5																(●)				
J1a	Weight fluctuation	✓																(●)				
J1c	Dehydrated	✓																(●)				
J1d	Insufficient fluid	✓																(●)				
J1f	Dizziness	✓													●						●*	
J1h	Fever	✓																●				
J1i	Hallucinations	✓																			●*	
J1j	Internal bleeding	✓																●				
J1k	Lung aspirations	✓																			●*	
J1m	Syncope	✓																			●*	
J1n	Unsteady gait	✓																			(●*)	
J4a,b	Fell	✓													(●)						(●*)	
J4c	Hip fracture	✓																			●*	
K1b	Swallowing problem	✓																			●*	
K1c	Mouth pain	✓																	●			
K3a	Weight loss	1														(●)						
K4a	Taste alteration	✓														●						
K4c	Leave 25% food	✓														(●)						
K5a	Parenteral/IV feeding	✓														●	●					
K5b	Feeding tube	✓															●	●				
K5c	Mechanically altered	✓														●						
K5d	Syringe feeding	✓														●						
K5e	Therapeutic diet	✓														(●)						
L1a,c,d,e	Dental	✓																	●			
L1f	Daily cleaning teeth	Not ✓																	●			
M2a	Pressure ulcer	2,3,4														(●)				(●)		
M2a	Pressure ulcer	1																		●		
M3	Previous pressure ulcer	1																		●		
M4e	Impaired tactile sense	✓																		●		
N1a	Awake morning	✓											②									
N2	Involved in activities	0											②									
N2	Involved in activities	2,3										●										
N5a,b	Prefer change in daily routine	1,2										●										
O4a	Antipsychotics	1-7																			★	
O4b	Antianxiety	1-7													●						★	
O4c	Antidepressants	1-7													●						★	
O4e	Diuretic	1-7																(●)				
P4c	Trunk restraint	1													●							●
P4c	Trunk restraint	2													●					●		●
P4d	Limb restraint	1,2																				●
P4e	Chair prevents rising	1,2																				●

MDS 2.0 10/18/94N

Discussion

Use the following nursing diagnoses to organize your assessment data and develop a nursing care plan for Mr. B.

1. Nursing Diagnosis: *Self-Care Deficit* related to confusion manifested by inability to perform ADLs independently secondary to Alzheimer's disease and fractured wrist.
   ADL FUNCTION/REHABILITATION
   POTENTIAL
   VISUAL FUNCTION
2. Nursing Diagnosis: *Injury, high risk* for related to altered mobility as manifested by unsteadiness and wandering, secondary to hip injury and Alzheimer's disease.
   FALLS
   BEHAVIOR PROBLEMS
3. Nursing Diagnosis: *Nutrition, altered: less than body requirements* related to lack of appetite as manifested by significant weight loss in last 30 days secondary to Alzheimer's disease.
   NUTRITIONAL STATUS
   DEHYDRATION/FLUID MAINTENANCE
4. Nursing Diagnosis: *Urinary Elimination, altered* and *Incontinence* related to confusion mobility as manifested by not going to the bathroom to void secondary to Alzheimer's disease.
   URINARY INCONTINENCE AND
   INDWELLING CATHETER
5. Nursing Diagnosis: *Thought Processes, altered* related to inaccurate interpretation of environment as manifested by inability to state season, date, remember names of staff members, inability to follow commands secondary to Alzheimer's disease, and possible use of antipsychotic and sedative medication.
   DELIRIUM
   COGNITIVE LOSS/DEMENTIA
   COMMUNICATION
   MOOD STATE
   BEHAVIOR PROBLEM
   PSYCHOTROPIC DRUG USE
   PSYCHOSOCIAL WELL-BEING
6. Nursing Diagnosis: *Skin Integrity, impaired* related to a fall and being restrained in bed during hospitalization manifested by hematomas, abrasions, blisters, and stage 2 coccyx pressure ulcer.
   PRESSURE ULCER
7. Nursing Diagnosis: *Constipation* related to decreased fluid intake as manifested by bowel movements hard and difficult to pass and use of suppository secondary to Alzheimer's disease, altered nutrition intake, and dehydration.
   DEHYDRATION AND FLUID
   MAINTENANCE
   NUTRITIONAL STATUS

STUDY QUESTIONS

Select the one best answer to each question.

1. The nursing process is:
   a. A type of standardized care plan
   b. A framework for providing nursing care
   c. A procedure that registered nurses use to make care assignments
   d. An instinctive method of providing care

2. The steps in the nursing process are:
   a. Admission, inpatient care, and discharge
   b. Assessment, intervention, and documentation
   c. Assessment, nursing diagnosis, planning, intervention, and evaluation
   d. Admission, physical examination, interview, nursing history, and planning

3. Nursing diagnoses differ from medical diagnoses because they:
   a. Address the problems of the older person

   b. Are written in language that nurses understand
   c. Are standardized for any person who is receiving nursing care
   d. Are designed to address the medical treatment plan

4. When setting priorities during the planning stage of the nursing process, it is important to consider
   a. The needs of the physician
   b. The needs of the family
   c. The needs of the nursing staff
   d. The needs of the resident

5. Evaluation of the nursing care plan is documented by means of:
   a. The nurse's notes
   b. The resident care plan
   c. The doctor's orders
   d. Revising the admission note

Mary Ann Anderson

chapter **5**

Legal and Ethical Considerations Regarding the Elderly Person

Learning Objectives

After completing this chapter, the student will be able to:

1. Compare and contrast the terms *legal* and *ethical.*
2. Define the guiding principles of a restraint-free environment.
3. Outline the role of the licensed practical nurse (LPN) in using advanced directives and informed consent.
4. Describe the legal definition of elder abuse and the LPN's role in reporting it.
5. Express an understanding of the ethical responsibility of working with older adults in meeting their sexual needs.

▶ INTRODUCTION

Health-care decisions that are made daily across the nation are based on the legal and ethical definitions of health care. Advances in technology, increased resources, newer drug therapies, and other modalities of treatment continue to bring with them both ethical and legal problems and solutions to the health-care system that are unprecedented. While the legislators and ethics committees of this country debate the merits of treatment approaches, health-care providers deliberate every day as to their role and often wonder if it is one of help or hindrance. As a licensed practical nurse (LPN), you will be involved in making ethical and legal decisions that potentially are very complex. This chapter will assist you in understanding ethical and legal issues that relate specifically to the challenges facing older adults and their care.

▶ ETHICS

Ethics is the study of moral actions and values. It is based on the principles of conduct that govern both individuals and groups. Many people envision ethics as dealing with principles and moral concepts that determine what is good or bad behavior. The problem with this concept is determining who decides what is good and what is bad. Is this decision one for the older adult, the nurse, the family, or an outside group like an ethics committee?

A broader definition of ethics considers the value system of a person and the relationship of those values in determining what is good for an individual or group. It is important for LPNs to understand their own value systems and the ethical framework underlying the work performance that springs from it. The personal values of all the persons involved in making health-care decisions for older adults form the most important aspect of the nurse's delivery of ethical health care.

PATIENT'S BILL OF RIGHTS

The Patient's Bill of Rights is a document published by the American Hospital Association in 1975 (Box 5.1). It outlines the ethical behavior that is seen as appropriate and proper for care of those who are patients in a hospital. The nursing home organization has a Resident's Bill of Rights for those people who

are in nursing homes. Other organizations, such as the American Nurses' Association, American Dental Association, and National Respiratory Therapy Association, have ethical codes that are based on the principles in the patient's and resident's bills of rights.

The bill of rights for any client is based on that person's individual right to make decisions regarding health-care treatment. It is designed to serve as a model that defines acceptable behavior toward those in your care. All work done with clients of every age and condition should be based on the principles in the Patient's Bill of Rights. Please read and review the Bill of Rights in Box 5.1. It should be the foundation for the work you do with clients, and it has a very special significance when dealing with the older adults who may be struggling with the stress of a new situation, poor short-term memory, or chronic disease.

▶ THE LAW

The legal system is based on rules and regulations that guide society in a formal and binding manner. These are human-made rules capable of being changed by the legislative and judiciary systems of this country. The law gives you, the health-care provider, a general foundation for guiding your work; it may or may not complement your personal value system.

Ideally, the care you give is both ethical and legal. However, it is possible for a legal approach to care to seem unethical to you because it conflicts with your value system. This is when ethical-legal dilemmas occur. For

BOX 5.1. A PATIENT'S BILL OF RIGHTS

1. The patient has the right to considerate and respectful care.

2. The patient has the right to and is encouraged to obtain from physicians and other direct caregivers relevant, current, and understandable information concerning diagnosis, treatment, and prognosis.

   Except in emergencies when the patient lacks decision-making capacity and the need for treatment is urgent, the patient is entitled to the opportunity to discuss and request information related to the specific procedures and/or treatments, the risks involved, the possible length of recuperation, and the medically reasonable alternatives and their accompanying risks and benefits.

   Patients have the right to know the identity of physicians, nurses, and others involved in their care, as well as when those involved are students, residents, or other trainees. The patient also has the right to know the immediate and long-term financial implications of treatment choices, insofar as they are known.

3. The patient has the right to make decisions about the plan of care before and during the course of treatment and to refuse a recommended treatment or plan of care to the extent permitted by law and hospital policy and to be informed of the medical consequences of this action. In case of such refusal, the patient is entitled to other appropriate care and services that the hospital provides or transfer to another hospital. The hospital should notify patients of any policy that might affect patient choice within the institution.

4. The patient has the right to have an advance directive (such as a living will, health care proxy, or durable power of attorney for health care) concerning treatment or designating a surrogate decision maker with the expectation that the hospital will honor the intent of that directive to the extent permitted by law and hospital policy.

   Health-care institutions must advise patients of their rights under state law and hospital policy to make informed medical choices, ask if the patient has an advance directive, and include that information in patient records. The patient has the right to timely information about hospital policy that may limit its ability to implement fully a legally valid advance directive.

5. The patient has the right to every consideration of privacy. Case discussion, consultation, examination, and treatment should be conducted so as to protect each patient's privacy.

6. The patient has the right to expect that all communications and records pertaining to his/her care will be treated as confidential by the hospital, except in cases such as suspected abuse and public health hazards when reporting is permitted or required by law. The patient has the right to expect that the hospital will emphasize the confidentiality of this information when it releases it to any other parties entitled to review information in these records.

7. The patient has the right to review the records pertaining to his/her medical care and to have the information explained or interpreted as necessary, except when restricted by law.

8. The patient has the right to expect that, within its capacity and policies, a hospital will make reasonable response to the request of a patient for appropriate and medically indicated care services. The hospital must provide evaluation, service, and/or referral as indicated by the urgency of the case. When medically appropriate and legally permissible, or when a patient has so requested, a patient may be transferred to another facility. The institution to which the patient is to be transferred must first have accepted the patient for transfer. The patient must also have the benefit of complete information and explanation concerning the need for, risks, benefits, and alternatives to such a transfer.

9. The patient has the right to ask and be informed of the existence of business relationships among the hospital, educational institutions, other health care providers, or payers that may influence the patient's treatment and care.

10. The patient has the right to consent to or decline to participate in proposed research studies or human experimentation affecting care and treatment or requiring direct patient involvement, and to have those studies fully explained prior to consent. A patient who declines to participate in research or experimentation is entitled to the most effective care that the hospital can otherwise provide.

11. The patient has the right to expect reasonable continuity of care when appropriate and to be informed by physicians and other caregivers of available and realistic patient care options when hospital care is no longer appropriate.

12. The patient has the right to be informed of hospital policies and practices that relate to patient care, treatment, and responsibilities. The patient has the right to be informed of available resources for resolving disputes, grievances, and conflicts, such as ethics committees, patient representatives, or other mechanisms available in the institution. The patient has the right to be informed of the hospital's charges for services and available payment methods.

   These rights can be exercised on the patient's behalf by a designated surrogate or proxy decision maker if the patient lacks decision-making capacity, is legally incompetent or is a minor.

   Patient's Bill of Rights was first adopted by the American Hospital Association (AHA) in 1973. This revision was approved by the AHA Board of Trustees on October 21, 1992.

example, the law recognizes the right of a competent patient to refuse therapy. The patient has that right regardless of the health-care system's agreement or disagreement with the decision. For example, an older adult has the right to refuse to have a pacemaker replaced. Such replacement is essentially a benign procedure with minimal risk, and not to have it done amounts to a death sentence. However, it is the person's right to accept or refuse the therapy. Your values do not change the principles of the law.

Another example is shared by Dr. Jean Watson, nurse theorist. Dr. Watson's theory is the Science of Human Caring and is explained in detail in her book *Nursing: Human Science and Human Caring—A Theory of Nursing*. In it she emphasizes the importance of valuing patients as individuals and avoiding objectifying them. She explains that a nurse gives legal care when going into a patient's room to perform a complicated dressing change and assesses the wound site, removes the old dressing, and replaces it with a new dressing. The law does not indicate that the nurse needs to talk to the patient or to explain the procedure or the healing process. However, for that care to be ethical, the nurse must take the time to talk to the patient and treat the person as a human being rather than an object with a wound to dress. Another very simple example is that of bathing persons with dementia. Federal law requires that persons in nursing homes be kept clean. However, it is possible for a nursing assistant to give a resident a bath that is abusive; allowing no protection of modesty, not waiting for the water to warm, and being verbally abusive. This could be described as a legal, but unethical, bath. In the midst of the time pressures of health-care's complex world, one must be careful to determine the difference between legal and ethical care.

As an LPN, you are required to function under the mandates of the nurse practice act in your state. You are not allowed to practice nursing outside of the law as it is outlined in the practice act. An important consideration or rule of thumb to keep in mind, as you administer care, is to always consider "What is reasonable under the circumstances?" If you have the knowledge to answer that question whenever you have doubts, you should be able to make a legal and ethical decision. If you do not have the knowledge to answer that question, you need to go to someone with

more knowledge or education than you have to assist in making the right decision. If you were ever on trial for a decision you made in your practice as a nurse, the question "What is reasonable under the circumstances?" would be the main question the judge would want answered. The judge would possibly interview expert witnesses to determine what other LPNs would do in the same situation. The assumption is that most LPNs act in a reasonable manner, and if your behavior agrees with that exhibited by other LPNs in similar situations, you are being reasonable in your care administration.

ACTS OF NEGLIGENCE AND OMISSION

There are two very specific legal concepts that you should be familiar with as a licensed nurse: negligence and omission. Lawsuits frequently are based on these two principles.

Negligence is failure to exercise adequate care. The determination of negligence is based on the level of performance that is expected of an LPN as determined by the state nurse practice act, the policies and procedures for the facility where the LPN works, and what is considered safe and prudent care by other LPNs. For example, if you start an intravenous (IV) procedure even in an emergency situation, and you are not IV-certified, you have broken the law, as outlined in the nurse practice act, and you are liable for your behavior even if there is a good outcome from your actions. Why? Because you broke the law. Even if the outcome is good, you could be sued because you have broken the law.

The second example refers to following the policies and procedures in your workplace. Imagine that you are working the night shift and a nursing assistant calls in sick. You are responsible for the care that is given regardless of the number of people who report to work. After a great deal of effort, you are still unable to replace the sick assistant, and the entire shift is short one person. On the unit, you have a resident who is notorious for wandering at night. Without the additional nursing assistant, you do not have adequate staff to watch the resident and keep him from falling, so you restrain him. The night goes well, and you feel that you have successfully used good judgment. However, the restraint is still on the resident when his daughter comes to assist him with breakfast. She approaches you with an angry look and states that her father has been unlawfully restrained. She leaves the unit to contact other family members and eventually an attorney. The policies and procedures for your nursing home will determine if the family will win this case or not. If your unit has a policy of a restraint-free environment that requires resident or family permission to restrain (as required by the Omnibus Budget Reconciliation Act [OBRA]), or has a policy of calling the administrator whenever there is not adequate staff, you will lose the case. The policies and procedures in your work environment are the law of the facility and must be obeyed carefully to protect clients as well as your licensure.

Safe and prudent care is what most LPNs would give in the same situation. If you were being sued for putting the restraint on the nursing home resident described earlier, your attorney might ask three or four qualified LPNs to testify about what they would do. This is the same principle as that used with the question "What is reasonable under the

circumstances?" This legal concept should force every nurse to think in terms of safe and prudent care with each activity performed. The question is, "Would another LPN do the same thing under the same circumstances?"

The concept of omission is very straightforward. It occurs when you omit something that is either ordered or expected as a normal part of treatment for a client. Classic examples of omission involve treatment or medication. Omission also could involve failure to notify a supervisor or physician of a situation with a client. Many lawsuits are based on omissions of care.

There are many issues within the realm of nursing that are profoundly affected by both ethical and legal concepts. The purpose of this chapter is to discuss issues closely associated with nursing care of older adults, such as the use of restraints, advanced directives, informed consent, and elder abuse.

▶ USE OF RESTRAINTS

The long-practiced tradition of using restraints has been an accepted aspect of nursing care of the elderly until recently. It is important to note that the use of restraints in this country is significantly higher than in European countries. Only 4 percent of nursing home residents are restrained in Scotland and England, and the numbers are fewer in Sweden and Denmark. Fortunately, the numbers have changed regarding restraint use in nursing homes during the past few years. Current literature now shares research and information on how to work with older adults in an effort to avoid use of restraints. This is a positive sign. Even so, health-care statistics still indicate that 500,000 persons a day are restrained for some reason while in the care of health-care providers.

Thoughts about the ageism that exist in our society have been shared in Chapter 1 of this book. One of the premises of this author is that restraints are allowed as a care modality with older adults because of ageism. The fact that society allows the use of restraints for frail older people and refers to that intervention as nursing care should be appalling to anyone who reads this book. The feeling of being appalled over something is a feeling based on ethical thinking, structured after the value system of you, the person with the feeling.

The use of restraints on elderly people is the result of ageist thinking and old nursing traditions.

The implementation of OBRA in 1987 had a positive impact on decreasing restraint use in nursing homes. The OBRA regulation states that the resident has the right to be free from any physical restraint imposed or psychoactive drug administered for the purposes of discipline or convenience and not required to treat the resident's medical symptoms. Federal statistics state that the use of restraints has declined by 50 percent since 1987 because of the implementation of OBRA.

The OBRA Interpretative Guidelines define physical restraints as any manual method or physical or mechanical device, material, or equipment attached or adjacent to the resident's body that the individual cannot remove easily that restricts free movement or normal access to one's body. Physical restraints include leg restraints, arm restraints, hand mitts, soft ties or bed rails (Bandman & Bandman, 2002).

The nursing home industry is successfully striving to reduce the use of restraints and to make restraint alternatives the standard of care. Current federal laws clearly create a strong reason not to use chemical or physical restraints. The law places, on the nursing home that uses restraints, the burden of justifying their use as the least restrictive alternative available. Many LPNs work in nursing homes and have to deal with the ethical and legal concerns surrounding the use of restraints on a daily basis.

What are the laws that govern the use of restraints in hospitals? These laws are written by the individual state legislatures and are not managed under the umbrella of a federal law. They also are controlled by current nursing home or hospital policy. This makes the use of restraints in hospitals not only a legal issue but an ethical issue of great importance. It is often true that where there are less restrictive laws written, there is a need for a higher ethical awareness and concern. Generally, the laws regarding the use of restraints on older adults in hospitals are less defined and the decision to apply restraints is the decision of the nurse who is responsible for the person's care. How does a nurse make the decision to apply restrictive devices on a person, generally without that person's permission? And what theory of nursing or nursing principle allows that to happen without being questioned by other health-care providers?

WHY ARE RESTRAINTS USED?

The main reason restraints are used on older adults is to prevent injury from a fall or a wandering episode. They also are used in acute care settings like an intensive care unit (ICU) to keep the person from pulling tubes such as a catheter or IV line. These are a laudable reasons; however, in the current environment of resident or patient rights, the use of restraints should be re-examined. Other than the desire to prevent injury, the decision to use restraints comes from two recognizable sources. The first is nursing tradition. Before the 1960s and the invention of the antipsychotic drugs, severely mentally ill people were placed in state hospitals and often were securely restrained to avoid hurting themselves or others. Once drugs were invented that managed their psychotic behavior, most of these people were released from restraints and actively participated in psychotherapy. Those who did not respond or did not respond sufficiently to the drugs continued to be restrained.

How did this nursing tradition of protecting psychotic people from themselves and each other become translated to a standard of care for the elderly? As the citizens of this nation have aged, there are more and more "old-old" people who demonstrate the normal losses of aging. The percentage of old people with dementia has increased simply because more people are living to be older. Somehow in this scenario, nurses and other health-care providers have decided that a treatment modality for psychotic individuals is acceptable for frail older adults. It is important to question the ethics of that decision. Does it demonstrate the art of nursing, the science of nursing, the value system of nurses in general, or does it represent a misplaced, outdated nursing tradition?

The second reason many nurses use restraints is the fear of litigation. Often when given a viable option for care that does not require a restraint (e.g., validation therapy, as described in Chapter 13), nurses still use a restraint to avoid being sued. The most frequently cited reason for using restraints is to prevent the elderly person from falling. Yet, few nurses recognize that 200 deaths of institutionalized elderly clients per year are attributed to the use of restraints. Choking on a vest restraint is the most common form of death while restrained (Bandman & Bandman,

2002). Study results show that older adults are injured, sometimes fatally, while becoming agitated and trying to escape from their restraints. Examples from these studies include climbing over the siderails, strangling and suffocating with a restraint that has slipped or been improperly applied, and the failure of staff to monitor and adjust restraints at regular, timely intervals. The use of chemical restraints often results in confusion or personality alteration.

It is time for nurses to examine themselves professionally and consider whether the behavior of applying restraints is based more on a paternalistic bias toward the elderly, is done for staff convenience, or derives from a desire to control client behavior. The motivation for this practice needs to be strongly examined both in terms of legal and ethical principles.

I believe that if restraints were removed from the standard repertoire of the LPN, creative and effective nursing care strategies would surface. Care would be based on the individual needs of each older adult, and each person would be treated as an individual of value. The objective of care could and should be a restraint-free environment. Once restraint-free environments are in place for a period of time, a new and improved nursing tradition will have been created.

A RESTRAINT-FREE ENVIRONMENT

One of the important concepts for you, the licensed nurse, to understand is that there is no scientific basis to support the use of restraints to protect elderly people from injury. The exact opposite is true. Careful scientific research has shown that restraints can reduce a person's functional capacity and create problems with most body systems. With that in mind, the development of a restraint-free environment should be a priority for health-care providers who sincerely care about the physical and emotional condition of older people. How is that type of environment established?

USE OF LEAST RESTRICTIVE DEVICES

You, the caregiver, should always be thinking in terms of the least restrictive device possible for each person. The truth is that you do not want a resident to fall and sustain an injury, or to wander out of the building and become lost, or worse. The least restrictive approach would include the use of pillows, wedge cushions, pads, and lap trays. The criterion for each of these items is that they can be removed by the elderly person. The devices should serve as a reminder rather than a restraint. The concern over wandering can be dealt with in numerous ways. There are many commercial alarms available that will warn the employees when a resident walks through the doorway. Placing a rope or Velcro strip across doorways that should not be used by confused residents will work as a reminder in some situations. Having well-educated and caring volunteers available at peak activity times enhances both the safety and enjoyment of most residents. The use of validation therapy (see Chapter 11) often reduces the anxiety and, therefore, pacing behavior of some people.

When establishing a restraint-free environment, it is important to see each resident as an individual with rights and a history. Do some people pace or wander at a specific time each day because of a lifelong habit? A recurring concern? An unresolved life event? It is important to determine whether the resident's history is the cause of the wandering behavior.

OTHER CONSIDERATIONS

The staff in either a hospital or nursing home should have some common strategies for managing confused older people. There may need to be a policy of placing mattresses on the floor or of lowering the bed near the floor to keep a night wanderer from falling out of bed. If wandering occurs more frequently at night or in the late afternoon, then they are the times the staff should be increased so residents can be closely monitored. At present in most facilities, evening and night shifts are times of minimal staffing.

Implementing a restraint-free environment requires the education of everyone on staff, including ancillary people, to the principles of working in a restraint-free environment. Along with the education program, it is important to assist staff to focus on their personal values regarding care for the elderly person. This should help in establishing desirable approaches to care. A restraint-free environment is an innovative care strategy that also requires thought by bright and creative people who feel a commitment to the rights of all people, especially older adults.

▶ INFORMED CONSENT

Another very similar legal and ethical concern is the concept of *informed consent*. The Patient's Bill of Rights clearly outlines a person's right to information before giving consent to treatment. The law says that there needs to be a signature on the consent form. The ethical aspect of this situation is that the client has the right to all the information available on the treatment or procedure for which consent is being given. Again, the nurse assumes the role of patient advocate. Would you stop a patient from going to surgery if, as you were assisting him or her onto the cart, the patient asked, "Tell me again, what it is the doctor is going to do?" Legal and ethical knowledge says you should.

Obviously, there are better ways to manage this type of situation than to postpone the scheduled surgery. One is to simply be sure ahead of time that the patient has the information needed to make decisions about the health and treatment plan. This can become challenging when the patient is a frail elderly person who is experiencing behavior that ranges from forgetfulness to dementia. Is it enough just to get the signature when you know the person will not remember the instructions? The answer to that question must come from your value system, that ethical aspect of yourself. Do you value the patient and the patient's rights as outlined in the Patient Bill of Rights? Do you value the principle behind the informed consent rule? It is hoped that you do. If that is so, you have a great deal of work to do to protect the rights of all clients. That work may involve reporting the forgetfulness or dementia to the nursing manager. In a nursing home environment, it would be important to share that information at the interdisciplinary team (IDT) meeting. Talking to the family may be something you do or that is delegated to the social worker. The priority is to ensure that the elderly person has complete information when asked to make a decision regarding health care.

▶ ELDER ABUSE

Occurrences of elder abuse are on the increase in this country. It is estimated that 5% of older adults are abused each year, most often by a close family member. Abuse exists in family homes, nursing homes, and hospitals. It is done by family members, paid caregivers, and strangers. It seems to be a consequence of life in Western society, which moves faster and faster, with more and more demands. Into this scenario comes an increasing number of older people who, as a natural consequence of aging, move more slowly and experience mental changes that require patience from caregivers. This country has never had so many older citizens, and society does not seem adequately prepared to adapt to them and their needs.

Because of this lack of emphasis on understanding and meeting the needs of the elderly, caregivers tend to experience burnout. Accompanying this phenomenon is the tendency to abuse the elder for causing the feelings of burnout and frustration. I believe that elder abuse is the most extreme and destructive form of ageism that can be demonstrated. Elder abuse is against the law.

Every state in this country has laws against elder abuse. Again, it is your responsibility, as a licensed nurse, to determine what the law is in your state, as well as the policies and procedures for handling abuse in the organization where you work. Whatever the particulars of the law are, it will state that you are responsible, under the law, to report all suspected cases of elder abuse.

Elder abuse can occur in many forms. Some of them are:

- Inflicting pain or injury
- Withholding food, money, medication, or care
- Confinement; physical or chemical restraint
- Theft or intentional mismanagement of assets
- Sexual abuse
- Threatening to do any of the above

The composite picture of the person most likely to be abused is a female, 75 years old, who lives with a relative. She is physically, financially, or socially dependent on others. For LPNs who work in home care or in daycare centers, this description should be one to keep in mind. Do any of your patients have unexplained bruises or other markings? Do they seem unusually hungry or frightened? Are they unwilling to talk about their family member, or do they act fearful when you mention the family member who is responsible for their care? Any of these behaviors could be indications of abuse and deserve your attention.

If you are an LPN in a nursing home or hospital, it is critical to be alert for staff members who treat clients in negative and degrading ways. If a confused client is even more confused or is screaming and crying after receiving "care" from a particular staff member, be on the alert. Another cue is when residents have more bruises after a particular staff member has worked, than at other times. Residents who are complaining of things being lost may actually be victims of theft. An older adult should not have a fearful countenance when a family or staff member comes near; be on the lookout for such behavior.

It is critical that all cases of suspected abuse be reported to the proper authorities. In all settings, it is proper for you, the LPN, to report suspected abuse to your supervisor. If nothing is done to prevent the behaviors that seemed suspicious to you, it is both an ethical and legal mandate that you find the proper avenue for reporting your information to a legal authority. You will determine the proper protocol for reporting abuse by reviewing the abuse laws in your state and the policies and procedures in your work setting that govern this situation.

In most situations, that elderly person will be moved to a safer environment, or the employee who was performing the acts of abuse will be put on probation, terminated, or arrested. If the abuse is occurring in the home, the situation becomes very complex. The

The social worker is an excellent resource when dealing with suspicions of elder abuse.

family that allows elder abuse is obviously dysfunctional. Perhaps the abuse is occurring because of parental abuse of the child when the child, now turned caregiver, was younger. Perhaps it is simply a response to the distress of caring for an aging parent. Sometimes, the abused elder does not want to be moved out of the situation because of concern over being moved into a nursing home or other facility. This is a choice the older person is allowed to make. However, in most situations, the family members will be required to receive counseling in an effort to alter abusive behavior.

▶ SEXUAL NEEDS

Another ageist concept in our society is that old people are asexual. Biologically, this is simply not true. Sexual needs are as basic as eating and socializing. The aging process does not remove that need from the physiological schema of your clients. The question is how do you provide for the fulfillment or manage the needs of older adults for whom you are responsible?

Older people need love, too. I recall attending a conference many years ago in which the presenter, a music therapist, made the statement that every person needs 14 hugs a day. I do not believe that she had any scientific data to validate her point, but when she said it, I believed her! She continued to say that most of society finds old people very unlovable and, therefore, unhuggable. I immediately began a lifelong quest to provide as many hugs to older people as I could give in a lifetime. Older people in our society are touch starved; often people do not readily touch or hug them. Does this flash of unscientific insight bring to your awareness that you can do something positive about meeting this need for older adults in your care? It would be very exciting to see a care plan that said: 14 hugs a day evenly distributed over 24 hours. This approach to the elderly would be positive in assisting them to meet their normal, physical needs identified as sexual.

A myth that needs to be dispelled is that dirty old men are always reaching and grabbing inappropriate parts of the female body! When this accusation is made, it generally is directed at an older, confused man. Instead of restraining or isolating that individual, you should assess him on a professional level.

Sitting with him and asking, "You miss your wife, don't you?" to provoke a discussion of his sexual feelings would be very appropriate. After your discussion with this client, you may learn strategies that will help him manage his sexual feelings in a more appropriate manner. Perhaps he needs a picture of his deceased wife that he can keep with him at all times, for instance, in the dining room, or when he is in the hallway in his wheelchair. It may take something as simple as teaching the nursing assistants to point to the picture of his wife and ask him to tell them about her to ward off his confused attempts at meeting his sexual needs. Perhaps the solution is more complex, and the nursing assistants need to be taught how to stop his inappropriate behavior in a respectful manner that recognizes sexual needs as normal and confusion as a reality. It is your responsibility, in an ethical framework, to determine the approaches and strategies that will provide for effective management of the sexual needs of your clients.

Another problem that occurs at times is that of masturbation. Masturbation is a normal sexual outlet for people who are experiencing sexual frustration. Teenagers generally masturbate as part of their sexual experimentation. Adults often masturbate as part of their sexual relationships with other persons. It is not abnormal for older people to masturbate. It is something they have either done intermittently or have worked hard at suppressing throughout their lives. It is not wrong for an older adult to masturbate; however, because of different levels of cognitive ability, a client may be participating in this activity in an inappropriate place. Masturbating in the day room or in any environment in front of others is not appropriate behavior. If this should occur, it is your responsibility to gently and kindly stop the activity and take the client to his or her room. It is appropriate to leave the person alone there to do as the person wishes. This approach is an effective one to use if the client is acting out for attention or is forgetful or confused. If you walk into a client's room and the person is masturbating, just excuse yourself and close the door.

Often in nursing home settings, there is controversy about allowing married couples to room together or to have time for conjugal visits. Sometimes, it is not wise to have couples room together because one may need more care than the other, and the stronger person becomes worn out trying to administer to every need of the ill or degenerating spouse. Abusive behavior brought on because of dementia could be another reason. But only reasons that would jeopardize the health of one or both of the people involved are valid for keeping a married couple separated. It is normal for married people to live together. It is normal for married people to have sex together. The facility that recognizes that normalcy and individual right is to be commended.

Another situation that can occur is that of unmarried, consenting adults having intimate moments. You have the ethical and legal responsibility of protecting demented, developmentally disabled, or mentally ill clients from the sexual advances of others. If that person does not have the ability to make day-to-day decisions, neither does the person have the ability to make the normal, everyday decision to have an intimate relationship. As a licensed nurse, you are responsible for protecting such a person from what could be defined as sexual abuse.

What of those who are not cognitively impaired? Counselors do not go around the halls of high schools or universities to keep teenagers and young adults from holding hands or kissing. Why does society think it is necessary to do that for older adults?

Sexual feelings and expressions are a normal part of living even if one is old, handicapped, or confused. Every dependent human being has the right to expect protection from sexual abuse; but by the same token, every human being has the right to express sexual feelings within the framework of society's norms.

▶ CONCLUSION

This chapter covers several diverse topics that have legal and ethical ramifications in giving care to older adults. Every topic is one of importance and needs to be addressed by you as a gerontological nurse. Older people have rights, and when these people come into the health-care system, you, the licensed nurse, are the unofficial advocate for them. Their legal and ethical rights are your responsibility. The concepts explained in this chapter should help to provide you with a strong foundation for fulfilling that role.

CASE STUDY

As the 11–7 charge nurse on a 20-bed unit at Cherry Dale Nursing Home, you have had concerns over the staffing on your shift. Often, you have found the nursing assistants restraining residents for their own good without telling you. You have discussed the problem with the nursing assistants and have taught them the rules for restraint application at Cherry Dale. In spite of your efforts, there still is one old-time nursing assistant who does not follow the facility's rules and regulations, and clearly ignores your instructions.

This is your first charge nurse position as an LPN. You recognize that the nursing assistants see you as an inexperienced nurse. This is especially true of the older nursing assistant. During your first 6 weeks on the job, you believe you have made progress in earning the trust you need from the nursing assistants. However, one or two are still restraining residents at night without telling you or without trying other alternatives.

You discussed this problem with your nurse manager, and she simply told you that you were a charge nurse now and it was your responsibility to follow the policies of the facility. The policy indicates that restraints are not used for the convenience of the staff and are not applied without a written order from the physician and permission from the resident or the resident's guardian.

What are the ethical and legal ramifications regarding your current dilemma?

How will you resolve the problem?

Discussion

Because you are the licensed nurse responsible for what occurs on your shift, you are both legally and ethically accountable for the behavior of the nursing assistants who work with you. Because they are violating facility policy, it is as if you were actually performing the act.

It is both unethical and illegal to restrain people without their permission. When this occurs, and it also breaks the rules and regulations of the facility, your legal accountability is compounded. It is important you realize that the law is being broken every time the residents are restrained. It does not matter if you know about it or not. The point is that, as the charge nurse, you are supposed to know about it! Reporting the situation to your supervisor does not release you from responsibility either. She gave you clear instructions as to what to do; you are to follow the facility's policy regarding restraints. The ethical problems of restraining residents are as serious as the legal ones.

Solution

There is more than one approach that could resolve this problem. The truth is that you may have to use them all before you find an appropriate solution.

Make it perfectly clear to all the nursing assistants that the law is being broken and the act of restraining residents on your shift is a criminal offense. Then . . .

- Use the experience and wisdom of the nursing assistants to process different solutions to the problem of residents wandering or potentially falling at night. The nursing assistants will appreciate being asked to assist in solving the problem rather than being told what to do. Try all ideas that do not go against the policy of the institution, the law, or your ethical standards.
- Share your creative solutions with the nurse manager. Let her know how prudent and safe the care is on your shift. (Remember that prudent and safe care is the care that most LPNs would give in the same situation.) You also should build a case for additional staffing on your shift, if that is the problem.
- Document the unique approaches of care you use on your shift and share them with the other shifts by means of verbal report and the nursing care plan.

STUDY QUESTIONS

Please select the one best answer.

1. Ethics is the study of moral actions and values. One of the dilemmas within ethical thinking is concern over:
   a. Who decides what is right and what is wrong.
   b. Whoever pays the bill deciding what is ethical.
   c. Ethical and legal behavior being the same.
   d. The rules of ethical behavior changing daily.

2. Although you were not IV-certified, if you were to find a client bleeding and in need of immediate fluids to save his life, one of the following defines your legal role. Mark the correct answer.
   a. Under the Good Samaritan Act, you are required to do all you can to save the person's life, so you would start IV fluids and call the doctor.
   b. Call the RN and have her handle it. After all, she has the advanced license.
   c. Call an ambulance for immediate transport.
   d. Administer first aid, leave a nursing assistant with the resident, and call the physician or the RN.

3. The legal concept of omissions in care applies when
   a. The physician has missed a diagnosis and, therefore, you have omitted treatment for it because nothing was ordered.
   b. You have intentionally or unintentionally missed an antibiotic dose.
   c. Residents are given baths only every other day.
   d. The RN does not work the weekend.

4. A restraint-free environment consists of an environment in which
   a. Many of the residents fall or wander, but they do not sue the facility because they want to be without restraint.
   b. Mattresses are placed on the floor so residents will not fall out of bed.
   c. The least restrictive device is used on each resident.
   d. Restrictive devices are not used for any reason.

5. Elder abuse is a growing concern in modern society. Which of the following statements is correct?
   a. It is against the law to threaten abuse as well as perform abusive acts.
   b. Elder abuse includes inflicting pain or injury but not confining an older person.
   c. Elder abuse is likely to happen to a male client, over age 85, who lives with a relative.
   d. It is the legal responsibility of the RN to report all suspected cases of elder abuse; this is not the responsibility of the LPN.

Emily Ravsten

chapter **6**

End-of-life Issues in the Elderly Client

Learning Objectives

At *the completion of this chapter, the student will be able to:*

1. Define the essential characteristics of a hospice organization.
2. Identify the five stages of grief as outlined by Dr. Elisabeth Kubler-Ross.
3. List the qualities necessary for a nurse to give end-of-life care.
4. Express an opinion on assisted suicide.
5. List the eight signs of eminent death.

▶ INTRODUCTION

My only living grandparent is Margrette Romer, an 83-year-old woman who keeps on kicking! She gave birth to six daughters, is the grandmother to 16 children, and the great grandmother to nine children, with one on the way. She lived her entire life on a farm in rural, Northern Utah, until 1998 when she fell and broke her hip and femur. She now lives with one of my aunts who is her caregiver.

Grandma celebrated her 80th birthday party with her friends and family, and was hospitalized that evening for her fractures. The family thought she was going to die. Fortunately months before, my mom had sat down with Grandma and filled out a "Living Will," a document that expressed my Grandma's desires to live or die if she were in a hospital. This preparation was helpful to my Grandma and to her daughters. At the time of her hospitalization, the family realized that she might not live. However, her health gradually improved. When she was asked why she was fighting to live, she seriously stated that she still had quilts she needed to finish for her grandchildren! Three years later, Grandma is quilting and living a peaceful and pleasant life with her children and grandchildren all around.

I have a deep love for older people. My mom, the author of this book, practically raised me in nursing homes as she traveled from one nursing home to another evaluating the facilities and teaching the staff. Through such experiences, I learned that older adults are very wise and experienced. In addition, as they approach the end of their life, they have the courage to face the multiple, serious decisions that need to be made. The focus of this chapter is to explore how to assist older adults to die well through the excellent care and support you provide them as they approach the end of their lives. Some terms related to end-of-life care include the following:

- **End-of-life Issues, or EOL for short:** EOL care is a vital issue in health care throughout this country. Americans want to experience a "good death" without being burdened by symptoms or technology. Nurses have an essential role in maximizing EOL care by improving symptom management, communication and education about choices, referrals, and psychosocial treatments. You, as the care provider, will have

the responsibility to explain to older adults and their family members all of the options, referrals, and resources available. It is very important that, as you review some of the options in this chapter, you examine your individual attitudes, values, and beliefs. You need to consider what happens if your personal beliefs conflict with the choices and decisions made by the older adult in your care.

- **Palliative care** is the term used to describe care no longer aimed at a cure or active treatment of a certain medical condition (Matzo and Sherman, 2001.) Instead, the goals of palliation are to provide older adults with comfort and to be able to manage their symptoms. This type of care is the art and science of quality EOL care. It is your opportunity, as an licensed practical nurse (LPN), to take the initiative in providing palliative care that will ensure comprehensive, holistic EOL care for all older adults who are experiencing life-threatening, progressive illness and their families. It is the opportunity to be sensitive and respectful to the older person's values, religious beliefs, family traditions, individual cultures, and beliefs. It is a tremendous amount of responsibility.

- **Terminal restlessness (TR)** is another term for agitated delirium. This is a common occurrence for individuals nearing the end of their life. It may appear as involuntary muscle twitching or jerks, thrashing or agitation, tossing and turning, or yelling and moaning. These symptoms may not appear to be that different from those experienced by residents in long-term care situations. However, delirium at the end of one's life is usually multifactorial and intensified by the progressive shutdown of numerous body systems.

- **Hospice:** The term "hospice" comes from the term hospitality and can be traced back to medieval times, when there was a need to find a place of rest for weary and ill travelers. Today, hospice organizations are located all over this country. A large hospice organization attracts 100's of people each year with diverse diagnoses. However, more than 50% of all other hospices report being underused. This is poor utilization of a potentially tremendous service.

Often, referrals to a hospice come "too little, too late" in order to be most effective. An example of providing successful care is that of Alzheimer's disease (AD) patients.

These five brothers enjoy each other, their families, and fishing. In spite of their healthy and positive lifestyles, they each will die.

Providing them with palliative care may be the primary long-term mode of care. However, once death is imminent, generally around the last 6 months of life, a hospice team should be called on to provide their specialized knowledge to the palliation plan of care for the transition from dying to death.

▶ THE MYSTERY OF DEATH

Normally, more than 70% of annual deaths occur in people 65 and older. By the year 2020, 2.5 million individuals older than age 65 will die annually in the United States. Dying is an unpredictable event. People never know the exact moment or situation in which someone will die. Therefore, as the caregiver to older adults, you, as a nurse, need to be prepared to be a positive influence for appropriate EOL issues. First, you need to be educated in EOL issues and learn to communicate them. Then provide the older adults in your care with a high quality of life and a good death. You need skills in working as a team with other caring professionals, families, and the dying person. Finally, you need to maintain a positive work environment. Without skills in these areas, the quality of EOL care for older adults in your care will be diminished.

As all people know, death is an inevitable and natural human experience. However, death has been shrouded in mystery, envisioned as an experience of great suffering, and generally is contemplated with fear. The early settlers in this country had a different perception. They had a welcoming relationship with it, one that desired a release from pain as well as recognition of the cycles of nature. For them, there was a time to live and a time to die. They were able to accept death as a transition into an afterlife and a reward for a life well lived. Somehow modern society has lost that important concept. What has been the cause of this transition in thinking?

As I watched my Grandmother on the acute unit in the hospital, I saw how different members of my family reacted to the possibility of her death. There were many emotions ranging from acceptance to denial, as well as fear and anger, or joy and confusion. Those emotions were real and will be emotions that you, the nurse, will experience as you encounter family members of a dying person. People need to be allowed to cope with death in their own way, even if it is to deny death's reality until the end.

▶ THE STAGES OF GRIEF

Grief is the normal reaction to a catastrophic loss. What defines the catastrophe? The person experiencing the loss has that responsibility. A catastrophe to one person may not be to another. Understanding and compassion are essential when relating to people experiencing losses. Dr. Elisabeth Kubler-Ross, a Swiss psychiatrist, spent much of her life defining the stages of grief. Death, the greatest personal loss a person can have, was the focus of her grief work. If you understand the five stages of grief, you can recognize them within yourself, the older adults to whom you give care and their families. It is an important piece of knowledge to acquire.

Death is hard! It is a one-time experience for most people. That makes it a unique and powerful experience. When a person dies, that individual loses everything they ever had. The dying person loses friends and family members, home, pets, beauty, everything! Therefore, the stages of grief demonstrate the reactions, the normal human reactions, people can have when facing a loss. Perhaps the person grieving is a family member of the person dying. Their loss is also great. In addition to death, the stages of grief are valid with the loss of an extremity through amputation or a stroke, divorce, and, for some sweet, young girl the loss of a date to the prom can result in a brief grieving process.

CRITICALLY EXAMINE THE FOLLOWING:

Now that we have discussed various aspects of EOL issues, it is time for you to express some of your thoughts on the topic. Please take a few minutes to contemplate and consider *your perfect death*. The purpose of this exercise is to have you apply the information you have just read. Some of the questions you should answer are listed below. Answer them and then add more detail. Consider this a "free write," where anything you say will be respected. You will not have to submit this assignment to the faculty person. However, you will be better able to relate to other people who are dying if you thoughtfully complete this assignment.

How old you will be when you die?

What will be your general health condition?

Who will still be alive and be with you as you die?

How will you die?

Other comments you want to make.

Now consider your ancestors, and how and when they died. You have described your perfect death, but few people get to experience such an event. By looking at your parents' and grandparents' health and the death of family members, you will see your genetic predisposition. What do your genes indicate as a possible death?

Do you have any potentially dangerous hobbies like sky diving or car racing? Do you drive an excessive number of miles in a year? Do you have poor health habits? What do these lifestyle behaviors indicate about your eventual death?

You will die. By trying to understand your own death, you will be able to give better care to people who are at the end of their life.

Kubler-Ross identified the five stages as:

Acceptance
Depression
Bargaining
Anger
Denial

Think of these terms as steps in the process of resolving grief. The person experiencing the loss can go from one stage (or step) to another, and then move back up or down the stages. There is no exact formula or prescription to follow because people are individuals and manage their grief in very personalized

This mother and daughter are struggling with the feelings of denial and shock after the mother was told she had a terminal condition. Notice the seriousness and confusion on their faces. They are clinging to each other and have not moved beyond denial and shock.

ways. Nurses need to allow that type of independent grieving.

DENIAL

When a catastrophic loss occurs, a person's psyche has difficulty accepting it. Consider a young mother who leaves her aging and confused mom outside for "only a moment" while she goes in the house to get her baby. When the young mother comes out of the house, her beautiful, loving mother has wandered out into the street, was hit by a car, and eventually dies in the hospital. Some denial behaviors are shock, praying for it to not be true, walking about or standing and saying, "no, not Mom" over and over again.

Denial is the psyche's way of protecting itself from the harsh, bitter truth. It is as if the mother were wrapped up in a soft, protective cocoon. This psychological protection is there until the person's psyche can deal with the loss. You have heard of people who "were in a daze" during the funeral of a loved one. That is denial. There is no reason to try to force people out of denial. They will move to the

next stage when they are able. During this time, people need to be protected from neglect, injury, and financial abuse. Family members need to understand this stage of the grief process, and be willing to take care of other children, prepare meals, and protect the grieving person.

ANGER

Once the psyche has developed the strength to face the situation, it comes out in a way that tends to keep people away, which saves the person a great deal of energy. What else does it do? This is the one time anger should be encouraged in a person, and supported as a healthy behavior when it occurs. Did you think of some of the advantages of the grieving person showing anger?

Anger demonstrates an awareness of the loss and its consequences. This is one step toward adjusting to the loss. It is also an outlet for the outrage the person feels. Assist the grieving person not to hurt himself or herself or others with the anger. Again, the family needs to understand the advantages of the anger so they can accept what is happening and support the behaviors that occur.

CRITICALLY EXAMINE THE FOLLOWING:

List three reasons why anger is a healthy behavior in the person who is experiencing grief:

1.
2.
3.

I will share my answers with you. Perhaps you thought of some reasons that did not occur to me. Compare your list with mine, and come to class prepared to share your thinking.

It means the psyche is healthier because the person is no longer in denial.

It keeps the people away who say things like: "You'll always have your memories of your Mom." or "She is at peace now." Comments like these disrespect the loss and the grief being experienced. People who make such comments often are not comfortable with anger. Their purpose is to "make everything all right," which is not congruent with angry feelings.

BARGAINING

The anger is as if the psyche wants to "scare away" the bad thing that has occurred. However, as we know, that does not work. Once the grieving person realizes that the "bad thing" will not go away, people often turn to God or other supernal powers. This behavior often is demonstrated by bargaining.

Bargaining is seen as something like prayers to God stating that the person will donate a great deal of money to a charitable organization, will never sin again, or will actively do good for others. The thinking is that if one trades something of value, like goodness with God, then God will perform a miracle. This is very heartbreaking for family and friends. Many say they prefer anger over the wrenching episodes of bargaining. The negotiation with God is the final chance to change the situation. If God cannot "fix things," then no one can. This time in the grieving process requires both patience and gentleness. People are often exhausted in their efforts to support the grieving person. They do not have much more to give. Yet, more is asked of them. When you teach families about the bargaining stage, assure them this is often near the end. Praise them for staying with the grieving person throughout the entire experience. Try to give them strength and the courage to see the experience to its conclusion.

Not everyone believes in God or a higher power. Work with grieving people with whatever way they are bargaining. The principles are the same for all forms of grief bargaining.

DEPRESSION

Depression never is an easy condition. But in the grieving process, it definitely shows progress. When the grieving person is depressed, it means that the individual does not accept the loss but accepts the fact that nothing can change it. Neither the denial, anger, nor bargaining worked. It makes sense that the grieving person would be depressed.

As with all forms of depression, actively assess for suicidal thinking. If you identify it, keep someone with the grieving person, and contact the registered nurse (RN). Suicide is a preventable outcome, so be sensitive to its possibility. Depressed people cry, they sleep a great deal, and they have low energy. Teach this to the family members. Ask them to once

again support the grieving person through this last hurtle to acceptance.

Depressed people do not need to be told "everything is all right." For them nothing will ever be all right again. They need quiet love and support while they find a way to continue on with their life.

ACCEPTANCE

Once the grieving person reaches acceptance, there is a sense of relief. The individual still is searching for life structure without the loved one who died. The point is that the grief process is over and living has started again. The grieving person still may call out the name of the deceased person, be found crying after finding a piece of clothing of the loved one, or just sit quietly contemplating the life of the person who died. This is normal.

The grieving process is difficult for the person experiencing the loss and the family members. The management of the experience can be improved when you, the LPN, know the stages of grief and readily share them with appropriate people.

▶ QUALITIES FOR A NURSE TO BE A PROVIDER OF END-OF-LIFE CARE

Many nurses have difficulty talking about EOL matters with patients. That makes it necessary for you to learn new skills and acquire new knowledge in order to improve the care of older adults who require palliative care (Box 6.2). Some of the new knowledge you need may be communication skills and knowledge of resources and available services.

You, as a nurse, have a tremendous potential to change the care of dying older adults and the support given to their families. It is critical that you understand human nature as you give care to people who are dying. You need to be able to identify the stages of grief, for example, and translate those stages to family members. Because the stages are expressed individually by different people, you need to be able to comprehend the impact on specific individuals, or understand the nature of the people involved. Another critical aspect of what you need to know in order to be an effective palliative nurse is the ability to identify and meet the holistic needs of individuals, families, and communities.

TOLERANCE AND EMPATHY

Each individual who you come across in your work is unique and different. This means that you, as the care provider, will need to gain an understanding of people and their differences. This requires that you learn to become tolerant and empathetic to those with whom you associate. Synonyms of tolerance are "compassion," "endurance," "patience," "impartiality," and "open-mindedness." Synonyms of empathy are "understanding," "sympathetic," "identifying with the patient," and "providing insight and feeling in your care."

In order to provide appropriate tolerance and empathy, you must strive to provide an environment that meets the physical, emotional, social, and spiritual needs of each dying person. This includes, but is not limited to, allowing people to die in their communities with loved ones, in their own homes.

SENSE OF HUMOR

Having a sense of humor with the dying person is a simple way to assist in relieving, reducing, and soothing the symptoms of a disease. Of course, you must know the personality and mood of the older adult in your care

before making jokes about the situation. You must make sure that it is done at the right time and in the right situation. Please think about a time and place when you were suffering and laughter helped with the cure.

COMMUNICATION

Communication seems to be the key to most situations. When it comes to death and dying, this situation has the possibility of being discussed in a context of hope, meaning, and opportunity. With strong communication skills, uncertainty is replaced with certainty, hopelessness is replaced with faith, and despair is replaced with empowerment.

GOOD LISTENING SKILLS

Being a good listener is the greatest skill any nurse can have. Take time to listen to the older adults' stories about their children and grandchildren, stories about falling in love, and possibly losing their loved ones. Older people enjoy sharing their life experiences. It is important to remember, when talking to an older person, that you need to speak in a voice that he or she can hear. Move in close to the person, touch their shoulder, smile, and really listen to what he or she has to share.

To listen, you must be fully present and attentive to the other person. You are not listening if you:

- Are in a hurry

- Are thinking about yourself
- Interrupt
- Ask the same question twice
- Do not ask any questions
- Assume that you know what the other person is going to say

The good listener is one who does not think about what to say until after the other person has finished speaking.

▶ CULTURAL ACCOUNTABILITY

In addition to the above-mentioned qualities that are needed to care for those nearing the end of their life, it also is important to be familiar with the cultural diversities of the older adults in your care. A person's culture will influence the decision-making process toward various treatments.

In many cultures, a family's interdependence, harmony, duty, and obligation to a "senior" family member are quite obvious. Some cultures believe that it is inappropriate to tell someone that they are dying because it will create a sense of hopelessness and sadness. Some cultures believe that a sick individual should not be allowed to make any decisions about their EOL care, but rather have the family or the eldest son make those decisions. Cultural needs should be addressed immediately on admission to any facility in order for you, as the LPN, to be aware of the family and the individual's diverse needs.

▶ END-OF-LIFE DECISIONS

As a care provider for those individuals who are nearing the end of their life, it is critical that you recognize the importance of being aware of the decisions a person has made about their current and future medical care, and to honor his or her preferences. According to a study report in the RN magazine (August, 2000), 25% of nurses have seen other health-care providers deliberately disregard a patient's advance directive, such as a durable power of attorney, a living will, or a health-care proxy document. Therefore, to help protect the patients' right to make his or her own health-care choices and to avoid getting yourself or your facility into legal trou-

ble, you need to understand the various laws, your individual duties to the person dying, and the individual wishes of that person.

Gaining an understanding of all of the issues surrounding EOL care is a daunting task. You will run into challenges about knowledge and skills in assessing and managing pain in cognitively impaired older adults. You will experience frustration about physicians being unwilling to consider a nurse's assessment and recommendations. You will find it difficult to deal with the strong emotional attachments that are formed with older adults at the EOL stage. These are all reasons to learn and study EOL issues.

▶ ADVANCE DIRECTIVES

One of the most difficult situations health-care professionals face when caring for the older people is how to assist patients and families trying to make decisions about whether to start, continue, or stop life-sustaining treatments. Elderly people, as a group, comprise 73% of deaths each year, making EOL treatment decisions far more prevalent among them. Documents that assist the health-care team in making such complex decisions are advance directives. There are two types of advance directive documents available: the durable power of attorney for health care (also called health-care proxy) and living wills.

The health-care proxy has the authority to make health-care decisions if the individual loses the ability to make decisions or communicate personal wishes (Box 6.3). The proxy can make decisions as the need arises and is not restricted to a decision that was made previously without knowledge of the current situation.

The other type of advanced directive is known as a living will (Fig. 6.1). This is a legal document that allows individuals to share their opinions and wishes regarding their death. The legal statutes that govern the use of advance directives vary from state to state. You, as a licensed nurse, must clearly understand the advance directive laws where you work.

Advance directives came into use when legal cases such as those involving Karen Ann Quinlan and Nancy Cruzan surfaced in the

Pennsylvania Declaration

——————————————

I, _____, being of sound mind, willfully and voluntarily make this declaration to be followed if I become incompetent. This declaration reflects my firm and settled commitment to refuse life-sustaining treatment under the circumstances indicated below.

I direct my attending physician to withhold or withdraw life-sustaining treatment that serves only to prolong the process of my dying, if I should be in a terminal condition or in a state of permanent unconsciousness.

I direct that treatment be limited to measures to keep me comfortable and to relieve pain, including any pain that might occur by withholding or withdrawing life-sustaining treatment.

In addition, if I am in the condition described above, I feel especially strongly about the following forms of treatment:

I ( ) do ( ) do not want cardiac resuscitation.

I ( ) do ( ) do not want mechanical respiration.

I ( ) do ( ) do not want tube feeding or any other artificial or invasive form of nutrition (food) or hydration (water).

I ( ) do ( ) do not want blood or blood products.

I ( ) do ( ) do not want any form of surgery or invasive diagnostic tests.

I ( ) do ( ) do not want kidney dialysis.

I ( ) do ( ) do not want antibiotics.

I realize that if I do not specifically indicate my preference regarding any of the forms of treatment listed above, I may receive that form of treatment.

Other instructions:

Fig. 6.1.

APPOINTING A SURROGATE

PRINT THE NAME, ADDRESS AND PHONE NUMBER OF YOUR SURROGATE

PRINT THE NAME, ADDRESS AND PHONE NUMBER OF YOUR ALTERNATE SURROGATE

PRINT THE DATE

SIGN THE DOCUMENT AND PRINT YOUR ADDRESS

WITNESSING PROCEDURE

YOUR TWO WITNESSES MUST SIGN AND PRINT THEIR ADDRESSES

Surrogate decisionmaking:

I ( ) do ( ) do not want to designate another person as my surrogate to make medical treatment decisions for me if I should be incompetent and in a terminal condition or in a state of permanent unconsciousness.

Name: _____

Address: _____

Phone: _____

Name and address of substitute surrogate (if surrogate designated above is unable to serve):

Name: _____

Address: _____

Phone: _____

I made this declaration on the _____ day of _____.
                            (day)   *(month, year)*

Declarant's signature: _____

Declarant's address: _____

The declarant, or the person on behalf of and at the direction of the declarant, knowingly and voluntarily signed this writing by signature or mark in my presence.

Witness's signature: _____

Witness's address: _____

Witness's signature: _____

Witness's address: _____

Courtesy of **Partnership for Caring, Inc.**   6/96
1620 Eye Street, NW, Suite 202. Washington, DC 20006 800-989-9455

BOX 6.3. HEALTH-CARE PROXY

I, _____ , of _____ , this day of , _____ ,
being of sound mind, willingly and voluntarily appoint _____ , as my
agent and attorney-in-fact, without substitution. This gives my proxy lawful authority to
execute a directive on my behalf under Section 75-2-1105, governing the care and
treatment to be administered to or to be withheld from me at any time after I incur an
injury, disease, or illness that renders me unable to give current directions to attending
physicians and other providers of medical services.

I have carefully selected my above-named agent with confidence in the belief that
this person's familiarity with my desires, beliefs, and attitudes will result in directions to
attending physicians and providers of medical services that would probably be the
same as I would give if able to do so.

This power of attorney will remain in effect from the time my attending physician certi-
fies that I have incurred a physical or mental condition rendering me unable to give
current directions to attending physicians and other providers of medical services as to
my care and treatment.

_____

Signature of Principal

State of _____

County of _____

On the _____ day of _____. _____, personally appeared before
me, _____ who duly acknowledged to me that he/she has read and fully understands the foregoing power of attorney, executed the same of his/her own volition and
for the purposes set forth, and that he/she was acting under no constraint or undue
influence whatsoever.

_____

Notary Public

My commission expires: _____

Residing at: _____

judicial system. Both were situations in which a young woman was kept alive on life-support equipment but had no quality of life at the time and no possibility of improvement in the future. In both cases, the family members decided to remove the life-support equipment and allow their daughters to die. In both cases, the health-care facility refused to remove the equipment and the parents sued.

In 1989, the U.S. Supreme Court ruled that not even the family should make decisions for an incompetent patient without "clear and convincing evidence" that indicated the person's desire was to die if incompetent. In a five-to-four decision by the U.S. Supreme Court, the following rights were listed for states (Cruzan v. Director, 1990):

- The state has a right to assert an unquali-fied interest in the preservation of human life.
- A choice between life and death is a very personal matter.
- Abuse can occur when incompetent patients do not have loved ones available to serve as surrogate decision makers.

After this court ruling, the majority of state legal systems began requiring an advanced directive on admission to health-care facilities to predetermine the actions that should be taken if a patient became incompetent. As an LPN, you need to determine what the law is in your state regarding advance directives. If they are required on admission, you need to know where they are and what they say regarding your clients. It is the role of the nurse to be an advocate for the people to whom care is given. Knowledge about the advance directive and the state laws that govern its use is very important to you.

When one is working with advance directives, there is more involved than just knowing the law. The law represents legal responsibilities. These are serious responsibilities and should not be ignored; however, as in every issue, there is also an ethical component. It is the ethical responsibility of every nurse to be sure that the person signing the advance directive is not coerced and has full understanding of what is being signed. In most states, the nurse is not allowed to witness this document. It is important that outsiders who would not wield undue influence act as witnesses.

Whenever you are giving care to a patient who is in a terminal condition, it is important that you listen as the person talks and give them honest answers to their questions. If someone feels concern over what was written in the advanced directive, you should bring that to the attention of the nurse manager. The instructions for completing a living will are provided in the Appendix of this book. In all situations, it is necessary to keep in mind the primary objective of the advanced directive: to follow the wishes of the person who wrote it.

▶ DURABLE POWER OF ATTORNEY

Durable power of attorney is another legal document about which you need to know. Durable power of attorney is used in cases in which an individual is incompetent. The law allows a competent individual to make all (health care, financial, disposition of personal items) legal decisions for the incompetent person. The classic example is someone with AD. Before the person with AD becomes incompetent, he or she can identify someone they trust and who knows their wishes and assign them durable power of attorney. Then when the dementia increases, the individual's wishes are met.

Not everyone knows that they will eventually become incompetent. When a person becomes incompetent because of, for example, undiagnosed AD or a car accident that causes brain damage, the family may seek a durable power of attorney and the older person is unaware of what is happening. The forms for durable power of attorney need to come from a qualified attorney to ensure their legality in the state where the older adult resides.

To ensure protection of the older person's rights, you, as the nurse, need to recommend to families and patients that they seek legal council. Once a durable power of attorney has been established, you have a responsibility to identify the type of decision-making authority each person possesses.

▶ IMMINENT SIGNS OF DEATH

It is important for you, as the LPN, to know the imminent signs of death. It is easy to assist someone in their preparation to die if they have been diagnosed as terminally ill. A terminal diagnosis allows individuals to realign their priorities, mend various relationships and say good-bye to loved one. In addition, a terminal diagnosis allows staff the opportunity to prioritize their care and assist persons in meeting their goals and achieving a peaceful life closure.

When death is near, bodily functions will slow and certain signs and symptoms will occur, including the following:

- Rapid, weak pulse
- Decline in blood pressure
- Dyspnea and periods of apnea
- Slower or no pupil response to light
- Profuse perspiration
- Cold extremities
- Bladder and bowel incontinence
- Pallor and mottling of skin

CRITICALLY EXAMINE THE FOLLOWING:

Have you considered what you would like written in your living will? Do you want to be pain free? What about antibiotics? A ventilator? Food? Xerox a copy of the living will in this chapter and complete it for yourself. Add the details that are important to you and be prepared to submit your living will to the faculty person or discuss it in class.

- Loss of hearing
- Remember that one of the last senses lost is that of hearing.

One clear sign of eminent death is that of TR. Reports indicate that more than three fourths of dying patients experience this condition. TR happens in the last hours of life. It is the spiraling down of physiological functions and can be very distressing to the older adult who is dying, and family and staff members. At this time so close to EOL, there is a crucial need for careful and thoughtful intervention to provide the dying person with comfort and to be able to control his or her symptoms (Forbes, 2001).

If the dying person in your care has not been diagnosed with a terminal illness, various assessments or interviews can occur at the bedside in order to be prepared to assist the individual. Formal assessments will be done by the assigned RN, however, you, as the LPN, are giving the bedside care and need to be prepared to respond to questions that are asked following an official assessment. The goals of your assessment are to be able to gain a clear understanding of the older persons' experiences with their illnesses. In addition, you need to be able to identify distressing symptoms that need management, convey your concern and empathy to the persons involved, and to evaluate any risk that may be expressed due to current distress or feelings. It is important for you to take immediate action when a problem is detected.

To begin an appropriate assessment or interview with the dying person, you should ask various questions about discouragement or distress. For example, "What hurts or distresses you most, and how can I help?" Another good opening question to ask is what the person worries about most when the illness is at its worst, and what has been most difficult throughout the process? Your assessment should review the older adults various abilities to cope with stress and anxiety. For example, "During periods of discouragement, some people wish all this suffering were over. Have you felt this way? Tell me about it." "You seem as if life is not worth living. Are you thinking of doing something to hasten your death? Tell me about it." "No one thinks about ending their life without a reason, tell me how you are feeling." (Valente, 2001)

▶ ASSISTED SUICIDE

Approximately 2% to 5% of terminally ill people choose to hasten their own death (Valente, 2001). The reasons for this include poor quality of life and failed requests for treatment withdrawal. People have the right to refuse treatments, food, or fluids if they wish to do so. The Patient's or Resident's Bill of Rights assures people of that right (see

CRITICALLY EXAMINE THE FOLLOWING:

Please comment on the questions posed below. They are questions that require you to ponder their significance. Perhaps you do not believe that you have enough experience to make such decisions. Remember that you will soon be part of the nursing work force, and the need to make some of these decisions will come to you. This exercise is an effort to prepare you for them. Please be prepared to discuss your decisions in class.

How do you feel about assisted suicide?

Would you be a part of such a decision?

Would you work for a facility that supported "slow codes," by not getting to a patient on time or a facility that openly participated in assisted suicide?

These are questions that you will be confronted with as you continue to provide care to patients nearing the end of their lives.

Chapter 5). To make a rational decision about ending life, the older adult needs a clear mind, communication with others, knowledge of alternative treatments, and an understanding of the long-term consequences of actions. The difficulty for most health-care providers is to differentiate between a person's refusal of life-sustaining treatments or providing support to a dying person.

In Oregon, terminally ill people have the right to hasten their deaths by physician-assisted suicide (PAS). By the second year PAS was legal in Oregon, 27 people chose this option. Their median age was 71, 16 were men, 26 were white, and 12 were married (Valente, 2001).

▶ CONCLUSION

Now that you have read this chapter, I hope you will understand the importance of giving meaningful EOL care to all people but especially to older adults. Dying is a unique experience for everyone. The hallmark of a professional nurse is one who can support the dying person and the family in their personal uniqueness of that special event.

I admire your desire and passion for working with older adults. They are at a fragile time in their lives when they are in need of people who care about them. You are that individual, the LPN who will provide older adults who are dying with positive, EOL experiences.

CASE STUDY

Please take some time to focus on the following case study situation. Let us say that you have recently moved to the state of Oregon, where assisted living has been legalized. You were surprised on your first day when a patient on the unit was going to receive some assistance in their own suicide.

1. Before you moved to Oregon, what resources did you use to learn about the legality, rules, and regulations related to assisted living?
2. Every nurse has a right to his or her personal ethical framework of practice. What does your personal framework of practice dictate about what you will do regarding the woman who is assigned to you for assisted suicide?

Solution

1. If I were moving to Oregon and had the potential of working with assisted suicide patients, I would initially contact the state board of nursing for specific Oregon laws. I would also contact the hospital where I would be working and have them send me a packet on their specific protocols regarding assisted suicide. I also may spend some time on the Internet just to see what information is available about the specific topic. You may have additional ideas around gathering specific information. Please list them and feel free to discuss your ideas with your class.
2. I do not know how you would respond to this situation. The answer to this question is based on individual standards and beliefs. Take some time to ponder thoughtfully giving this kind of nursing care, in terms of your personal ethical framework. Consider your knowledge and acceptance of the death and dying process, your personal reaction to assisted suicide as a health-care principle, and explain your responses in writing. Follow through by sharing those ideas in class, in a way you feel most comfortable.

STUDY QUESTIONS

1. When an elderly client experiences TR, he or she will display symptoms such as:
   a. Involuntary muscle twitching or jerks
   b. Extreme fatigue
   c. A sudden energy for life
   d. A calm affect causing the body to have no reactions

2. Palliative care is described as:
   a. The type of care aimed at a cure or active treatment of a certain medical condition
   b. The type of care that provides comfort and management of symptoms
   c. The type of care that allows the family to make all of the decisions
   d. The type of care that provides bereavement support to the family for 1 year after death

3. The stages of grief in order are:
   a. Denial, anger, bargaining, depression, acceptance
   b. Denial, communicate, pain, sadness, joy
   c. Denial, affection, bartering, acceptance
   d. Denial, anger, acceptance, joy, peace

4. When speaking to an elderly, dying patient it is important to:
   a. Never talk to the patient, but rather communicate all decisions through family members
   b. Communicate clearly, possibly with a sense of humor, in a manner that the patient will be able to hear what is being said
   c. Explain your frustrations with the patient and his or her care in front of the patient and the family
   d. Be sympathetic rather than empathetic with the patient and the family

5. Four of the eight signs of eminent death are:
   a. Increased blood pressure, warm extremities, bowel and bladder incontinence, pallor, and mottling of the skin
   b. Loss of hearing, dyspnea and periods of apnea, increased bowel and bladder control
   c. Increased sexual drive, slow pupil response to light, increased awareness of surroundings, more communicative
   d. Rapid weak pulse, profuse perspiration, loss of hearing, decline in blood pressure

Mary McCarthy Slater
Kathleen R. Culliton

chapter 7

Environments of Care

Learning Objectives

After completing this chapter, the student will be able to:

1. Discuss the role of the licensed practical nurse (LPN) as an environmental manager.
2. Describe at least two components of the physical environment that nurses need to consider.
3. Discuss the aspects included in a climate of caring.
4. Identify at least four settings in which nursing care for older adults is provided.
5. Describe how nurses, in various care settings, meet the needs of older adults.
6. Discuss relocation stress and ways in which a nurse can help an older person adjust to a new environment.

▶ INTRODUCTION

One of the most important tasks for a nurse is to manage the patient-care environment. Florence Nightingale saved the lives of hundreds of soldiers during the Crimean War simply by cleaning the wards, opening the windows, and providing the soldiers with daily hygiene. Miss Nightingale and her nurses also provided direct, caring, "hands-on" nursing to the soldiers under her care. Before Miss Nightingale's interventions, there were more soldiers dying in the hospitals because of the lack of hygienic conditions than there were dying in the actual battles. Improved health for the men dying during the Crimean War required both environmental management and quality nursing care.

The role of a nurse is not that of a housekeeper but that of an environmental manager. To be effective caregivers, nurses must be aware of the influence of environment on the health and functioning of the patient. Nurses are responsible for the manipulation of environmental conditions to improve patient care. In Miss Nightingale's era, environmental management included such tasks as opening windows to clear the patient's room of stale, potentially illness-producing air; managing raw sewage because plumbing was not available; and controlling the population of mice and rats in the hospital. Modern nurses also must understand the effect that the environment can have in enhancing or impeding the progress and functioning of older adults.

▶ ENVIRONMENTAL MANAGEMENT

Providing care to older adults must include environmental management. Assessment of the environment is the first step. As an LPN, you need to examine the total environment starting with where the older person is living. Remember that there are multiple environments of care where an older adult might live. If the person lives at home, you may want to ask: What is the neighborhood like? Is it a safe neighborhood for an older person? Is there a security system in the home or building?

If the older adult lives in a nursing home or in a hospital, you may want to ask: What Is the staffing ratio? Is the environment clean and

free of odor? Is there a place where the older adult can socialize with family and friends?

Assessment of the physical environment includes all aspects of the older adult's living situation that can be seen, heard, touched, or smelled. Each of the physical items in the environment can either contribute to or detract from the optimal functioning of the older person. A room that is too hot may make the older person tired, lethargic, and unwilling to participate in personal care activities. A room that is too cold may likewise result in lack of activity because the older person is unwilling to get out of bed or to come out from under the cover of an afghan.

A critical question to ask throughout the assessment of the physical environment is how well the older person functions in the living areas. Is the environment as barrier free as possible? Can the older person walk unencumbered or wheel a wheelchair through the entire setting? Are there features in the environment to promote physical function? These may include grab bars in the bathroom by the commode, shower, or bathtub seat, and handrails by stairs. When assessing the older person carrying out activities of daily living, be aware of possible alterations that may improve function. Lowering a mirror or moving a storage area below shoulder level may improve both safety and convenience. The risk of falling can be decreased with adequate room lighting and the use of night-lights. The room where the older person reads should have high-intensity illumination.

CLIMATE OF CARING

Another important part of the environmental assessment is evaluating the climate of caring. The climate of caring involves the people in the environment, and the environmental tone and atmosphere. The people in an older person's living environment may include family members, neighbors, friends, and paid caregivers.

The people in an environment are extremely important to the older adult's potential for improvement and optimal function. Families, staff, and visitors can be encouraging and uplifting or depressing and discouraging. A climate of caring includes persons who present a positive but realistic outlook. The older adult's personal space is respected in a caring climate. Such an atmosphere also affords opportunities for privacy, encourages activity and involvement, and facilitates independence.

SAFETY

In any setting, safety for the older person is a primary concern. Are there any environmental hazards, such as frayed extension cords, malfunctioning equipment, or broken furniture? Falls among elderly people are common, and not all of them can be avoided. One thing that can be done is keep the environment free of fall risks. Such risks include clutter, throw rugs, wheelchair leg rests, and poorly fitting shoes or slippers. Sometimes, a pet can be a fall risk as well.

STIMULATION AND PERSONALIZATION

Opinions vary on whether environments for older adults with cognitive impairment should be very stark and nonstimulating or should contain eye-catching and stimulating compo-nents. More important, however, is a personalized environment for the older person. Personalized items help older adults relate to the environment and maintain a sense of identity. A special picture can be displayed in the hospital room as well as in the nursing home. In some settings, such as nursing homes and retirement communities, the entire bedroom or apartment can be personalized with cherished furniture and decorations.

A climate of caring facilitates optimal independence and autonomy for each older person living in the setting. There are times when the routines and regulations necessary to operate a large health-care facility, such as a hospital or nursing home, cannot accommodate the individual needs or desires of older adults. The nurse must assess, however, which rules and routines are absolutely necessary and which are the result of a controlling institution or individual staff member. Although a nursing home may need to serve meals at particular times because of regulations and staffing, the rule that all residents must be dressed for breakfast may be unnecessary. This rule does not allow for each resident to take the time to personally do as much of the dressing as possible. Such a rule forces the resident to be dependent on staff for dressing. A climate of caring provides multiple opportunities for individual choice in the environment and encourages the older person to function as independently as possible.

PERSONAL SPACE AND TERRITORIALITY

Personal space and territory are important to every human being. Personal space is the area around a person. Some individuals define their personal space very close to their bodies, whereas others define it as a broader area. It is viewed as an intrusion for someone to invade another person's personal space. In providing nursing care, nurses must frequently invade the personal space of the patient. Nurses must be conscious, however, that they do not do so unnecessarily.

Territory is the space used by a person and seen as owned by the person. Think about a current class. Do you, as students, tend to sit in the same seats during each class session. Technically, you and your classmates do not own the seats, but the tendency exists to define a territory and return to it habitually. The seating arrangement in a dining room in a nursing home or retirement community is frequently consistent for each meal. This tends to occur whether or not seats are assigned. Individuals will defend their territory if an unwanted person intrudes. An older person who has a favorite chair at home or in the nursing home may fiercely defend it from others.

PRIVACY

All human beings need time to be alone. People need to have opportunities for privacy as well as for human contact. At times, it is difficult for the older person living in a health-care setting to find opportunities for privacy. Many hospitals and nursing homes have multiple-occupancy rooms, so that the patient may never have a chance to be truly alone. As a nurse working with older persons in a congregate setting, you must be aware of the older person's needs for privacy. You should respect that right to privacy by knocking on the door before entering, pulling cubicle curtains during care, and arranging private time for the older adult.

ACTIVITY AND INVOLVEMENT

As a person ages, the number of social roles fulfilled tends to diminish. An older woman who was once a daughter, a mother, a wife, a neighbor, an accountant, a scout leader, and a bridge player may hold none of these social roles at 90 years of age. Owing to aging and disability, these roles may no longer be possible. Involvement with others, however, is still a need. A climate of caring affords each individual multiple and diverse opportunities for activity and involvement with others.

As a nurse working with older people in multiple health-care settings, you can help to provide important opportunities for active

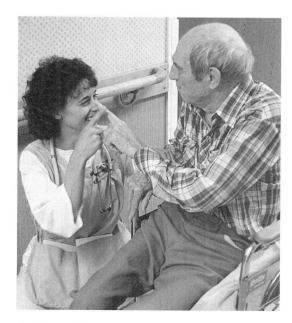

A climate of caring includes people who present a positive, realistic outlook.

involvement. It is important to find out the older person's prior social roles, particularly the ones he or she most enjoyed. Activities that include tasks associated with these roles should be encouraged. It also is important to create opportunities for social interaction. By introducing the older person to others in the setting who may share similar interests and by arranging seating for natural conversation rather than against walls, the nurse can be instrumental in encouraging social exchanges.

▶ RELOCATION TRAUMA

Moving from one environment to another is stressful. Anyone who has ever moved from one house to another or from one city to another can appreciate the stress of relocation. It takes time to adjust to and become familiar with a new setting. During times of crisis or illness, one has less energy available to deal constructively with stress. Older adults are particularly susceptible to being overcome with the stress of relocation. Such stress also is referred to as transitional stress. This refers specifically to the emotional stress that occurs during the time a person is changing from one phase in life to another.

Older people use a considerable amount of energy coping with chronic illness and disabilities. The onset of an acute illness or some other major crisis requires additional coping. If the crisis or illness results in the need to move to another living situation, the older person's coping abilities may be exhausted. A crisis, superimposed on the day-to-day stresses of living with disability and dysfunction, frequently leaves the older person with little coping reserve to deal with the stress of relocation and transition. When the stress is overwhelming, and the older person is unable to cope with the situation, there will be signs of decompensation. These may include disorientation, agitation, acting out, and hallucinations. It is not uncommon for an older adult, newly admitted to any of the health-care settings described in this chapter, to exhibit some of these signs. Thus, the movement from one environment to another can be extremely disruptive to the older adult; this disruption has been termed *relocation trauma*.

In addition to identifying and understanding relocation trauma, the nurse can help to relieve relocation stress. It is important to understand that relocation trauma is temporary, and the behavioral signs of decompensation should diminish as the older person becomes familiar with the new environment. You can, however, accelerate the process of adjustment.

Limit stimulation and the introduction of new activities and people on the older person's first day in the setting. Orient the older person to the environment slowly so that the person can incorporate new areas and routines gradually. On the first day, introduce only people and places that are absolutely necessary. For example, placing an older person in the dining room of a nursing home with 20 other residents shortly after admission may be overwhelming.

Look for ways to provide links between the old environment and the new one. The more familiar the new environment is to the older person, the easier the transition will be. Bringing favorite furniture and objects to the new setting will increase its familiarity to the older person. Including the older person in planning for the move is ideal. This is not always possible, however, if the move occurs because of an acute illness. If it can be arranged, involve the older person in selecting the items to take to the new location.

CRITICALLY EXAMINE THE FOLLOWING:

Review the following situation and devise a plan that would have minimized Mrs. G's relocation trauma. Be prepared to share your ideas in class.

Mrs. G. was moving from her home of 40 years to a retirement community. She had some short-term memory problems and walked with a slow gait. To expedite the move, Mrs. G's son packed for her and sorted through all of her belongings to identify what items to take and what to give away. Because many of her things were very old and worn, her son decided to purchase all new furniture and decorations for her new apartment. The new apartment looked beautiful. After moving, Mrs. G. became extremely disoriented and paranoid, and she accused everyone of stealing her belongings. As the nurse in the retirement community, what would you have taught Mrs. G's son about preparing his mother for relocation?

▶ ENVIRONMENTS OF CARE

There are a variety of settings in which older persons may receive health-care services. This chapter does not discuss all such settings or services but reviews some of the most commonly used environments of care.

DAY CARE

A number of communities now have adult day-care centers available to provide supervised activities for older adults. Day treatment centers for older people with psychiatric problems and day hospitals for older persons with considerable physical disability are available in many localities. Day treatment centers and day hospitals focus on a particular type of older person and provide specific services to meet their physical and psychiatric needs. Many day-care centers provide transportation for the older person to and from the center. Fees for day care may be charged on a sliding scale, according to the ability of the older adult to pay. Few insurance policies, including Medicare and Medicaid, cover the cost of day care. Generally, the older person or the family must pay for these services personally.

A typical day in this care setting includes planned activities, such as group discussion, current events, exercise, snacks, and lunch. Volunteers often visit a center to speak on community affairs, health-promotion topics, or to present entertainment programs that encourage group participation. Many centers have activity directors who plan and schedule events that are appealing, offer a variety of choices for the older adult, and promote group interaction.

Nurses working in a day-care setting provide a number of services, according to the needs of the individual. Assessment of the older person's physical, psychological, and emotional functioning is a critical component of the nurse's role in the day-care center. Health teaching to older persons and their families and ways to administer medication also may be included in the nurse's role.

Some older people may need assistance with mobility, toileting, or eating. Other older adults may need help in taking medications, whereas, still others simply need encouragement to participate in center activities. Nurses in day-care centers need a solid foundation in gerontological nursing to help them in their daily interactions with older people. Such a foundation ensures that subtle physical or emotional changes are not disregarded or blamed simply on "old age."

Acute illnesses in older adults can present themselves in atypical fashion. The nurse who knows and appreciates normal aging is better prepared to assess subtle changes in older persons and to be alert to the possible implications of these changes. Because so many older adults have chronic illnesses, medication administration often becomes a major responsibility for the nurse in a day-care center. The nurse needs to be skillful at administering medications and needs to know their expected effects and possible side effects. The nurse also can use knowledge of medications to teach the older person and family members the importance of safe and accurate medication use. Do the older adult and the family know which medications are being taken and why they are prescribed? Are the older adult and the family aware of possible side effects, potential drug interactions, and the necessary steps to take if problems are suspected? The nurse, as teacher, has an important role in this setting.

Ongoing assessments of the day-care participants are especially important. Frequent contact with the older person allows nurses to see subtle changes in function that may signal serious underlying physiological problems. The nurse's powers of observation and knowledge of the aging process are critically important in detecting actual or impending illness. Is an older person experiencing mobility changes? Are you seeing decreased participation in formerly active participants? Has an older person had changes in weight or affect? If you are making these types of observations, the next questions becomes, "Why are you seeing these changes?" Good communication skills may uncover a change in family living conditions, changes in medica-

CRITICALLY EXAMINE THE FOLLOWING:

Read the patient care situation below before reading the author's comments. Ponder what you would do and make some notes. Compare your thinking with that of the author. Be prepared to discuss your thinking in class.

You are the licensed nurse at the Golden Ages Adult Day Care Center. Mrs. Y. attends the center every Monday, Tuesday, and Wednesday until after lunch, when her husband picks her up. This Tuesday you notice, for the second day in a row, that Mrs. Y. has been unsteady when she walks. She stops to rest frequently when moving around the center and has been falling asleep during group activities. These behaviors are unusual because Mrs. Y. normally ambulates well, participates enthusiastically in center activities, and often encourages others to "join the fun." What further assessment do you now want to make?

Author's comments:

Certainly, vital signs will provide some basic information. It also would help to ask Mrs. Y. if she has noticed any changes in the way she feels or functions. When you speak with Mr. Y., you ask him about changes in Mrs. Y.'s routine and medications. He tells you, "She was so upset and restless last weekend, I had to give her one of my sleeping pills to help her calm down and get some rest Sunday night." By using your powers of observation and problem solving, you are able to uncover the need for medication administration teaching for Mr. Y.

tion, or exacerbation of the effects of a chronic illness.

Day-care centers provide opportunities for socializing and staying involved in the world. Many families use day care to give respite to the main caregiver for the older adult. The stresses of caregiving can have a strong effect on the older person, caregiver, and family. Respite allows caregivers some time to attend to their own needs. Grocery shopping, housekeeping, socializing with friends, and participating in enjoyable activities for the caregivers can often mean the difference between continued home care versus institutionalization for an older adult. Nurses in day-care centers are able to use their assessment skills to identify the older person's strengths and weaknesses, help elders to continue to participate in daily living activities, and provide information for older persons and their families about community resources.

Although day-care nurses may perform few technical nursing procedures, they use a variety of different nursing skills. Day-care nurses must have particularly strong physical and psychological assessment skills. They also must be adept in communication and teaching. The day-care nurse also must have a thorough knowledge of community resources and be able to refer the older person and family to appropriate services in the area.

With the increasing awareness and concern about care for people with dementia, there are some programs now available to provide day care specifically for older persons with cognitive impairments. These day programs are designed to give care that takes into account the abilities and safety needs of individuals with Alzheimer's disease or other dementias.

HOME CARE

Home health-care agencies provide a number of services for older adults in the home. Such agencies provide nursing services given by licensed nurses and nursing assistants, and therapy services, such as physical, occupational, and speech therapy. Many agencies also provide medical supplies and equipment. Most agencies are licensed and, therefore, eligible for state or federal reimbursement for services. Medicare, Medicaid, and community funding may pay for limited home health-care services if the older person qualifies for such reimbursement.

Home care may be provided on a daily basis or intermittently, according to the needs of the patient. Nursing care provided in the home has become more complex in the past two decades. It is not unusual for people who need help during their recovery to be discharged from the hospital "quicker and sicker." Chronically ill older adults may be receiving home care to avoid frequent hospitalizations.

The LPN in home care works under the instructions of the registered nurse case manager. In the home-health role, the LPN will be assigned basic nursing care, medications administration and teaching, dressings and wound care, and may be asked to spend 4 to 24 hours in the home to provide respite

CRITICALLY EXAMINE THE FOLLOWING:

Read the patient care situation below before reading the author's comments. Ponder what you would do and make some notes. Compare your thinking with that of the author. Be prepared to discuss your thinking in class.

As an LPN for a visiting nurse group, you are assigned Mrs. E. Mrs. E. is 75 years old and lives with her husband in their home. Mrs. E. was just discharged from the hospital following surgery to pin her broken right hip. She is not capable of weight bearing, and the physical therapist is scheduled to visit her at home twice a week. Mrs. E. has mild dementia and frequently forgets that she is not permitted to walk. Her husband, Mr. E., wants to keep her in bed to remind her not to walk. What care do you need to teach Mr. E.?

Author's Comments:

It would be appropriate to talk with Mr. and Mrs. E. about the hazards of immobility and the need for Mrs. E. to be out of bed. Together with the physical therapist, you should teach Mr. E. how to safely transfer his wife in and out of bed and on and off the toilet. With Mr. E., you work out a system to remind Mrs. E. that she cannot walk alone. This may include posted notes and frequent verbal reminders. You also suggest that Mr. E. try to keep his wife in the same room with him as much as possible. Finally, you teach Mr. E. how to do skin checks and observe his wife's bony prominences for signs of redness or breakdown.

care to the primary caregivers. The LPN often is asked to work with the certified nurse assistant (CNA) in coordinating care for the patient.

A certain amount of creativity is needed in home-care nursing owing to limitations in the type of equipment and supplies that are available. As in other settings, it is helpful for the nurse to be aware of resources available to the older adult and of ways to gain use of those resources. Nurses who choose home-nursing care can expect a variety of older persons and conditions. Caring for older adults in the home can be very rewarding and challenging. Because the home-health nurse generally visits the older person on a less-than-daily basis, patient and family teaching is very important. Teaching may be needed to help the family ensure a safe environment for the older adult. Educating older persons and families about fall prevention, medication safety, positioning, and transferring techniques may be needed. A family also may need to learn more complex procedures, such as how to change dressings or give injected medications.

The amount of time spent with older persons is often limited by the nurse's workload and the reimbursement for care given. The nurse is responsible for assessing and documenting care needs and providing prescribed treatments. Good communication skills are important to ensure that all members of the health-care team are aware of the older person's needs and progress.

COMMUNITY-BASED CARE

Nursing opportunities are available in a variety of settings not linked to formal institutions such as hospitals or nursing homes. LPNs may provide care for older adults in a community clinic, dialysis center, or physician's office. In these noninstitutional settings, the nurse may practice under the direct supervision of a physician rather than a registered nurse. Practice in these settings often includes assisting with physical examination and treatments, and nurses in these settings are frequently an important source of information and clarification for patients. The nurse uses assessment skills and provides information on resources available in the community to meet the older person's needs. Contact with older adults in these settings may be more infrequent than in other care settings.

CRITICALLY EXAMINE THE FOLLOWING:

Read the patient care situation below before reading the author's comments. Ponder what you would do and make some notes. Compare your thinking with that of the author. Be prepared to discuss your thinking in class.

You are the office nurse for Dr. Agnew, a geriatrician. Mr. M., a patient of Dr. Agnew's, is 74 years old and recently retired. On this day, Mr. M has an appointment with the doctor for a complaint of stomach upset. You notice that Mr. M. is quieter and more withdrawn than usual. What additional assessment would you make?

Author's Comments:

While you are waiting for Dr. Agnew, you ask Mr. M. if he has had any changes in routine lately. In reviewing his sleeping, eating, and activity patterns, you note that he said he is getting up early in the morning and not eating well. In the course of the conversation, Mr. M. tells you that he is tired all of the time and does not feel like living. You suspect depression and share your observations with Dr. Agnew. before he examines the patient. Dr. Agnew assesses Mr. M. further and identifies a clinical depression with suicidal thoughts and prescribes an antidepressant. When he is leaving, you ask Mr. M. if he would mind if you call him in a few days to see how he is feeling.

HOSPICE

Hospice care is designed to provide care for the dying patient and the family. A team approach is central to the hospice concept. Team members include physicians, nurses, social workers, and nursing assistants, as well as other ancillary workers. The goal of hospice is to help dying persons remain at home, if possible, with all the support needed to ensure a "good death." In this case, "good" means that the older person is kept comfortable and able to receive the support of family and loved ones in a familiar setting.

Hospice work allows nurses to give direct patient care and develop a close relationship with the patient and family. As in the care settings previously discussed, the nurse's role as a teacher is especially helpful. Most families are not prepared to meet the needs of a

Licensed practical nurses working in community-based care perform a role that does not exist in other environments.

dying family member. The hospice nurse can teach family members how to provide for the comfort of their loved one. The nurse also can identify hospice resources available to help families and older persons cope during this extremely demanding time. Nurses who have not worked in a hospice setting may be reluctant to try this type of nursing because all of the clients are terminally ill. Talking with nurses who work in a hospice, however, often shows that the team support and the closeness to patients and families provides a high degree of job satisfaction.

RETIREMENT COMMUNITIES

As people age, there is a tendency to simplify lifestyles and living space. The size of the home needed to provide adequate living space for a family can become more of a burden than an asset to older adults. Retirement communities are an increasingly popular way for the elderly person to have a home without homeowner responsibilities. Not having yard work and other maintenance tasks associated with a large home relieves a number of burdens. The communities offer a variety of living spaces and services. Apartments, duplexes, or individual homes

may be located within the boundaries of a retirement complex. The goal for these retirement communities is to appeal to a broad range of older adults by offering security and a variety of conveniences and services. Although communities for retirees have been popular for quite a while, retirement complexes that also provide services for older adults with physical care needs are now increasingly common.

The goal of assisted living units in retirement communities is to provide older persons with help in performing activities of daily living. Frail older persons who do not require continuous care are able to have help in such activities as meal preparation, grooming and bathing, laundry, and housekeeping. Most assisted living programs require that the older person be ambulatory and fairly independent.

Much of the care provided is done by nursing assistants rather than LPNs. The practical nurse in an assisted living program often provides supervision for nursing assistants, medication administration, basic documentation of care given, and assessment of the older person's ability to function.

The assisted living nurse also must use creative talents to ensure that the environment is as homelike as possible. This means the nurse must be flexible in tailoring care to the individual needs of each older adult. The nursing assistant in assisted living may be called a resident assistant and perform many functions that do not relate directly to activities of daily living. Assisted living nurses and nursing assistants often are very involved in activities and social planning for residents.

Continuing-care retirement communities are designed to meet the needs of older adults along a continuum from complete independence to total dependence. The centers offer not only apartments or cottages for independent older persons and assisted living services but also nursing home care.

For many older adults, the appeal of a continuing-care retirement center lies in the fact that clients are able to stay in a familiar environment regardless of their health status. Nursing in a continuing-care retirement center offers many opportunities. Home visits, health promotion, or screening activities (such as blood pressure monitoring clinics), health teaching, or direct bedside care to nursing home patients are a few of the opportunities available to nurses in continuing-care communities. As in assisted living situations, supervisory ability is a valuable asset for the licensed nurse. Retirement community nursing allows nurses to work with older adults who have a variety of needs and abilities. The ability to apply your knowledge of the aging process in this setting helps you enhance the quality of life for older persons in the setting.

NURSING HOMES

The nursing home is an area of practice that has been available to practical nurses for a number of years. With the growing number of frail elders as well as the old-old (85 and older), the need for nursing home care remains high. Some nursing home residents need a full range of nursing care; others may

CRITICALLY EXAMINE THE FOLLOWING:

Read the patient care situation below before reading the author's comments. Ponder what you would do and make some notes. Compare your thinking with that of the author. Be prepared to discuss your thinking in class.

As a center staff nurse, you have been invited to the Evergreen Retirement Center's Monday Morning Coffee Club. The center's activity director has asked you to talk with club members about home safety. Make a list of at least four safety concerns for older adults. What suggestions would you give regarding these concerns in speaking to the Coffee Club Group?

1.

2.

3.

4.

Author's comments:

Your talk might focus on the following areas:

Problem	Solution
1. Unable to read dials and gauges on thermostats	Bright, nonglare lighting to enhance visual ability
2. Potential for falls when walking into the home, while using the toilet, and getting in and out of the shower	Handrails and hand guards
3. Potential for falls through tripping over items or slipping on unsecured scatter rugs	Uncluttered environment
4. Hazard of living alone and falling or losing consciousness	Daily networking with family or friends

be independent physically but have cognitive changes that require a high degree of supervision to maintain their personal safety. In discussing nursing home care, there are two categories of care defined by federal regulation. The first category is the skilled nursing facility (SNF) and the second is the nursing facility (NF). The nursing facility level was previously referred to as intermediate care.

All nursing homes must be licensed by the state in which they operate. If they wish to receive reimbursement from Medicare or Medicaid for the services provided to residents, they also must meet additional federal requirements and be certified by the federal government. A nursing home may choose not to accept Medicare and Medicaid funding and admit only private-pay residents. Medicare, the federal health insurance program for older and disabled individuals, has two parts that can pay for some services in the nursing home. Most persons over 65 years of age have Medicare Part A. This will pay for up to 100 days of care in an SNF if the older person is being discharged from the hospital after a stay of at least 3 days and requires skilled nursing or therapy services. The requirements for skilled services are very specific; do not assume Medicare will pay for nursing home care after a hospital stay. Medicare Part B is a voluntary insurance program that many older persons purchase. It will pay for some physician and therapy services and some medical equipment, but it does not pay the daily fee for the nursing home.

Medicaid is a welfare program that pays for more than 50 percent of the nursing home care in this country. Older people must have a very low income to qualify for Medicaid. Many older persons pay for nursing home care privately at the beginning of their stay until they have spent all of their savings. They then can apply for Medicaid. The Medicaid program pays for all medical services in the nursing home.

In an SNF, care is provided by licensed nurses around the clock, and a registered nurse is present at least 8 hours a day, 7 days a week. A SNF unit also offers the services of allied health professionals, such as speech, physical, or occupational therapists, at least 5 days a week. An NF generally does not have the same level of staffing by registered nurses or therapists as an SNF.

Regardless of category, long-term care facilities offer a team approach to meeting the older person's needs over time. Facilities that receive federal funds are required to offer the services of a social worker as well as an activity director and dietetic consultant. Licensed nurses can gain input from a variety of sources in planning and delivering care by being actively involved with the interdisciplinary health-care team.

The practical nurse, in long-term care, has traditionally been responsible for supervising the nursing assistants who give hands-on care to residents. In many facilities, practical nurses mainly give medications or do treatments.

The nurse interested in long-term care has the opportunity to get to know residents well over a long period of time. Owing to the changing needs and physical condition of residents, the long-term care nurse needs very good assessment skills. Skills such as monitoring resident responses to treatments, observing for signs of decreasing function, and assessing subtle changes in condition are used by long-term care nurses on a daily basis. Accurate documentation, skillful use of

CRITICALLY EXAMINE THE FOLLOWING:

Read the patient care situation below before reading the author's comments. Ponder what you would do and make some notes. Compare your thinking with that of the author. Be prepared to discuss your thinking in class.

Mrs. H., an 85-year-old widow, was recently admitted to Sunny Acres Nursing Home after falling in her apartment and breaking a hip. She had surgery for a hip replacement and can walk short distances, but she is unsteady and tires easily. She is underweight, eats poorly, and does not want to be in the nursing home. Her family lives out of town and is not sure she can live on her own any longer. You are the nurse in charge at Sunny Acres. What are some of the most important areas you would want to assess for Mrs. H.?

Author's comments:

Because Mrs. H. was functioning independently before her fall and she does not want to be in the nursing home, the first area you assess is her potential for discharge. What is the prognosis for improvement in function? With what does she need help? Could she return to her own apartment with additional services in the home? Will she fit appropriately into an assisted living program? In addition to discharge planning, your assessment includes mobility function, eating patterns and ability, and evaluation for signs and symptoms of depression.

the nursing process, and good interpersonal skills in working with residents, staff, and family members are valuable tools in long-term care.

Care in a nursing home differs from hospital care in many ways. The skills required of the nursing home nurse are no less challenging and the tasks no less difficult than those of the hospital nurse. The goal for the hospital patient is to cure illness in a brief period of time. For the nursing home resident with multiple chronic conditions, cure is not possible. In the nursing home, care rather than cure is the primary focus. When you make the care given to residents transpersonal caring, the quality of care will improve remarkably.

ACUTE CARE

The final clinical site for working with older adults is the acute care setting. Most admissions to hospitals comprise people aged 65 years and older. In fact, depending on the source used, it is estimated that 40 to 65 percent of hospital admissions include older adults. Nursing practice in a hospital setting presents a number of opportunities and challenges. Usually, practical nurses are given responsibility for a set number of patients, and depending on policy, they may perform a variety of procedures. Most patients are hospitalized only briefly. The emphasis on cost containment and federal mandates mean that reimbursement for care is often limited to a set period of time. The concept of diagnosis-related groups (DRGs) has allowed reimbursement for hospital treatment to be based on a specific number of hospital days for specific conditions. Hospital-based practice requires all the basic skills the practical nurse possesses. Acute care also involves brief contact with a large number of patients.

There are a number of challenges in giving nursing care to older adults in the hospital setting. They include establishing a trusting relationship over a short period of time, dealing with problems secondary to relocation stress or medications, and resisting the tendency to stereotype patients because of their age. In addition, a major challenge for the nurse working with older people in the hospital setting is to create a safe and caring environment that facilitates independence. This must be done while the tasks required for the cure and treatment of the patient are

Forty to sixty percent of all admissions to acute care hospitals are people 65 years of age and older.

CRITICALLY EXAMINE THE FOLLOWING:

Read the patient care situation below before reading the author's comments. Ponder what you would do and make some notes. Compare your thinking with that of the author. Be prepared to discuss your thinking in class.

Mr. W. is a 90-year-old resident of a nursing home who was admitted to your floor at Hoover Medical Center for treatment of congestive heart failure. He has a significant dementia, is incontinent of bowel and bladder, and is very unsteady on his feet. As his primary nurse, what can you do to make his hospital environment more like home?

Author's comments:

You call the nursing home nurse and talk with her about Mr. W.'s habits at the nursing home. You also ask her to send to the hospital any familiar items Mr. W. may appreciate having in the hospital. The nurse tells you that Mr. W. likes to stay up late and is accustomed to remaining in bed until after breakfast. You write this routine into the care plan and pass the information on to the night shift.

accomplished. Environmental management, as discussed earlier in this chapter, is the most difficult task to accomplish in the hospital setting. The short time frame and the urgency for treatment in many situations cannot accommodate the slowed responses and abilities of older persons. It is your challenge to slow things down so the older adult can manage them.

As a gerontological nurse, it is important to understand the special needs of older adults. They have difficulty seeing and hearing. They move much slower, and they need clear explanations as to what Is happening. Now that you recognize these needs, you have a responsibility. That responsibility is simple; it is to meet the needs of older adults, and assist others to slow down and focus on their needs as well.

▶ CONCLUSION

This chapter has provided a brief overview of the nurse's role in environmental management and the various settings where older adults receive health care. Of special significance for the older adult is the opportunity to receive care from a nurse who is familiar with the aging process and uses that knowledge when giving nursing care in any setting.

CASE STUDY

Your neighbor, Sally, asks your advice about finding good care for her 80-year-old grandmother. The grandmother, Mrs. G., lives at home alone in an isolated section outside the city limits. She recently was discharged from the hospital after injuring her right arm in a fall at home. The arm is in a cast, which makes it difficult for Mrs. G to cook and perform other self-care activities. Your neighbor is unable to visit her grandmother daily because of work and child-care commitments, and is worried about her grandmother's ability to remain at home. She wants her grandmother to move in with her for at least a month. However, Mrs. G. insists on staying in her own home. Sally asks for your advice. She ends the conversation with the statement, "I just don't know what else we can do to make sure Grandma is safe and taken care of in her home."

Discussion

Based on the above situation and your readings from this chapter, what advice would you offer Sally?

Solution

Considering Mrs. G.'s location and her desire for independence, Sally could look into home-care services. The assistance with bathing, grooming, and food preparation could be addressed by the home-health agency team and a plan for home care could be developed. There are no indications that Mrs. G. needs the type of care offered by the other agencies or facilities mentioned in the chapter.

STUDY QUESTIONS

Please select the one best answer.

1. Mr. D., 75 years old, is discharged from the hospital after a right-sided cerebrovascular accident. He requires at least 6 weeks of further nursing care and physical therapy. The facility most likely to meet these needs is:
   a. A continuing-care retirement center
   b. Hospice care
   c. An intermediate care facility
   d. A skilled nursing facility

2. Hospice care provides a multidisciplinary approach to caring for people with:
   a. A chronic illness
   b. An acute exacerbation of a chronic illness
   c. A terminal illness
   d. A contagious illness

3. The major benefit of living in a continuing-care retirement community is:
   a. Low household maintenance requirements
   b. Services available for a continuum of health-care needs.

   c. A safe environment for older adults
   d. The presence of a hospital in the complex

4. Mr. J., 83 years old, has Alzheimer's disease and has wandered from home on several occasions. Mrs. J. is concerned for her husband's safety and desires some respite services. You recommend that she investigate:
   a. A local nursing home
   b. The local senior center
   c. A home health-care agency
   d. Adult day-care center

5. In the home health-care setting, the licensed nurse can expect:
   a. A limited amount of equipment and supplies to be available
   b. Intermittent contact with patients
   c. To care for clients discharged from the hospital with a number of physical care needs
   d. All of the above

unit **TWO**

Clinical Practice

Judith Pratt
Kyle Cannon

chapter **8**

Common Infectious Diseases

Learning Objectives

After completing this chapter, the student will be able to:

1. Identify causes of common infectious diseases in older adults.
2. Use appropriate environmental and hygienic measures that will reduce infectious diseases.
3. Identify measures that will assist older adults maintain a healthy immune system.
4. Identify appropriate immunization protocols.
5. Identify infections that can be precipitated by chronic medical conditions and by the aging process.
6. Discuss the role of the licensed practical nurse (LPN) in the management of infections in older adults.

▶ INTRODUCTION

Everyone wants to be healthy. Even the simple head cold is an irritating and inconvenient event in our lives. As a nurse, you know that there are many more serious infectious diseases than a head cold. When these infections attack older adults, the problems can be grave. This chapter is a challenge to you, the bedside nurse, to knowledgeably protect older adults from the harsh reality of infectious diseases.

Natural immunity toward infectious diseases may not be affected by aging in healthy older adults (Norman, 2001). Yet some infections tend to increase with the process of aging and are major health problems in the older population. Older patients' physiological responses during an infectious illness differ from that of younger or middle-aged adults. In addition, the course of illnesses leading to recovery or death is different.

This chapter provides information on the prevention of infectious diseases and the treatment of infections when they occur. Items to be discussed are as follows:

- Maintaining a healthy immune system by participating in health promoting activities.
- Preventing infections with scheduled immunizations, keeping a clean environment, and following good hygiene.
- Common infections caused by food or water, other people, animals, or insects.

Infections can effect all the systems of the body and may be precipitated by chronic medical conditions such as diabetes. In this chapter respiratory, genital and urinary, intra-abdominal, and integumentary infections are addressed.

The nursing role in the management of infection in older adults includes recognizing, reporting, and documenting signs and symptoms of infection; complying with medical direction for care; and preventing the spread of infection.

▶ MAINTAINING A HEALTHY IMMUNE SYSTEM

One of the purposes of the immune system is to protect the body from the invasion of harmful bacteria, fungi, viruses, parasites, and other microorganisms. As the body ages, lymphocyte function and antibody immune responses become delayed or inadequate and put the older adult at risk for infections. The following are ways to support the health of the immune system.

NUTRITION

The LPN is responsible for assessing and monitoring the client's nutritional status. This is an important aspect of maintaining a healthy immune system. (Review nutrition and the reasons for poor nutrition in Chapter 2.) It is important to identify nutritional deficits and potential reasons for these deficits. The LPN must determine, through questioning and observing the person's nutritional patterns, why there may be deficits in eating. There often are problems with older adults and the food they eat. Food may be too expensive, or it may not taste good. Perhaps there is no a desire to prepare food or the older person may be unable to eat or digest food properly. These are just a few reasons for poor nutritional patterns. You, the LPN, are an important team player when reporting nutritional concerns and potential solutions to members of the interdisciplinary health care team (IDT) for management.

FLUID INTAKE

Another nutritional challenge is for older adults to maintain adequate fluid balance for wellness. Dehydration following outside activities, an illness, or not drinking enough fluid during the day can lead to potential problems. Fluid intake should be assessed, along with nutritional intake and deficits.

LIFESTYLE

The need for exercise, rest, stress management, avoidance of cigarette smoke, and alcohol usage are discussed in Chapter 2. Compliance with these activities heightens the abilities of the immune system. As an LPN, you will need to frequently assess compliance or noncompliance with these activities and educate the patient as necessary. Knowing the older adults' lifestyle, living conditions, and economic situations are important when endeavoring to assist them in maintaining a healthy immune system.

CHRONIC MEDICAL CONDITIONS

Chronic medical conditions have an effect on the older adult's immune system. Chapter 9 discusses chronic medical conditions and the potential for infections. A classic example is the person with diabetes. You need to educate the diabetic person to take precautions to prevent infections by wearing appropriate shoes, observing for lesions that do not heal, and caring for skin cuts and abrasions.

URINARY TRACT INFECTIONS

Preventing urinary tract infections is an important aspect of preventive nursing. Older adults should be encouraged to drink adequate fluids and to empty their bladders frequently. If incontinence occurs, older patients should have their skin cleansed and soiled clothes replaced. Older adult's skin is sensitive and can break down, which invites infection. Catheters often are a source of infection; the LPN needs to follow agency protocols in an effort to prevent them.

RESPIRATORY INFECTIONS

Respiratory infections may have a significant effect on the older adult. Older people need to be encouraged to receive influenza and pneumococcal vaccines to prevent severe respiratory infections. Increased fluids will keep the secretions thin and allow the pathogens to be coughed out of the respiratory tract.

INTRA-ABDONIMAL INFECTIONS

Intra-abdominal infections are common in older adults. Signs and symptoms of infections may be difficult to differentiate from other chronic diseases in the older patient. Laboratory results and uncharacteristic complaints may confuse the findings. Older adults may have coexisting conditions or be mentally confused, making history and physical examination difficult or misleading. Cholecystitis, diverticulitis, and appendicitis are examples of intra-abdominal infections that may be difficult to diagnosis in older people. The LPN is able to help gather verbal information, note signs and symptoms, and evaluate vital signs to assist in diagnosing the condition.

INTEGUMENTARY SYSTEM

With age come changes in the integumentary system. Many factors influence changes in the course of aging. Exposure to the sun, diet, heredity, and general health affect the skin. Pressure ulcers and their potential for infection are discussed in Chapter 9. The LPN needs to be aware of other skin infections. Redness, swelling, pain, lesions, and discoloration are among the signs and symptoms of skin infections. As an LPN, you will report all signs and symptoms of a skin infection to the registered nurse (RN). If requested, you will obtain a specimen for culture. Culture and sensitivity tests may be necessary to identity the organism causing the infection and to treat it appropriately.

The following microorganisms are listed to give an overview of skin pathogens:

- Staphylococcal bacterial infections are impetigo, boils, carbuncles, and cellulitis.
- Streptococcal bacterial infections are impetigo and erysipelas.
- Fungal infections are the cause of "athlete's foot" and thickened nails on the fingers and toes.
- Viral infections are herpes zoster and herpes simplex.
- Scabies and lice are examples of parasitic infections.

It is impossible to protect people from the invasion of harmful microorganisms, but an older adult with a healthy immune system will have a better recovery if an infection occurs. Adherence to wellness activities plus additional measures to prevent infections should be used for a positive outcome.

▶ PREVENTING INFECTIONS

IMMUNIZATIONS

Immunization recommendations change as people age and health conditions affect immune responses. Unfortunately, the need for the older adult to be immunized is not always recognized. Immunization histories may not be part the patient's medical record or the information simply may not be noted. The older adult's immune system may need to be "boosted" for the body to continue to have the ability to resist certain infections. The LPN must consider the need for the older adult to have continued protection from preventable disease.

DIPHTHERIA-TETANUS

Diphtheria-tetanus (DT) vaccine is probably the most overlooked immunization. Once the initial DT series have taken place, a booster is required every 10 years for life. The LPN should evaluate the DT status for all older adults and determine the need for a booster. Often, it is discovered that some older adults have never had a DT series. All the men going into the military during World War II were given DT immunizations, but during this time period, women were not routinely immunized. Not all adults who lived during the 1940s were immunized. The LPN should report the need for the DT series if a patient is identified who has never had it.

INFLUENZA VACCINE

The influenza or "flu" vaccine should be given each year to all adults older than 65 years, unless contraindicated. Older adults who have lung disease, diabetes, kidney disease, or other diseases that affect the immune system should be particularly encouraged to get the vaccine. The flu virus changes each year, so the formulation of the vaccine changes each year. Vaccines should be given starting around mid-October. The vaccine is generally available in physician offices, senior centers, home-health agencies, public health departments, and certain places of business.

PNEUMOCOCCAL VACCINE

Pneumococcal vaccine provides protection against pneumonia. Generally, only one dose is needed if it is given after the age of 65. When chronic health conditions such as lung disease, heart disease, diabetes, kidney disease, alcoholism, liver disease, cere-

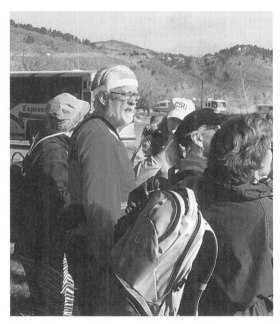

This older man has spent the day with a group of younger people building walking paths in a park. The young woman he partnered with has a baby at home with chickenpox. What disease can this man potentially get from such an exposure?

brospinal fluid leak, or cancer are present, the vaccine should be considered before the age of 65 years. If pneumococcal vaccine is given before age 65, a second dose would be required after age 65. The second dose would need to be given at least 5 years after the first dose. The physician or primary care provider will make the determination as to when the vaccine should be given. The vaccine is available from a physician's office, hospital, or public health department.

HEPATITIS A

Hepatitis A vaccine arrived on the market during the past 10 years. Hepatitis A is recommended for people traveling to global areas where Hepatitis A prevalence is high. In the past, people traveling to some countries would request immune globulin or the "gamma shot." Now, getting the first dose of a two-dose series of hepatitis A 2 weeks before traveling will provide significant protection against this disease. For the best protection, the older adult should receive both doses. Immune globulin "gamma" will not be necessary after the hepatitis A vaccination series has been completed. The vaccine will provide protection for many years.

Hepatitis A is prevalent in some areas of the United Sates as well, and a hepatitis A vaccination may be warranted. Local health departments should be consulted as needed. The vaccine is available at public health departments.

HEPATITIS B

Hepatitis B continues to be problematic throughout the world. Older adults traveling to areas of the world where hepatitis B is present should consider being vaccinated. If the person is planning on staying in the country longer than 6 months, hepatitis B immunization should be strongly encouraged. The vaccination is given in a three-part series over a 6-month period. Patients on kidney dialysis or requiring transfusions for clotting problems are candidates for hepatitis B vaccine. Older adults who provide services to developmentally delayed persons, health-care workers, or safety workers should consider being vaccinated. Hepatitis B has not been specifically categorized as a sexually transmitted disease, but it is a blood-borne pathogen. The LPN may be asked to evaluate the patient's sexual history to help the primary health-care provider decide whether or not to vaccinate against hepatitis B. The vaccine may be available at hospitals, the physician's office, or at the public health department.

MEASLES-MUMPS-RUBELLA

Measles-mumps-rubella (MMR) is thought of as a childhood immunization. The vaccine may be recommended for persons who travel internationally. Health-care workers and older adults who are actively working with or volunteering to help "high-risks groups" should be considered for MMR immunization. Even if a MMR has been given during the person's lifetime, a second dose MMR is recommend for

people in the above-mentioned groups. The LPN will assess the immunization status and report the findings to the primary care provider, who will determine immunization needs. The vaccine is available at hospitals, the physician's office, or the public health department.

MENINGOCOCCAL VACCINE AND HAEMOPHILUS INFLUEN-ZAE TYPE B

Older patients with compromised immune systems, organ transplants, cancer treatments, or splenectomy should be considered for meningococcal and *Haemophilus influenzae* type B (HIB) immunizations. The immunizations also are recommended for older adults who travel to areas of the world where these diseases are prevalent. The LPN will assess the immunizations and report the findings. The primary health-care provider will determine if the immunization is needed. The vaccines are available from the public health department.

Immunizations should be continued throughout life for vaccine-preventable diseases. A report from the United States Centers for Disease Control and Prevention claimed that approximately 70,000 American adults die from diseases that could have been prevented by vaccine or complications as a result of not being immunized. Immunization histories are an important part of the assessment you, as the nurse, will perform. New vaccines are being developed, and when completed, they will be added to the list of available treatment options.

▶ SAFE FOOD AND WATER

Food-borne diseases are very common in the United States. Each year millions of people become ill due to contaminated food and thousands die. Microorganisms find food a great place to live and breed. The signs and symptoms of food-borne diseases may resemble a bad case of "stomach flu" and the older adult may delay seeking medical care. Most food-borne diseases have common signs and symptoms, which are sudden onset, abdominal pain, fever, and vomiting and diarrhea.

Laboratory testing is required to identify the infecting organism. The LPN will need to instruct the person on collecting a stool specimen.

CAMPYLOBACTERIOSIS

Campylobacter infections are the most common food-borne diseases. Foods most commonly associated with *Campylobacter* infections are undercooked poultry, unpasteurized milk, and contaminated water (campylobacteriosis is also known as travelers' diarrhea). Inadequate cleaning of food preparation areas and poor hand washing before food preparation can lead to infection. Symptoms of *Campylobacter* infection are diarrhea, abdominal pain, fever, nausea, and vomiting. These symptoms occur within 2 to 7 days after exposure. A stool specimen will be required for an accurate diagnosis. The older adult is at risk for dehydration complications due to the diarrhea. The LPN needs to encourage the elderly client to drink more fluids. *Campylobacter* infections may resolve without medical treatment, but dehydration and delayed recovery need to be referred to a health-care provider. The LPN will need to educate all household members about hand washing to prevent the spread of the infection to others.

CHOLERA

There are sporadic outbreaks of cholera in the United States that are related to eating raw or undercooked seafood from contaminated waters. In addition, cholera can be spread by the people preparing foods and by foods that have been washed with contaminated water. The main symptom of cholera is diarrhea and may appear in a few hours or up to 5 days after exposure. Stool specimens are required for diagnosis and treatment. Increased fluid intake needs to be stressed because diarrhea will put the older adult at risk for dehydration. Medical intervention may be required. Travel information is available for people who plan to visit global areas where cholera is present. The travelers should be particularly aware of food preparation, water, and certain foods being served (Chin, 2000).

SALMONELLA

Salmonella bacteria can be found in many foods such as custards, milk, eggs, salad dressing, and shellfish. Contaminated water and food handlers are the causes of many salmonella infections. Symptoms of infection are diarrhea, fever, and abdominal cramps that usually occur within 12 to 72 hours after exposure (Lundy & James, 2001). A stool specimen is required for the diagnosis of salmonella. The concern of salmonella infection in the older adult is dehydration from the diarrhea. Again, the LPN needs to educate the person to increase fluid intake. As in all cases of food-borne illnesses, the LPN needs to educate household members to practice good hand washing and to keep food preparation places clean.

SHIGELLA

Shigella infections are found in many foods and are usually due to contaminated water or poor hygiene practiced by food handlers. Symptoms of infection are vomiting, nausea, cramps, and diarrhea, with blood and or mucus in the stool. Symptoms may occur from 12 to 96 hours after exposure. Shigella may require medical intervention in the frail elderly client and other older adults. Increased fluid intake is important, and the LPN needs to give instructions to family members on hand washing and sanitary food preparation.

There are other food-borne infections that are not mentioned in this chapter. Signs and symptoms of food-borne infections are similar, and diagnosis can be made only by a laboratory test. You, in your role as the nurse, will want to note the following in a suspected food-borne illness: the time that signs and symptoms occurred, what the person ate in the last few days, where the food was served, and did other people become ill. This information should be reported to the local health department. The health department investigates all potential food-borne diseases, and they will take appropriate actions.

Food-borne infections can be prevented by good hand washing, using safe foods, and keeping food preparation areas sanitary. You need to instruct those preparing food to:

- Store food correctly
- Protect food from insects, rodents, and animals
- Cook food thoroughly
- Eat cooked food immediately
- Refrigerate uneaten food immediately
- Reheat cooked foods thoroughly

- Wash hands frequently
- Keep food preparation areas clean

▶ ENVIRONMENTAL CLEANLINESS

HOUSEHOLD PETS

Household pets are a source of friendship and
companionship for older adults. Older people
need to be aware that pets also can become a
source of infection. Pets may become infected
and transfer their disease to household
members. Animal's waste can become a
source of infection if it is not properly
handled. Pets need health and medical
consideration to protect the older adult from a
disease carried by a pet. An assessment of the
home always should include mention of
household pets and how the care of the pet is
managed.

KITCHENS AND BATHROOMS

Kitchens and bathrooms are great harbors for
infections. Household assessments need to
include bathroom inspection of towels, tooth
care items, sinks, tubs and toilets.
Instructions by the LPN include not sharing
personal hygiene items such as razors and
tooth care articles. Kitchen assessments

involve reviewing food preparation and food
storage, as has already been mentioned.
Personal cleanliness and hygiene may need
frequent instructions. When instructing older
adults about hand washing, the LPN should
include cleaning under the fingernails. Older
adults who love and care for others in the
household would not want to be the cause of
a loved one's illness.

▶ SEXUALLY TRANSMITTED DISEASES

Many health care providers are uncomfortable
when considering sexually transmitted
diseases (STDs) in older adults. One of the
myths of aging is that older people do not
participate in enjoyable sexual activity. The
reality is they can and many do! The development of new medications, such as sidenafil
(Viagra) and various vaginal creams, have the
potential to increase sexual activity, as well
as sexually transmitted diseases, in older
persons.

Some people who have lived in monoga-
mous relationships and have lost their
companion may have sexual relations with
one or more persons who have an uncertain
sexual history. This factor can have a strong
impact an older adult's overall health. There
are several STDs about which you, as the LPN
in the community, should have a working
knowledge. These STDs include syphilis;
gonorrhea; chlamydiosis; hepatitis A, B, and
C; genital warts; lice; and other viral and
bacterial infections. These diseases generally
are discussed in basic medical/surgical
classes. Their impact on and treatment for
older adults do not differ from that of younger
adults.

As the nurse, you need to teach older
adults, who are sexually active with more than
one partner, the signs and symptoms of STDs
and to seek medical treatment for them immediately. Older adults tend to not discuss
sexual matters with younger people. This is a
barrier you need to overcome through caring
and sensitive communication skills. Older
adults need to realize the variety of STDs and
the symptoms of the most common ones.
They should be able to report their symptoms
clearly so the appropriate tests can be
performed for accurate diagnosis. Common
symptoms are pain, discharge from the penis

or vagina, abdominal pain, and genital lesions. Your responsibility is to teach the older adults in your care about STDs, their signs and symptoms, how to get appropriate care, and how to have safe sex.

OBTAINING A SEXUAL HISTORY

Prevention of STD infections in the older population is the reason for obtaining a sexual history from the patient. Some older adults are at little or no risk for STDs, whereas others may be at high risk. Health education, appropriate treatments, and stopping the transmission of STDs begin with the identification of at-risk behavior.

A sexual history is an integral part of a complete patient history profile. The right questions need to be asked to elicit responses that give key information about risk factors and patient behaviors. Open-ended questions are more likely to give responses that have the most pertinent information. "Tell me about your sex life" will give much more information than simply asking, "Do your have sex?"

Patients must be reassured their responses are confidential. Developing a confidential relationship will aid the LPN in building a rapport of trust and confidence with the older adult. It is important to remember that the patient's values regarding acceptable sexual behavior may differ from yours, and you should not make personal judgments.

Some specific questions need be asked and may cause you, as the interviewer, to be uncomfortable. Questions such as "How many sexual partners have you had in the past 3 months?" or "Do you prefer to have sex with men, women, or both?" can seem intrusive. However, the answers can be very important when identifying potential risks for STDs. A complete sexual history should be included on the history form.

HUMAN IMMUNODEFICIENCY VIRUS AND ACQUIRED IMMUNODEFICIENCY SYNDROME

The CDC (2002) is concerned about the rise of HIV/AIDS in people older than 50 years of age. Florida has the highest rate of HIV/AIDS in people over age 50 in the United States. There are approximately 87,000 people (CDC, 2002) with HIV/AIDS in the 50+ age group in this country, which constitutes approximately 10%

of all persons with HIV/AIDS nationally. The increase in the disease in the older age group is attributed to the lack of education of HIV/AIDS directed toward older persons, as well as the performance-enhancing drugs that have increased sexual activity for older people.

The initial intervention you, as the nurse, need to do is sex education. People in their 60s, 70s, 80s and beyond generally have not had the benefit of sex education on any level. They did not have the friendly chat with their mom, high school gym teacher, or a sex counselor. An intensive, but sensitive interview may indicate that the older adult does not have a full working knowledge of his or her own reproductive system even after having multiple children. This is the place to start if your assessment indicates that there is a knowledge deficit in this area. Be careful to not patronize older adults, or in other words, do not treat them as though you are the "all-knowing" parent. Be a colleague and a friend. Explore the information together. Share only what is essential for good health unless the learners indicate a desire for more information. Allow them to share the wisdom that comes through experience in having and raising children, often under very dire circumstances.

The second educational concept you need to teach sexually active older adults is safe sex. Many older people no longer feel a need to protect themselves sexually because they

HIV/AIDS is on the increase in older adults. One reason for this increase is that the education has been focused on younger adults, not older people. This young woman is an HIV/AIDS counselor who specializes in treating older adults and meeting their particular needs.

are not concerned about becoming pregnant. Your responsibility is to teach them that safe sex also means protection against STDs, most critically HIV/AIDS. Many older adults have never used a condom. It may be uncomfortable to teach someone old enough to be your grandparent how to use one. The easiest technique may be practicing putting a condom on a banana. It is acceptable to laugh and make the teaching fun. That will assist the older adult who is uncomfortable with the exercise to relax and learn better. Make the point that the only truly safe sex is absti-nence or monogamy. Then emphasize that condoms are next in terms of safety and should always be used. Again, older adults often associate condoms with birth control, something about which they no longer feel concern.

Another point that needs to be explored with sexually active older adults is the type of disease HIV/AIDS really is. In this, the 21st century, many people view HIV/AIDS as a chronic disease. The common association is with diabetes mellitus. People recognize diabetes as a disease for which there is not a cure and one that requires a careful medication regimen. It also is seen as something with which millions of people live successfully. People like "Magic" Johnson, a former national basketball star with HIV, helps perpetuate the chronic disease myth.

It is critical that the older adults you teach understand that HIV/AIDS is a killer disease, not a chronic disease. The medications that keep people with this disease alive must be taken every 4 to 6 hours around the clock. It requires setting an alarm during the night because doses cannot be missed. Those who think of HIV/AIDS as a chronic disease do not see the gastrointestinal distress and emotional agony that accompanies this disease. It is a tragic process.

The patient care for hospitalized older adults with HIV/AIDS is similar to other fragile patients or residents. Be gentle and do not rush the care given. Listen to the needs of the older person, and take the time to demonstrate genuine caring.

When caring for someone with HIV/AIDS, always use universal precautions. It is critical that you follow the medication regimen closely and report any adverse reactions immediately. Good nutrition and hydration also are important. You can encourage this by sitting with the older adult in a nonrushed manner and providing encouragement to eat and drink. The intake and output on older adults with HIV/AIDS should be carefully noted.

The person with HIV/AIDS is a person who is dying. Review Chapter 6, "End-of-Life Issues for the Elderly Person," and evaluate how you can apply the information to the person with HIV/AIDS. Do not judge the person to whom you are giving care. Some people are critical of HIV/AIDS persons and believe that they "deserve" the disease. That simply is not true. Do not be taken in by such thinking.

The responsibility you have as the nurse is to educate the sexually active older adult in an effort to promote avoidance of all STDs, especially the growing numbers of individuals with HIV/AIDS. If you are caring for a person with HIV/AIDS, you have a responsibility to assist him or her with management of the disease and delivery of quality palliative care.

HUMAN PAPILLOMAVIRUS INFECTION

There are many types of human papillomavirus (HPV) that can infect the genital tract and anus of both women and men. Generally the resulting genital warts are not painful and if visible, have a "fleshy" cauliflower appearance. The warts easily can be spread and increase in frequency with an increase in the number of sexual partners. A patient can be infected with multiple types of HPV at the same time. The LPN must be aware that some cancers of the genital tract are associated with HPV infections. Medical treatment should begin as soon as diagnosis is made.

TRICHOMONIASIS

Trichomoniasis is a condition caused by a protozoan pathogen. Generally, symptoms are characterized by a foul-smelling yellow-green discharge. Women may complain of intense vaginal itching, especially at night. Pain and burning upon urination are common complaints with this STD. Redness and swelling may be present. Women more often have complaints with this STD than do men. All sexual partners should be treated.

GONORRHEA

Gonorrhea is caused by the bacteria *Neisseria gonorrhoeae*. In this disease, symptoms are much more pronounced in men than in women. Symptoms in men are large amounts of green discharge from the penis, as well as burning during urination. Testicular pain is frequently reported. Often, women present with abdominal or pelvic pain. Treatment needs to begin at once after diagnosis is made. All sexual partners need to be identified and treatment given.

CHLAMYDIA TRACHOMATIS

Many patients who are infected with gonorrhea are coinfected with chlamydia. Signs and symptoms of chlamydial infections are similar to gonorrheal infections. As the nurse, you need to assist in identifying sexual partners for treatment.

SYPHILIS

Syphilis is a complex disease and can manifest itself throughout the life span if it is not detected and treated. Generally, the description of the disease is based on signs and symptoms at the time the diagnosis is made. The first symptoms appear about 3 weeks after exposure. A chancre, or open painless sore, appears. The chancre can appear anywhere on the body. It is the classic symptom of primary syphilis. The sore resolves without treatment, but that does not mean the disease has disappeared.

Secondary syphilis is marked by a classic rash most prominent on the palms of the hands and the soles of the feet. You, as the nurse, should report these unique symptoms as soon as they appear so treatment can be started. These symptoms may last a few weeks or a year without treatment.

If syphilis is not treated in the primary or secondary stage, latent syphilis symptoms will present as neurological impairment, mental retardation, and memory problems. Syphilis may not be identified until the latent stage when an older adult exhibits the symptoms of latent syphilis.

Treatment for syphilis is stage dependent. Fortunately, testing techniques are advanced and detection is usually made early, in the primary stage, when cure is likely to be successful. The exacerbating and remitting nature of the disease, moving from an acute phase to dormancy, makes this a difficult disease to diagnose. That is why a good sexual history is so important.

GENITAL HERPES

Genital herpes is caused by a virus, which is unfortunate because treatment options for virus infections are limited. Herpes usually present with blisters on the genital area. These blisters are fluid filled and very painful. Besides the blisters, other symptoms include itching, tingling, burning, or even achy joints. Transmission of the virus can occur with or without symptoms. As the LPN, you can educate the older adult about the transmission of the virus that causes genital herpes. Antiretroviral therapy is not curative and seems to only shorten the duration of symptoms and infectiousness.

HEPATITIS B

Hepatitis B is transmitted sexually as well as by exposure to infected blood. A unique characteristic of hepatitis B is that a person can be in a "carrier" state. The carrier is always considered infectious. Fortunately, a vaccine against hepatitis B has been available for several years and provides excellent protection against exposure. You, the LPN, will need to instruct the patient about the availability of vaccine and to use condoms or abstinence to prevent transmission. A small percentage of carriers will go on to develop cancer of the liver.

HEPATITIS A

Hepatitis A is usually considered a disease caused by food or water, not by a sexually transmitted disease. Men who have sex with men are at risk for hepatitis A. Hence, hepatitis A is mentioned here as a STD in gay men. As mentioned earlier, hepatitis A vaccine is available, and you should encourage those at risk to receive the vaccine to prevent infection.

▶ TUBERCULOSIS

In the early part of the 20th century, tuberculosis (TB) was a major cause of death in the United States. In the 1940s new drugs became available to treat TB. The United States, unlike many poorer countries, had the resources to treat all cases of TB, and the disease almost was eliminated in this country before the 1980s. Worldwide, TB is the cause of many deaths and illnesses. Resources for TB treatment have been lacking in poorer countries and continue to be problematic for world health organizations.

Few new cases of TB were reported in the 1970s in the United States because of the use of the national "push" to treat the disease. That resulted in government funding sources being cut for TB services in the 1980s. Suddenly, new cases of TB began to occur. Human immunodeficiency disease (HIV) was identified at that time, and TB was diagnosed in some of the HIV patients. Was lack of funding for treatment a reason for an increase in TB? This question continues to be debated by the public health service because treatment protocols for TB have been complicated by a TB strain that is drug resistant. This occurred after the period of TB minimal treatment in this country.

Older adults have a high probability for exposure to TB from when they were younger. In many cases, they were exposed but never developed the disease. The TB bacterium may lay dormant in the body for many years and never cause an active disease unless the immune system weakens. This can happen as people age.

Tuberculosis screening should be conducted on all nursing home residents to identify undiagnosed cases for treatment. Staff and other residents need to be protected from TB, if a case is identified. Chapter 16 addresses TB skin testing; you may want to review it. Sputum smears also will confirm a case of active TB. The LPN may be asked to collect a sputum specimen. The protocols at your facility dictate how the specimen should be gathered. Review the protocols, and ask questions if you are unsure of the procedure.

As the TB nurse, you will need to follow the medical orders closely and watch for signs and symptoms of complications with the drug protocols. It is possible you will be asked to watch the patient take the medications to ensure that the pills are actually consumed. The medications may cause some side affects in the older person, which is why there could be attempts at avoiding them. Direct observed therapy (DOT) has been found to be successful in ensuring that the medications are being taken as directed. The LPN may do this or choose a responsible family member to observe the medication therapy.

The following are the medications given, along with commonly used doses, times given during the day, and possible side affects:

1. **Isoniazid (300 mg PO QD):** May cause liver toxicity. Liver function profiles should be performed monthly. Signs and symptoms of liver toxicity are dark urine, yellow skin and sclera, and light gray stools. The LPN will need to monitor and report any of these signs and symptoms.
2. **Rifampin (600 mg p.o. q.d.):** Body fluids may become reddish orange. This is normal but may be alarming to the patient. The LPN will need to reassure the patient that this symptom is normal.
3. **Pyrazinamide (1000 mg p.o. q.d.):** Watch for generalized rashes, hypersensitivity, and shortness of breath.
4. **Ethambutol (800 mg p.o. q.d.):** May cause red-green color blindness. Baseline color vision testing is required as the damage is irreversible. The LPN will need to instruct the older adult on watching for visual color changes. The patient may notice changes in the red and green on stop lights. This should be reported to the RN or physician.
5. **Pyridoxine (50 mg p.o. q.d.; vitamin B$_6$):** Watch for generalized rashes, hypersensitivity, and shortness of breath.

You need to teach older adults with TB to wear a mask when in public or with people. The LPN will need to support the patient because the mask is uncomfortable to wear, difficult to use, may cause an imbalance in blood gases, and may cause the person to be sensitive about needing to wear the mask. The mask will need to be worn until sputum smears confirm that the person is no longer infectious.

Hospitals have special ventilation rooms for patients with TB to prevent the pathogen from being spread to other areas of the hospital. If the patient is at home and weather permits, windows and doors should be opened to ventilate the home. Sunlight destroys the TB bacteria so excursions outside on a sunny day should be encouraged.

▶ WEST NILE FEVER

West Nile fever is a new infection that has caused older patients to become very ill. A few older adults have died in New York and Florida. This infection has been confined to states on the East Coast and is thought to have been brought to the United States by birds traveling on the wind currents from Africa. The mosquito is the vector that transfers the infection from the bird to the human. Symptoms are fever, headache, malaise, and muscle pain. Meningoencephalitis is a complication of West Nile fever. The LPN should advise older adults to protect themselves against mosquito bites (Chin, 2000).

Worldwide, mosquitoes are the cause of many serious diseases such a malaria and dengue fever. The older adult should take precautions when planning to travel to countries where mosquito-borne diseases exist. You will need to advise the older person to wear proper clothing when in a mosquito environment. The physician can advise on proper insect repellants and the use of insecticides.

▶ ANTHRAX

Anthrax has been suggested as a potential bioterrorism infectious agent. The anthrax bacteria has existed in the United States for centuries, and except in a few populations that are exposed to infected anthrax animals, there has not be an outbreak of this disease. Anthrax can be found in wild and domestic animals. The general population is not at risk for anthrax infection except in the case of bioterrorism. Anthrax infections can occur on the skin, in the lungs, or in the intes-

tinal system. Skin infections may present as a depressed black eschar at the site of infection. Lung symptoms are similar to a respiratory infection. Intestinal infections resemble food-borne illnesses. It may be necessary to treat the infected person with an antibiotic.

▶ CONCLUSION

This chapter has discussed infectious diseases that have the potential to cause illnesses, even serious illnesses leading to death. The LPN has an important task to perform by assessing signs and symptoms of infectious diseases. The immune system changes with aging and may make it more difficult to recognize an infectious process. The LPN often is responsible for assessing older adults. Remember to consider the subtle signs and symptoms that could indicate an infectious process. They are elevated temperature, lesion, redness, swelling, and pain, among other possibilities. The LPN will need to consider other changes the older adult may demonstrate such as becoming confused, demonstrating lethargy, and being anoretic. It is important for the LPN to be a critical thinker while performing an assessment on older adults.

CASE STUDY

Mrs. B. is 95 years old and was recently widowed. Mrs. B. and her husband immigrated to the United States from Germany 45 years ago. She has been in generally good health and is being treated for osteoporosis and a mild elevation in blood pressure. Mrs. B. has reported a persistent dry cough for 1 month. Her health history does not reveal any other health problems. Mrs. B uses a walker to help her ambulate. She enjoys a close association with her daughter and church friends. She has lived alone for nearly a year, because her husband resided in an extended care facility until his death. Mrs. B. insists on being as independent as possible but does allow family and friends to visit her and help her with some personal and household tasks. Mrs. B. prefers speaking in her native language, which is German.

Just before his death, it was discovered that Mr. B. had infectious TB. Mr. B. was plagued with a persistent cough and recurrent pneumonia for the last 5 months of his life. A full-scale contact investigation was initiated at the extended-care facility and among close family members.

A PPD (Mantoux) skin test was done on Mrs. B., and she was found to have 16 MM of induration. A chest x-ray scan revealed right upper lobe fibronodular calcification. It was suspected that Mrs. B. had a case of infectious TB. Medical orders were written for a sputum test to confirm the suspicion of TB, a liver function profile laboratory test, and for medical treatment to be started. Results of the liver function test were normal. The sputum test came back 4+ for acid-fast bacilli. Mrs. B did have active tuberculosis. Five medical drugs were started immediately to treat the disease.

The protocol for treating Mrs. B.'s TB follows:

Isoniazid 300 mg p.o. q.d.
Rifampin 600 mg p.o. q.d.
Pyrazinamide 1000 mg p.o. q.d.
Ethambutol 800 mg p.o. q.d.
Pyridoxine 50mg p.o. q.d.

Mrs. B. is to wear a high-efficiency particulate air (HEPA) filter mask when in public places or anytime she is with other people. The mask will be necessary only until her sputum smears become negative for acid-fast bacilli. You are the LPN assigned to Mrs. B. as her home health nurse.

Discussion

1. What nursing care should the LPN implement?
2. How can the LPN help Mrs. B. maintain social contact with family and friends?

Solutions

What nursing care should the LPN implement?

1. The LPN should incorporate appropriate respiratory isolation measure until this patient is no longer infectious. The HEPA filter mask should worn for personal protection. If the weather permits, windows and doors should be open for sunlight and ventilation. It is important to note the sunlight will kill the TB bacterium and the ventilation can disperse any airborne bacteria.
2. The LPN should observe Mrs. B. taking all her medication. This is called DOT, or directly observed therapy. It means that the LPN would need to visit the home daily or designate a reliable family member or neighbor to ensure the medications are taken correctly. The objective of DOT is to ensure compliance with the medical regimen and, thereby, avoid building any drug-resistant TB bacterium.
3. The LPN will need to continually educate Mrs. B. on the importance of taking all the medications. You will need to teach Mrs. B. about the side affects of the medications.
   a. Isoniazid can be toxic to the liver. Liver toxicity can be particularly problematic in older adults, so liver function profiles will need to be performed monthly. Mrs. B should be taught to avoid using alcohol and medications that contain acetaminophen. You will need to instruct the patient to monitor her urine for dark yellow color and report any changes. Ask Mrs. B. to notify you if her skin or sclera becomes yellow, or if her stools become light gray. These are symptoms of liver damage and need to be reported immediately.
   b. Mrs. B. will need to know that rifampin is always started with isoniazid when treating TB. Rifampin will change the color of body fluids to a reddish orange. This is normal but can be alarming if Mrs. B. has not been prepared ahead of time.
   c. Ethambutol can cause red-green color blindness. A baseline color vision test is

required for Mrs. B. The color blindness will be irreversible if it occurs. Therefore, it is critical that you teach Mrs. B. to report any difficulty discriminating between red and green.

d. As with any medication, you need to watch for generalized rashes, hypersensitivity, and shortness of breath that are associated with medication dosing. You are responsible for medication compliance and for observing for complications. Immediately report all changes to the RN case manager.

How can the LPN assist Mrs. B. maintain social contact with her family and friends?

1. As the LPN, you will need to help Mrs. B. to not feel socially isolated because of the need to limit visitors for infection control measures. You do not want her to become depressed or lonely. Make your own visits unhurried and pleasant. Make the effort to bring stories that will interest her. Reinforce the fact that this is a temporary situation, and she can expect to return to her usual activities as soon as her sputum smears return negative. Once appropriate therapy begins, Mrs. B. could become noninfectious within 2 weeks.
2. As the nurse, you need to instruct Mrs. B. on how to wear a filter mask when in public or with others. The mask is uncomfortable when worn, even for short periods of time. It can impair ease of breathing and may promote feeling of claustrophobia. Changes in blood gases may occur when the mask is worn for any length of time. Mrs. B. may feel self-conscious when wearing the mask in public. She may prefer to stay at home until she is no longer infectious. As her nurse, you need to listen to her and support her in her feelings. Teach her the seriousness of wearing the mask in spite of the discomfort. Be sure she has access to the telephone and telephone numbers of her family and friends. (The numbers may need to be written in large print.) Does Mrs. B. have access to the Internet? E-mail is an effective way to communicate with people. If her communication needs are met, she will not have to wear the mask except minimally.
3. Mrs. B. may experience feelings of anger, loss, guilt, uncertainty or a host of other feelings associated with her disease. You need to be sensitive to her feelings. In many cultures TB is a "taboo" disease because it is seen as a disease of the poor. TB is an emotionally charged disease, and you are the person to give social support to Mrs. B. to assist her in managing her feelings.

STUDY QUESTIONS

Please select the one best answer.

1. The following are signs and symptoms of food-borne illness *except*:
   a. Sudden onset
   b. Abdominal pain
   c. Vomiting and diarrhea
   d. Cough

2. Which of the following items would not need to be taught to an older adult to prevent a food-borne disease?
   a. Store food safely.
   b. Maintain a clean kitchen.
   c. Wash hands before and during food preparation.
   d. Wear a HEPA filter mask when preparing food.

3. In assessing the immunization status of an older female, the LPN needs to ask:
   a. "Do you have trouble seeing red-green colors?"
   b. "Have you had a DPT immunization in the past 5 years?"
   c. "Have you had a pneumococcal vaccination?"
   d. "How many sex partners have you had in the past 3 months?"

4. Many older adult diabetics are at risk for infections because they are not eating correctly.
   T F

5. TB testing should be done on all long-term nursing home residents.
   T F

Mary Ann Johnson

chapter **9**

Common Medical Diagnoses

Learning Objectives

After completing this chapter, the student will be able to:

1. Identify differences between acute and chronic stages of common medical problems of older adults.
2. Describe at least two common physiological changes in each body system that are thought to be normal as the person ages.
3. Describe nursing care appropriate for chronic care of an older adult who has one or more of the common pathologies discussed in this chapter.

▶ INTRODUCTION

Congratulations! You now are at the point where you will learn how to enhance and personalize the bedside nursing care you will give to older people. Notice that the points of emphasis are specifically on the physiology and psychology of older adults. You will recognize what makes gerontological nursing a specialty after reading this chapter and those that follow. Be open to the uniqueness of giving holistic care (care that involves the entire person) to older adults. Frame the care you give within a transpersonal caring format. The knowledge you will learn will be valuable to you throughout your entire career.

Older people develop multiple health-care and medical problems that often complicate the nursing and medical treatment plans. Older adults often have at least three chronic diseases or health-care problems by the time they reach 65 years of age. In contrast, younger people frequently see a physician or enter a hospital with a single health problem.

This chapter has been developed to provide information in three areas:

- The differences between the acute and chronic states of a problem or medical diagnosis. More emphasis is placed on problems related to chronic rather than acute situations because of the frequency of chronic problems in older adults.
- The differences between nursing care for acute and chronic medical conditions. For more detail regarding the acute phase of illness, the student is referred to the many texts that are available to explain signs and symptoms of the acute phase of medically diagnosed illnesses.
- The effect of the normal changes of aging on medical symptoms. These symptoms are discussed in terms of the specific effect that aging has on a health problem.

Five body systems have been selected for discussion in this chapter. The changes in these systems are commonly found with older adults in any setting. Frequently seen medical conditions are included as examples of the disorders that affect each system. Often, these conditions do not occur alone. For example, two or more cardiac problems may be present at the same time, and arthritis often occurs with other chronic conditions.

▶ ACUTE VERSUS CHRONIC CONDITIONS

Acute medical problems are those that develop rapidly. The person experiencing an acute problem notices symptoms for a few minutes to less than a month. The acute symptoms may be caused by some previous chronic condition, such as congestive heart failure (CHF), or the pathology may be caused by a change in body function that is related to aging. For example, changes in kidney function could induce acute renal failure. Conversely, an acute problem may be due to an infection.

Traditionally, chronic conditions exist for at least 6 months and create some disruption in biological, sociological, and psychological function. Examples include both physical and emotional conditions that are not limited to the older population. However, chronic health problems are common with older people. Approximately 80 percent of older people who live in the community have at least three chronic conditions. Arthritis, heart conditions (including hypertension), and sensory changes occur most frequently

There are a number of ways to distinguish between acute and chronic medical conditions. Acute conditions may be thought of as requiring more immediate and often more sophisticated or technical levels of treatment. The goal in an acute condition is to cure the problem.

Chronic conditions develop over time and often are not noticed by the client until major deficits become manifest. These conditions tend to require more help from the informal system of caregiving, specifically from the family or home-health nurse. Often the client develops a partnership with members of the informal system to gain more control over the chronic disease. Cure is not the goal with chronic conditions. From a nursing standpoint, the goal is to provide care that is helpful in managing the chronic condition. This should be focused on assisting the client to function at the highest possible level in the physical, social, psychological, and spiritual arenas of life. Achievement of this goal should provide a higher quality of life for the individual and decreased morbidity (disability). An alternative goal is to work with the client to enable the person to die with dignity, a realistic goal that needs to be acknowledged when working with people who have chronic, debilitating diseases. Chapter 6, which focuses on end-of-life care in the elderly person, will assist you in understanding this goal.

Nursing care requires observation of the patent's physical functioning, which makes this one of your responsibilities. In the acute phase of illness, it is essential that the nurse note responses to medical treatments such as medications or surgery. New signs and symptoms may arise because of such treatments. All changes must be reported, because the new symptoms may be critical in determining whether to continue treatment, or they may indicate complications.

Nursing care for people with chronic diseases also requires the nurse to observe the person's physical functioning. In addition, it is important to have the observations of informal caregivers. The most critical information comes from the chronically ill person's observation of personal symptoms and overall condition. For treatment to be most effective, the person must be tuned in to the body's responses to treatment or to changes in total body function.

Various stressors may exacerbate a chronic but stable disease both in the short and in the long term. Such stressors can include uncertainty about the future, such as relocation or transition stress, starting a new treatment, or the development of an acute condition. For example, a patient with emphysema may develop pneumonia, and although penicillin may cure the acute condition, the pneumonia may cause a flare-up of the previously controlled chronic emphysema.

Many nurses and other health-care workers have difficulty working with people with chronic conditions. There is a tendency to look for time lines, to place limits on how long the condition may last, or when it might get worse. It is critical for you, the licensed practical nurse (LPN), to recognize that each chronic condition has its own pattern. Some conditions, like cancer, may get progressively worse. On the other hand, for the person with a cerebrovascular accident (CVA), the recovery and return of ability depend on the part of the body affected. There is no accurate prediction or measure of recovery because of variable factors that differ from person to person. Other conditions may not change over months or years. This situation can be seen with multiple sclerosis, in which a person goes through a period of remission or absence of symptoms that lasts for a prolonged period.

Patients with a chronic health problem, such as hypertension, may have to learn to cope with a disease in which there are no visible signs of pathology. Some patients may not realize the disease is even present. Medications for hypertension often have side effects that cause patients to stop taking the drugs. Other patients stop taking their medication for hypertension when they feel good or believe the condition has been cured. This can occur with both physical and emotional conditions and is something that the knowledgeable nurse frequently assesses and works to deter. Chronic diseases require chronic (or long-term) treatments.

Working with people with chronic conditions is a challenge for the nurse. It is common for people with chronic diseases to become discouraged. This type of nursing care calls on your creativity to assist the older person to conserve time and energy to participate in activities that have meaning for the individual. Fatigue should be prevented and ways must be found to help the chronically ill person learn to cope with loss and change. Use of a self-care model in providing nursing care can help patients maintain their remaining abilities. The nurse, patient, and family form the team that is needed to encourage self-care. A crucial part of the team's function is maintaining good communication. This begins with an understanding of the past history of the older person. One part of that past history comes from a review of systems.

▶ REVIEW OF SYSTEMS

To determine pathology and functional ability, a review of systems is used as part of the history and physical examination. This review covers all the body systems in an orderly fashion. One purpose of the review is to uncover symptoms that may be associated with the current health problem.

Another goal is to identify chronic conditions that may have persisted for years and to learn how the person has managed those conditions over time. The review also is a method of gathering data that can help in deciding on the appropriate type of treatment. For example, some medications may not be appropriate if the person has problems with falling.

The review is especially useful for an older adult because:

This 96-year-old man lives at home alone with multiple chronic conditions. He finds it increasingly difficult to prepare his food, clean the house, and do the laundry. What type of assistance does he need?

- Older people frequently have nonspecific, atypical symptoms. The review helps to identify possible causes for present problems. It is a method of defining the usual and unusual for the individual.
- Changes of aging may affect two or more body systems simultaneously. The review can help to demonstrate how an interaction between systems occurs.
- Older people often have a complex history. Here, the review can help to tie the past into the present problem.

For the system review, each system and the usual questions asked are listed. Any positive response to a question is followed by other questions to determine the extent or duration of the problem and treatment, if any. It is desirable to have information about treatment used in the past and the effectiveness of those treatments. Treatments include medications bought over the counter (OTC), as well as those prescribed by a physician.

PULMONARY SYSTEM

- History of frequent colds or upper respiratory infections?
- Cough? Productive or nonproductive of sputum?
- Appearance of sputum (not saliva)?
- Dyspnea whether on exertion, changing position (orthopnea), or during the night (paroxysmal nocturnal dyspnea)?
- Immunization history (pneumococcal vaccine [Pneumovax] and influenza)?
- Exposure to anyone with tuberculosis and knowledge about the purified protein derivative (PPD) test for tuberculosis?

CARDIOVASCULAR SYSTEM

- History of hypertension?
- History of murmurs, irregular heartbeat, or palpitations?
- Fainting or falls, especially when changing position?
- Chest pain (at rest or after exercising) or presence of edema?
- Easy bruising? Varicose veins? Anemia? Blood clots (if so, where)?

GASTROINTESTINAL SYSTEM

- Food and fluid intake (a typical 24-hour food intake, number and size of glasses of water and other fluids)? Who prepares the meals? Any food intolerances? Likes and dislikes? Vitamins taken? Use of alcohol or tobacco?
- Stomach or abdominal discomfort before or after meals?
- Problems with bowels and frequency of use of laxatives (what types)? Presence of hemorrhoids (any bleeding, pain, itching)?
- Nausea or vomiting (under what conditions)?

MUSCULOSKELETAL SYSTEM

- Pain, stiffness, or discomfort in joints (when or under what situations)?
- Pain or cramping in muscles (when and under what situations)?
- Weakness of arms or legs? Swelling in joints? History of broken bones or other injuries to muscles or bones?
- Ability to walk? Distance traveled before stopping and reason for stopping?

- Use of assistive devices such as cane or walker (if so, under what circumstances)?
- Type of daily exercise or activity?

GENITOURINARY SYSTEM

- Difficulty holding urine and under what conditions?
- Burning, pain, or bleeding on urination?
- Sense of fullness in bladder even after urinating?

Women

- Number of pregnancies? Any problems?
- Symptoms associated with menopause?
- Vaginal drainage? Itching? Burning?
- If sexually active, any pain or discomfort?

Men

- Nocturia? Dribbling after urinating or difficulty starting to urinate?
- If sexually active, any problems?

NEUROLOGICAL SYSTEM

- Falls or fainting with or without dizziness? Steady or unsteady gait?
- Periods of amnesia or forgetfulness?
- Inability to hold on to objects?
- History of stroke?
- Difficulty with vision or hearing? Ask to describe.
- Loss of feeling or numbness in legs or arms?
- Headaches?

ENDOCRINE SYSTEM

- History of increased thirst, urination, or hunger?
- Dry skin, loss of hair, or thinning of hair?
- Intolerance to either heat or cold?

This review of systems provides only a baseline of information. As a physical examination is performed, the client frequently remembers other symptoms or events to be added to the history. Often, the first contact with any client does not provide all the information that may contribute to an understanding of the person's health problems. The person may believe that symptoms were not important at the time, or the symptoms may simply have been forgotten, so that the review remains incomplete.

Consequently, the systems review is always left open for additional information that may help with both the planning and continuity of care.

▶ CHRONIC ILLNESSES COMMONLY FOUND IN OLDER ADULTS

This section provides some background information about chronic conditions frequently found with older adults. The primary focus is on continuation of care rather than on immediate treatment and nursing care.

CARDIOVASCULAR CONDITIONS

Coronary Heart Disease

The term *coronary heart disease* (CHD) indicates that the heart muscle is not receiving a blood supply adequate to meet its needs. Included under this category are angina pectoris, myocardial ischemia and infarction, arrhythmias, CHF, valvular diseases, and hypertension. Three of these conditions are discussed to show how some of the changes of aging may compound a person's ability to manage the condition. The first example includes angina and myocardial infarction (MI).

A heart attack (MI) may be the first indication of CHD for an older person. This condition is found in both men and women over 65 years of age. The morality rate for those older 70 years of age is about twice the rate for younger individuals. Cardiovascular disease is the leading cause of death and disability in older adults. The symptoms of an MI for the older person are often atypical. Instead of chest pain, there may be delirium or a change in behavior, fainting, stroke, dyspnea, or gastrointestinal symptoms such as nausea and vomiting. Chest pain occurs even less often in the person older than 85 years of age.

Because of the atypical symptoms, the diagnosis of myocardial ischemia or MI may be difficult in older people. For example, the electrocardiogram (ECG) may not be as specific in diagnosing an MI as for younger people because of age-related changes such as ventricular hypertrophy. The cardiac enzymes, especially creatine kinase (CK; also known as creatine phosphokinase, CPK) may not be elevated as much as in a younger person because of decreased muscle mass.

Therefore, nurses who work with older people need to be alert to the possibility of an MI even when the usual signs do not appear.

Medical management for the older person is essentially the same as that for a younger person. Coronary artery bypass surgery, for example, has been demonstrated to be effective in older adults. Decreasing risk factors such as obesity, smoking, and hypertension also help decrease the probability of a heart attack. One goal of medical care is to avoid complications. CHF, arrhythmias, thrombi and emboli, and extension of the infarction are common complications. These may be prevented by close monitoring during the acute phase after MI.

Some people restrict their activity following MI and become less capable of self-care. Decreased activity can lead to a situation called *deconditioning*. This may compound aging changes in the musculoskeletal system, such as decreased muscle mass and decreased muscle strength. The ability to balance activity and rest to avoid incapacity requires a strong cooperative effort among family, patient, and health-care personnel. Referral to cardiac rehabilitation may help the person to identify individual abilities and limitations, and thus avoid deconditioning. Older people are capable of recovery and may return to their usual lifestyles. At other times, however, alterations in lifestyle may be necessary.

Congestive Heart Failure

The majority of people with CHF are older than 60 years of age. This condition is defined as one of congestion in the circulatory system owing to cardiac malfunction. The common causes of CHF in older adults include hypertension, heart valve calcification, MI, cardiac hypertrophy, arrhythmias, thyroid disease, and anemia. An acute episode of CHF can be brought on by treatment for other conditions. For example, overaggressive intravenous fluid replacement (too much, too fast), or medications such as beta blockers (e.g., propranolol [Inderal]) are common causes for some

people. The symptoms of dyspnea and frequent nighttime wakening often lead to fatigue and decreased activity.

The goal of medical treatment is to reduce the workload on the heart and help the heart pump better. Older people are able to maintain a normal cardiac output unless they are under physical or emotional stress. The presence of CHF is a pathology that can decrease cardiac output. Use of drugs such as digoxin is still a primary treatment. Digoxin is most frequently used when atrial fibrillation occurs with the CHF. Some older people have taken digoxin for many years. Periodic blood level evaluation of this drug is necessary to prevent toxicity and ensure that the drug is still needed. Other drugs include diuretics and those that increase dilatation of the blood vessels. A side effect with these drugs is falling, which results from a drop in blood pressure with change in position (orthopnea).

Nursing responsibility in chronic CHF includes monitoring the older person for:

- Presence of edema in feet, legs, sacral area, lungs, abdomen, and around the eyes. Look for increased fluid in any dependent parts and weight gain, especially when appetite is decreased. Often, people gain weight because of fluid retention but lose actual body weight. This type of weight gain and loss can lead to decreased endurance and increased workload on the heart. A weight record is helpful to monitor fluctuations daily to weekly, depending on severity or level of control of the CHF.
- Blood pressure changes with change in position (postural hypotension). Blood pressure and pulse should be checked after 5 to 10 minutes of rest in a flat position, again within 1 minute of sitting, and again 1 minute after standing. Also ask the person whether dizziness occurs with these changes. A drop of 20 mm Hg in pressure on changing position is significant. Patients need to be taught how to control balance before walking and how to use support equipment, such as a cane. The medication may need to be changed, or the patient may

---

POINT OF INTEREST

When digoxin doses are too high, a common side effect is confusion. This often is not recognized as a cardiac symptom and, subsequently, is not always treated.

not be drinking sufficient fluid. Postural hypotension may result from a physiological change of aging in which the body does not respond to pressure changes due to changes in pressure receptors in blood vessels. The cause of postural hypotension may be any or all three of the preceding possibilities.

- Maintaining a balance between rest and activity is critical to prevent fatigue and accompanying inability in self-care. Most patients find that they benefit from a daily routine that allows for short periods of activity followed by rest. During the acute phase, activity should usually be minimal: possibly sitting in a chair for 30 minutes three times a day. As cardiac function improves, increased activity is possible. The activity level should be determined by the physician and closely monitored by the nurse.
- Maintaining an adequate diet to prevent loss of lean body mass. The person's appetite may be decreased, or fatigue may be so great that five instead of three meals a day are needed. A reduced-salt diet (2–3 g/d) may be prescribed, although many people do well on a diet with no added salt and no foods that are high in salt. Decreased sodium intake may make food unappetizing and can cause anorexia. Use of spices instead of salt (e.g., cinnamon, thyme, lemon) and commercial salt substitutes may improve the taste of some food.

Hypertension

A blood pressure over 160/90 is regarded as hypertension (HTN) for any age group. This condition is still the leading cause of death and morbidity in the United States. The prevalence of HTN increases with age, and about 40 percent of those over age 65 are affected. Men, African-Americans, and obese people tend to be at greater risk. Most research now supports the need to treat a systolic HTN above 160 mm Hg and diastolic HTN over 90 mm Hg. Several factors associated with aging may predispose the older person to HTN. For example, stiffening of the aorta, increased cardiac afterload (the force needed to pump blood from the ventricle), and increased peripheral vascular resistance may be present. Changes in the baroreceptor reflexes may be indicated by fluctuation blood pressures during physical activity or emotional experi-

ences. Other causes for HTN may include changes in the kidney and endocrine system due to aging.

Blood pressure measurement is one of the most important items of physical examination. The following are some guidelines for obtaining an accurate blood pressure reading in older adults:

- Allow the person to sit quietly for 3 to 5 minutes before taking a blood pressure reading. Older adults, especially when physically deconditioned, require more time to adjust to a baseline function even after a minor stress, such as walking into an examination area.
- Select the size of cuff appropriate to the person: the regular adult cuff may be too large or too small. Use of a pediatric cuff for small arms and a large adult or leg cuff for obese people is essential for accuracy. The cuff should be about 20 percent larger than the diameter of the arm.
- An auscultatory gap is often found with older adults. To avoid an inaccurate systolic reading, palpate the brachial artery and inflate the cuff in increments of 10 mm Hg while palpating. When the pulse disappears, inflate the cuff another 20 to 30 mm Hg, then listen for the sounds as you deflate the cuff. The first sound may be followed by a gap of 20 to 30 mm Hg before the sounds are again heard.
- If this is the first contact with the older adult, take readings on both arms to determine whether there are differences of more than 10 mm Hg. If there is an arteriosclerotic plaque in the right subclavian artery, for example, the blood pressure is lower in the right arm. The correct reading is then obtained from the left arm.
- Determination of orthostatic hypotension is needed, especially when monitoring the effect of antihypertensive drugs. (See previous note under Congestive Heart Failure regarding technique.)
- If you have difficulty hearing the last sound for diastolic pressure, take the reading of a muffled sound as diastolic pressure. Make a note of this in your recording. One technique that can facilitate the diastolic reading is to elevate the arm above heart level.

Another nursing care technique for someone with HTN is the monitoring of medications to ensure the maintenance of regular doses. This also will tell you the person's willingness to continue taking the drugs. The usual reason for a person to discontinue the drug or alter the dosage schedule is the experience of unpleasant side effects. The specific side effect varies with the class of drug (e.g., angiotensin-converting enzyme inhibitor, calcium channel blocker, diuretic). Examples of side effects that may cause the person to stop taking the drug include constipation, drowsiness, depression, cough, dizziness related to orthostatic hypotension, anorexia, and in men, impotence. In addition, some patients stop taking diuretic medications if frequent trips to the bathroom interfere with their sleep or their daily activities.

When a person has had consistent systolic pressure reading of 150 mm Hg or above and then has a normal reading (120/80), further checking may be required. The drop may be due to side effects of medication, or the person may have altered lifestyle preferences. It also could be an indication of a heart attack. The usual symptoms of an MI may not be present, but the person will be more fatigued and have less strength or energy to do things.

Teaching good health habits related to diet and exercise is also a nursing function. Some people may be placed on dietary restrictions, such as no added salt, reduced cholesterol, or reduced calories. Severe restrictions usually are not needed, but basic teaching is needed to alert the client and family to factors that can help control blood pressure. If these measures are successful, medications may not be needed.

Efforts to reduce blood lipid levels in people older than 75 years of age are still considered questionable by some practitioners. Measurements of fasting cholesterol and high-density lipoprotein (HDL) are minimal laboratory tests to determine lipid levels. The older person may have more difficulty than a younger person in changing a lifetime pattern of eating. Use of a food diary may help with this change. Periodic contacts with nursing staff should check not only adherence to the diet but also the person's reaction to the changes that have occurred. Emotional support provided in this way increases compliance with difficult dietary changes.

The use of regular exercise in controlling blood pressure is just as important for older people as it is for younger people. The physician may prescribe aerobic exercise, especially walking, as an adjunct to control blood pressure and weight. Regular exercise may be just as beneficial as medication for some people. When people do not exercise regularly, they tend to start too fast. Instructions should be given for a minimum of 5 minutes of warm-up and stretching, and a gradual increase in the amount of time spent in aerobic walking. Usually, the older adult can start with 10 minutes of aerobic walking two to three times a week. The time and frequency of aerobic activity can gradually be increased by 5 to 10 minutes each week. The person should be taught how to take a pulse to ensure that the pulse does not go beyond that person's maximum limit during the peak workout time. The maximum is based on resting heart rate and age. A cool-down period of at least 5 minutes also is needed following exercise.

CRITICALLY EXAMINE THE FOLLOWING:

Read the patient care situation below. Ponder how you would resolve the situation. Give it your best thinking. Make some notes regarding what you decide. Be prepared to share your thinking in class.

Mrs. Patrick is your new home health patient. She has been admitted and assessed by the registered nurse (RN), and your first visit is scheduled for this afternoon. Some of the things your think are significant from the RN's notes are that Mrs. Patrick is a 72-year-old, morbidly obese woman who underwent right total knee surgery 9 days ago (3 days hospital; 6 days nursing home). Lives alone. Home is on one level. Requires oxygen 24 hours a day because of right-sided heart failure with pulmonary hypertension. Has been on antidepressants for most of her life; finds them effective. Has HTN managed with medication. Knee replacement done because of severe degenerative osteoarthritis. Plans a second total knee within the next 3 months. Has joint pain in shoulders and hips as well. Admits to being deconditioned because of chronic joint pain. The RN has asked you to evaluate Mrs. Patrick and outline a plan to counteract her deconditioned state so her next knee surgery and her recovery from it will be easier on her. This requires some very creative critical thinking. Give yourself some time to consider this problem; ask others what they think would be effective; and think of Mrs. Patrick as a real person who really needs your help and knowledge.

Peripheral Vascular Disease

The maintenance of good vascular supply to the extremities is critical for older people. When blood vessels are affected by both arteriosclerosis and aging changes, the nutrition of tissues is impaired. Both arteries and veins may be involved at the same time. This results in a depleted oxygen supply and retention of waste products in the body.

Evidence of decreased vascular function is indicated by skin ulcers resulting from venous stasis. Venous stasis is marked by changes in the skin, such as thinning and dryness or overgrowth of epidermis. A permanent brown discoloration may appear because of small hemorrhages (petechiae). Any slight trauma to the area can break the skin and begin an ulceration. Prompt treatment is needed to avoid infection. Even when an ulcer is healed, the area is always at risk for further breakdown. Concern about the condition may cause the person to limit activity. Functional problems, for example, limited ability to ambulate, may result.

Prevention of further trauma and interference with blood supply is the guide for nursing intervention. Patients can be taught to:

- Keep the legs elevated when sitting, unless arterial insufficiency is also present.
- Avoid constricting clothing, such as hose with elastic bands.
- Avoid extremes of temperature (hot or cold).
- Keep the legs uncrossed when sitting.
- Use cotton socks or stockings and properly fitted shoes.
- Report any break in the skin as soon as possible.
- Avoid applying tape or any irritants (salves) to the area.

NEUROLOGICAL CONDITIONS

Cerebrovascular Accident

The third leading cause of death for older adults continues to be a CVA or stroke. This is true despite increasing emphasis on prevention. One risk factor for stroke is advanced age. Other risk factors include hypertension, diabetes mellitus, transient ischemic attacks (TIAs), and heart disease (such as a myocardial infarction or CHF). The mortality rate has declined over the past decade, yet about 40% of those who experience a stroke die within 1 month. About 60% of those who do survive must cope with some disability and physical impairment. Such coping may involve sensory or motor abilities, memory, or language and other communication skills.

There are several ways to classify strokes.

- By type: thrombosis (large vessel or small vessel, also called lacunar), embolism, or hemorrhage.
- Location of the ischemia or the infarction: the posterior or anterior circulation, such as the brainstem, pons, cerebellum, or medulla; or the cortex.
- Rate of development of the stroke: slow (sometimes called *stroke in progress*) or sudden and massive.
- Brain hemisphere: right or left hemisphere, or dominant or nondominant hemisphere. This last classification is used herein for the discussion of treatment and continuity of care.

Once the patient has been stabilized, usually in the hospital, planning for discharge and follow-up care is needed. Rehabilitation should begin as soon as possible, preferably in the hospital. Such an early beginning helps prevent the development of some of the physical complications of a CVA. Two common complications are contractures and skin breakdown. Continued care aids in regaining prestroke abilities, providing emotional support, and maintaining physiological defense mechanisms, such as resistance to infections.

Classification of stroke on the basis of the involved hemisphere is important because it points to the type of nursing care required. The goals for care and the way the nurse interacts with the patient are particularly affected. Frequently, the patient with a right hemisphere stroke:

- Has problems accurately determining level of abilities
- Has problems in learning owing to a shortened attention span
- Is easily distracted from tasks
- Is unable to transfer learning from one situation to another
- May show poor judgment about the lack of ability that occurred because of the CVA, and take risks leading to injury

Homonymous hemianopsia

FIG. 9.1. Homonymous hemianopsia results in the patient's ignoring the entire side of the body that he or she cannot see.

- Is unable to determine distance or rate of movement of people or objects because of poor spatial perception
- Retains language abilities and can convince others of abilities that do not exist, such as stating, "I can walk," when in reality, the person cannot safely do so.
- May have visible deficits such as weakness or paralysis on the left, or nondominant, side of the body

In contrast, the person with a left hemisphere stroke will tend to have more visible disabilities. These disabilities include:

- Problems with language and physical function.
- A need for adaptation of all activities of daily living if the dominant hand is affected.
- A tendency to be more cautious than those who sustained a right hemisphere stroke in their behavior. The tendency is to take few risks and deny the extent of their abilities (rather than extent of disability).
- A tendency to engage in repetitive behavior such as washing the same body part over and over again.

- May have weakness or paralysis on the right, or dominant, side of the body.

The goal of care for the person with a left hemisphere CVA is to improve his or her physical ability. Physical, occupational, and speech therapies should be included as part of the interdisciplinary team plan of care. Fatigue may require scheduled rest times, but a limit should be placed on the length of time allowed for rest.

Other losses also occur that are independent of the hemisphere involved. Neglect of one side of the body may first demonstrate itself in failure to eat food placed on one side of the tray or by failure to turn toward a visitor. Homonymous hemianopsia (loss of vision in the left or right visual field; Fig. 9.1) or bitemporal hemianopsia (loss of the peripheral and/or temporal area of vision) may cause each of these symptoms. Therapy to teach the person to consciously look at a "total picture" of the self and surroundings is needed.

Prevention of complications is a major component of poststroke care. After a stroke, the person is frequently at risk for infections (respiratory and urinary), falls, malnutrition, repeated strokes, and deconditioning due to lack of activity. Prevention of complications includes all of the following:

- At a minimum, immunizations for pneumonia, influenza, and tetanus
- Keeping a routine for urination
- Monitoring fluid and food intake
- Monitoring medications
- Maintaining mobility and independence at optimum levels

Older people tend to drink inadequate amounts of fluid. Teaching both the patient and family ways to ensure consumption of 1500 to 2000 mL of water per day is useful. Some people fill a quart bottle with water every morning and drink from that throughout the day, periodically refilling it. When encouraging fluids, however, be sure the client does not have difficulty swallowing. People with swallowing difficulties after a stroke frequently have more difficulty with fluids than they do while swallowing solids.

The client's appetite may be affected by an inability to use a knife and fork. Occupational therapy should help with instruction on new ways for self-feeding. Meal plans may need to be altered to help the patient lose weight, or control sodium or cholesterol levels. Medications often are used to control HTN, cardiac arrhythmias, and blood clotting. When a person begins to feel better, it is common to believe some medications are no longer needed. It is critical that compliance with medications is frequently assessed. Accurate determination of blood pressure in the home or physician's office is essential. Listening to the apical heartbeat instead of relying on radial pulse is advisable. Laboratory work to follow prothrombin time and international normalized ratio (PT/INR) is critical (see Chapter 16). Following a set schedule to maintain a balance between rest and activity helps to minimize fatigue and to promote activity. Many older people who live at home may need continued follow-up after discharge from the hospital or nursing home. Home-health care is important for the client to maintain optimum health.

Parkinson's Disease

Parkinson's disease (PD) is found more often in men than women. The condition can begin as early as the mid-40s, but usually appears

between 60 and 80 years of age. This is chronic, progressive disease that is marked by slow movement, rigidity, unstable posture, and tremors at rest. There are some known causes for Parkinson-like symptoms but no known cause for PD.

The primary treatment for PD is medication; most commonly carbidopa or levodopa (e.g., Sinemet). Selegiline hydrochloride (Eldepryl) has proved beneficial for younger people but not for older adults.

This condition also requires active involvement of the person affected by the disease as well as the family. Education of the patient and family should be a primary objective for every nurse. Important information to be taught includes:

- Defining the disease and its problems
- Side effects and individual reactions to medications
- Methods to promote independence and activity while providing for safety

Some people with PD become very depressed and withdraw from social contacts. The person with PD can help to prevent depression by identifying times when fatigue occurs. The beneficial effect of medication may "wear off" close to the time for the next dose. Activity planned around these times of fatigue and decreased drug effect will help to maintain physical and social function.

As the disease progresses, the person is at risk for several complications. Infections, gastrointestinal problems, and injury from falls are most common. Respiratory infections occur when swallowing is affected. Aspiration of food and fluids can lead to pneumonia and malnutrition. Urinary tract infections may result from urinary retention and from inadequate fluid intake. Eye infections may result from seborrhea (a dandruff-like skin problem).

Constipation is a common gastrointestinal problem due to a lack of bulk-type foods and fluids. Problems swallowing can lead to anorexia. Nausea and anorexia are common side effects of the medications. Consumption of semisolid foods or those with the consistency of pudding, and foods with a high water content, such as fruits, may help.

There is a tendency for the person with PD to be physically unstable. Many falls can be prevented by the use of a cane or walker. Safety devices should be installed in the home, such as handholds in the bathroom and banisters in the stairway. Floor coverings and furniture should provide a barrier-free route for walking. Shoes that fit well, are lightweight, support the foot, and do not cause either slipping or too much friction are needed.

The goal is to maintain the person's function for as long as possible. A secondary goal is to support the family as they help to manage the daily activities of the elderly person. Coping with the changes that usually occur is difficult for most families. Referral to support groups and helping with problem solving are two important nursing functions.

Sensory Losses

Many adults find that visual and hearing losses begin around 50 years of age. The eyeball changes shape for most people so they become farsighted and require glasses for near vision, for example, when reading. This aging change is referred to as *presbyopia*. Changes in the shape of the lens and a yellow discoloration may alter the person's ability to focus and to distinguish colors.

Three common pathological conditions experienced by older people include cataracts, glaucoma, and macular degeneration. Clouding of the lens resulting in cataracts is the most common pathology found with the eyes. Blurred vision and difficulty with night-time driving may be the first clues of cataract formation. Current techniques for 1-day surgery have relieved the problem for most people who experience cataracts. Other eye conditions, however, require more adjustment.

Glaucoma is still a major cause of blindness and results from increased pressure in the eye that destroys the optic nerve. Central vision is usually retained, but peripheral vision is lost. People speak of having "tunnel vision." This condition is generally controlled with medications instilled in the eye daily. All people older than 40 years of age should have a yearly examination for increased intraocular pressure (above 22 mm Hg).

Macular degeneration destroys the point of maximum sight—the macula. Blindness does not result, but the person losses central vision. Peripheral vision is retained around that central blind spot. Increased magnification helps many people. Some people learn to adjust head positions in order to use peripheral vision. Use of zinc and vitamin B supplements has been effective for some people in decreasing the extent of this degeneration.

Hearing loss increases with aging and is noted more among men then women. This condition may be due to an aging change called *presbycusis* that occurs without previous injury or other known cause. Hearing difficulties carry both social and emotional consequences because communication with others suffers. Many people tend to talk more loudly to those who are hard of hearing. Speaking loudly results in sounds' becoming more muddled, so that comprehension is worse. Some people are helped by the use of hearing aids, whereas others cannot be helped in this way because of the type or extent of hearing loss. Adjustment to a hearing aid may be difficult because of lack of finger dexterity. The inability to tune out distracting noises may discourage individuals from using the aid.

The person with either visual or hearing loss should be informed about available services. Centers for the visually impaired in large cities can provide teaching and materials to assist people to use their remaining vision. Often people can be taught ways to compensate for the loss. Audio amplifiers are available for the hearing impaired. These devices can provide greater amplification and are especially useful in open-room areas.

Some general guidelines for nurses working with visually or hearing-impaired older adults are listed below:

- Face the person before beginning to speak. Avoid sitting in front of a window or light so there will not be any glare. Glare reduces the ability of a person to read lips.
- Speak clearly and slowly so that words are distinct.
- Try not to exaggerate your speaking voice.
- If possible use a low pitch when speaking.
- Touch the person to indicate where you are.
- Identify yourself by name and explain why you are there.
- Keep the patient's glasses and hearing aid clean.
- Refer to local, state, or national resources for assistance (e.g., centers for the visually impaired, audiologists, Lion's Club for help with glasses).

PULMONARY SYSTEM

Chronic Obstructive Pulmonary Disease

Chronic obstructive pulmonary disease (COPD) is a pathological condition resulting from exposure to irritants (especially tobacco smoke) and is not limited to older people. Chronic bronchitis, asthma, and emphysema are included in this very broad category. Chronic obstructive pulmonary disease is the fourth leading cause of death for those older than 65 years of age. The primary signs and symptoms are cough and shortness of breath. The lungs become hyperinflated, and the diaphragm flattens. The person must use abdominal and intercostal muscles (accessory muscles) to breathe. Use of these muscles requires more energy than use of the diaphragm.

Some older adults who develop a barrel chest appear to have developed COPD. Their appearances may be due to increased residual volume of air because of destruction of the alveolar walls. In this condition, there is less lung surface for diffusion of gases. Alternately, the person may have a severe kyphosis of the thorax. This condition should not be confused with COPD.

Different forms of COPD have distinct symptoms; however, the end result for all forms is chronic lung disease that has a strong negative impact on physiological and emotional function. Often, there is one event, usually an infection, that causes the person to recognize the chronic nature of the condition. There is no typical pattern to the disease process, except that COPD is progressive and serious complications do occur, especially repeated infections. Hypoxemia may result with any form of COPD.

The adjustments a person with COPD has to make in lifestyle, habits, and work can be overwhelming. Prevention of complications is the primary goal of chronic care. Each person (and family member or significant other, when available) needs to have knowledge about the disease process and how to aid in self-care. Teaching self-care includes:

- Ways to prevent infections with balanced diet, balanced rest and activity, avoidance of situations in which spread of infection may occur, and use of influenza and pneumococcal immunizations.
- How to recognize signs and symptoms of infection, such as increased cough, change in sputum, and decreased tolerance for activity.
- Instruction in self-medication, including the use of oxygen, the purpose of each medication, and side effects to be expected.
- How to keep track of the medication schedule and medications to avoid, such as cough suppressants.
- Explaining the need for adequate hydration (2000 mL/d unless other conditions such as heart disease rule this out).
- How to distinguish between anxiety and airway obstruction on the one hand, and measures to control both, on the other.
- How to develop a support group or how to locate one.

MUSCULOSKELETAL SYSTEM

Osteoarthritis and Degenerative Joint Disease

Osteoarthritis is the major chronic condition reported by older adults. The incidence of arthritis increases with increasing age. Destruction of the joint cartilage occurs, often followed by overproduction of tissue at the joint margins. The result is a visible enlargement of the joint, especially in the knees and fingers. The most common form, degenerative joint disease (DJD) or primary osteoarthritis,

Use of a walker and other devices can decrease the pain and stress on joints while exercising.

develops from an unknown cause. Inflammation of the joint usually does not occur. Primary arthritis is permanent and progressive. However, it also can fluctuate or vary in intensity. Secondary osteoarthritis develops from a combination of physical stress on joints and a medical problem such as diabetes or inflammation. Gout and rheumatoid arthritis are examples of this form.

The person with DJD usually reports joint stiffness in the morning with limitation of motion and muscle aches, cramps, or spasms. The extent of these symptoms varies from person to person. Some people have very little joint pain or stiffness. Others may experience joint pain most of the day. There is no specific treatment. The goals for treatment include:

- Control of pain with nonsteroidal medications, such as ibuprofen
- Weight loss if the person is overweight
- Maintain activity
- Coping with physical and lifestyle changes

To reach these goals, it is usually helpful for the person to understand the nature of the condition and to avoid the use of ineffective ("quack") treatments. It also is important to learn to identify events or activities that increase and decrease pain in order to promote self-care.

Another critical aspect of care is to teach the older adult to use medications to prevent pain, rather than to control pain after it has started, for example, before activity or on a routine basis. Meal planning is another challenge. The meals should meet but not exceed caloric needs. (This can be a problem for those with low income, with minimal sources of emotional support, or lack of energy to change eating habits). The nurse should teach the client to plan activities around the time of day when the person feels best and there is less pain.

Learning the proper use of moist heat, physical therapy exercises, and equipment (e.g., a walker) to decrease pain or stress on joints can be done with a physical therapist. Keep in mind that the walker or other equipment may need to be examined to ensure that it is appropriate for the person's needs. The nurse should focus on teaching the client self-expression to maintain self-esteem, decrease depression, and promote social interaction. Referral to an arthritis support group and use of their teaching materials may be helpful to older persons and their families.

Osteoporosis

The term "brittle bones" has been used to describe this condition. Actually the bone is not brittle, but bone mass is decreased because bone is reabsorbed faster than it is formed. This results in greater risk for fractures. There are two forms of osteoporosis: type I and type II. Type I osteoporosis is found primarily with women after menopause and is thought to be related to lack of estrogen. White women with fair complexions and women (white and Asian) with small body build are especially at risk. Type II osteoporosis can occur in both sexes with increasing age. (See Box 9.1 for other risk factors.)

Type I affects the spongy (trabecular) portion of bone such as the ends of long bones. Type II affects both compact bone found in the middle portion (diaphysis) of long bones and trabecular bone. Regardless of type, the person may not be aware that he or she has osteoporosis until minimal trauma results in a fracture of a rib or wrist.

POINT OF INTEREST

The ways older people demonstrate symptoms of NIDDM are different from that of younger people. Older people tend to have anorexia, dehydration, confusion or delirium, incontinence, and decreased vision. In addition, it is not unusual for the older person to have high triglyceride and cholesterol levels along with high glucose level.

A major goal when working with someone with osteoporosis is to maintain safety. Injury due to a fall, especially a hip fracture, is one of the most frequent consequences. The resulting loss of mobility and restriction of activity creates emotional problems and places the person at risk for other physical problems such as skin breakdown and constipation. In addition, treatment is long and costly.

A major nursing responsibility is to teach the person and family to identify hazards in the home and community. Some simpler techniques that can be used to help maintain safety are the use of grab bars by the toilet in the tub or shower and the use of a sliding board or tub chair for bathing. The house should be carefully examined for safety hazards such as "trippers" (e.g., scatter rugs, electric cords, uneven pavement, and pets). The client should be taught to maintain postural balance by rising slowly and avoiding sudden movement or hyperextension of joints such as neck and hip. Another area in which teaching is beneficial is the identification of risk factors, for example, limiting use of caffeine sources to one a day. Limiting the use of tobacco and alcohol may help decrease the progress of osteoporosis. Increasing the consumption of sources of calcium, such as fortified low-fat milk, yogurt, and cottage cheese will also increase the intake of vitamin

D. Do not recommend cottage cheese to someone with CHF because of the high sodium content.

METABOLIC AND ENDOCRINE DISEASES

Non–Insulin-Dependent Diabetes Mellitus

Non–insulin-dependent diabetes mellitus (NIDDM) is more common with older adults than the insulin-dependent form. Although the pancreas continues to produce insulin, the amount is not sufficient for carbohydrate metabolism. The reason for this pathology is not clear. Some people believe that a virus is responsible for triggering the destruction of the beta cells that produce insulin in the pancreas. This view is consistent with the state of immunodeficiency that is present with aging. Others believe that the body becomes resistant to insulin as the percentage of body fat increases and lean body mass (muscle) decreases with aging. The latter belief has been supported by the effect of weight loss on control of hyperglycemia.

The main complication of NIDDM is hyperglycemic, hyperosmolar, nonketotic coma. In this case, the serum glucose level is elevated, but ketosis is not present as it is with insulin-dependent diabetes mellitus.

Hypothyroidism is common among older women. The symptoms are often ignored because they are confused with characteristics of aging.

There is no cure for NIDDM, but usually it can be controlled with diet alone. When the person is overweight, a reduced caloric intake coupled with regular exercise is recommended. Oral hypoglycemic drugs may be used if control is not achieved with diet and exercise. Some older adults may need insulin when control is not achieved. In most instances, medications should be avoided because they may cause hypoglycemia.

The usual precautions for diabetes are needed for people with NIDDM. The types of complications found in diabetes mellitus, such as skin lesions and renal and neurological problems, also may be typical of aging. Therefore, teaching about skin care, protection of the feet, periodic eye examination, dental care, and recognition of infections is just as important for people with NIDDM as for those who are insulin dependent. The nurse also needs to teach the client how to follow a regular schedule involving medication, diet, exercise, and blood glucose monitoring.

Hypothyroidism

This condition has been found to be common, especially among older women. The presence of a low thyroid level is often overlooked, because of the similarity between the symptoms of hypothyroidism and characteristics of aging. Symptoms of hypothyroidism, which are thought to be typical among older adults, are fatigue, memory loss, slowing of thought processes, slowed speech, intolerance to cold, loss of equilibrium, constipation, and sleep apnea.

The current belief is that older people benefit from treatment with thyroxine, even if they have subclinical hypothyroidism. Caregivers often attribute behavioral changes in an older person only to aging. Even small deficits of thyroxine or small increases in thyroid-stimulating hormone can result in slowed reactions. This should be a clear safety alert for every nurse.

Hypothyroidism is common among older women. The symptoms often are ignored because they are confused with characteristics of aging. People must be taught how to recognize signs and symptoms of overmedication or undermedication for this disease. It is especially important to monitor respiratory and cardiac function, as well. People usually begin to notice improved function within a few days of starting treatment.

▶ CONCLUSION

Although all these conditions have been discussed separately, you probably have noted that there are similarities in approaches that can be used. Involvement of the patient has been stressed throughout. The need for exercise, high-quality meals with lowered caloric intake, and prevention of complications are three common themes. The following case study serves as an example of thinking out a unified approach to the care of a person with chronic conditions.

CASE STUDY

Mrs. O. is an 82-year-old widow who has lived alone since the death of her husband last year. She was able to care for herself with all activities of daily living and had help with light house-keeping, shopping, and banking. During the past 6 months, her energy and endurance have less-ened, and she has gained 10 pounds. Her appetite has not changed, and her food intake is reported to be the same. Her social activities include church and contact with her three chil-dren and grandchildren at least once a week. Mrs. O. has been told she has beginning cataracts in both eyes, which need to be checked every 2 months. The only symptoms she has noted are blurring of vision and increased glare, especially at night. She has been treated for several medical problems including osteoarthritis, HTN, and CHF. Current medications include:

Ibuprofen	650 mg q.6h. to control arthritic pain
Hydrochlorothiazide	12.5 mg q.d. for hyper-tension
Digoxin (Lanoxin) and Lisinopril (Zestril)	0.125 mg and 20 mg QD, respectively for congestive heart fail-ure
Current weight	175 lb
Height	5' 6"

Her mental status has been intact, and she takes pride in her good memory.

An appointment with her physician resulted in hospitalization for 4 days. The following were reported on admission: BP 187/98; P = 90 (apical) irregular beat; R = 24 with some dysp-nea on exertion. The physician heard inspiratory crackling in both lower lung bases (posterior) up to the midscapular area. He made a tentative diagnosis of acute CHF with atrial fibrillation. After 4 days in the hospital, she was sent home. Lanoxin was increased to 0.25 mg q.d., and Mrs. O. was given a no-added-sodium diet and was told to decrease the amount of fat in her diet.

Discussion

1. What nursing approaches, especially moni-toring through home care or physician office visits, can you suggest that may have helped to prevent this acute attack and hospitaliza-tion?

2. What chronic health-care problems might interfere with total self-care? What activities needing increased assistance might you anticipate?

3. What positive characteristics of Mrs. O. could be used to help her monitor her own health condition?

4. What referral sources can you think of that could be of help to Mrs. O.?

Solution

1. You should consider the desired effect of the medications, the possible side effects of each, and whether there are any interactions among the medications. In addition, consider how frequently blood pressure needs to be checked (probably every 1–2 weeks after a medication is started; consider the use of a home-health nurse to monitor this, or use of a senior center if there is one where blood pressure monitoring can be done). Check for edema, especially in the lower extremities, sacral area, and lungs. The area of edema depends on whether heart failure is right sided or left sided: right-sided failure results in edema in the lower extremities, sacral area, and abdomen; left-sided failure results in fluid in the lungs. In each case, the location of edema is related to where the backup of pressure occurs. Monitoring also should include a review of food actually eaten: 24-hour diet recall, keeping a diary of food eaten, and looking at salt content as well as quantity of food and fluids. Even after a patient has been on medications for some time, reviews of diet, activity, ability to take medications as prescribed, even ability to pay for the medications (to avoid skipping doses) are needed. One critical factor to monitor is weight. People with CHF may increase in weight because of fluid retention and not because of an increase in lean body mass. They may look healthy because of that weight, but fluid accumulation decreases their ability to function by putting more stress on the heart; both cardiac output available for daily activities and endurance are, thereby, decreased.

2. You should discuss the effect of gradual loss of vision with possible development of cataracts: what does this do to the person's ability to take medications as ordered, to shop, to obtain transportation, to use the telephone, and to feel safe, especially at

night? When that person also is hampered by osteoarthritis, a vicious circle may develop. Chronic pain may limit activity, which, in turn, creates more stiffness and decreased range of motion; as a result, the person needs to exert more energy to do even simple housekeeping and leads a more sedentary lifestyle; so the cycle continues. When these limitations are superimposed on the chronic conditions of HTN and CHF, the person may gradually lose not only the ability but also the desire for self-care. These psychosocial losses are then added to the physiological losses, and the need for assistance with activities of daily living is increased. You also might want to discuss the differences between acute and chronic pain and the effect of chronic pain on daily activities, perception of self-care abilities, involvement in social activities, and the effect that complaints about this type of pain have on social interaction.

3. One could make some assumptions that would need to be checked out about involvement with family. The case history indicates that Mrs. O. has been able to be self-sufficient and that she has some support from family members. Family tends to be the first line of defense for older people and only if family help is not available, will they rely on community support or formal and governmental agencies. The history of the individual is usually a good indication of what that person will do as an older adult provided that there is some support when problems occur. Apparently Mrs. O. has good cognitive ability and is capable of learning. Therefore, teaching and helping her to establish a program of monitoring herself (such as weight, food intake, type of food, shopping for inexpensive food) and teaching her ways to simplify housekeeping, conserve energy, and develop a daily schedule to do energy-requiring activities when she has the most energy could be very effective. Involvement of the patient in developing this program of care is essential. Allow the patient to be part of the decision-making process.

4. Look at community resources in her area. Investigate the county agencies on aging, home-health agencies, nutrition programs, transportation resources, and availability of neighbors or friends as well as family. What help is available to assist with visual problems? Control of arthritic pain, such as water aerobics? Physical therapy? Talk about or visit some of these resources to determine if they will help Mrs. O.

STUDY QUESTIONS

Please select the one best answer.

1. Chronic health conditions differ from acute conditions in which of the following ways?
   a. Chronic conditions begin at an earlier age.
   b. Acute conditions tend to take time developing.
   c. Chronic conditions require active work by patient or family.
   d. Acute conditions occur only once and then disappear.

2. A review of systems helps the nurse identify which of the following?
   a. Possible interaction among health-care problems
   b. Whether the person has been taking care of his or her health properly
   c. How much the patient can remember about past health history
   d. To whom the patient should be referred based on a system need

3. When a person has a right-sided neglect due to a stroke, one way to ensure the patient's continued attention to both sides of the body is to do which of the following?
   a. Observe for equal length of both arms.
   b. Observe the condition of the skin and mucous membranes on the affected side.

   c. Continue to teach the patient to strengthen the unaffected side and to avoid overuse of the affected extremities.
   d. Continue to approach the patient from the unaffected side to encourage communication.

4. One of the major concerns with older adults who have chronic conditions such as osteoarthritis is lack of activity. Which of the following is an unwanted result of decreased activity?
   a. Diarrhea
   b. Poor hygiene
   c. Loss of sense of touch
   d. Deconditioning

5. An older person with a chronic condition such as HTN may not take prescribed medications routinely. The main reason for this is which of the following?
   a. Inability to remember a medication schedule
   b. Lack of symptoms that indicate blood pressure is high
   c. Fear of becoming dependent on the medication
   d. Conflicting information about the purpose of the medication

Kay Martin Grott
Kathleen R. Culliton

chapter **10**

Physiological Assessment

Learning Objectives

After completing this chapter, the student will be able to:

1. Describe two unique aspects of physiological assessment for the older adults.
2. Describe at least three normal aging changes for each body system.
3. List two tools that are commonly used to evaluate functional status.
4. Discuss the importance of nutrition to the physiological well-being of the older adult.
5. Describe at least two important components to include in a home assessment.

▶ INTRODUCTION

This chapter provides you with the opportunity to learn how to do a holistic assessment. Holistic assessments go beyond the physical assessment and include all aspects of the older person's life. The ability to perform a holistic assessment requires a high level of thinking and a sophisticated ability to process information. This is your chance to learn and then really do something significant for the older adults in your practice. This chapter outlines the parts of a physical, functional, discharge, and wellness assessment. The interrelationship of physical health, psychological well-being, and safety (Fig. 10.1) is highlighted. You, as the licensed practical nurse (LPN), need to be prepared to make a complete and thorough holistic assessment of the older adult in an effort to improve the person's overall health and happiness.

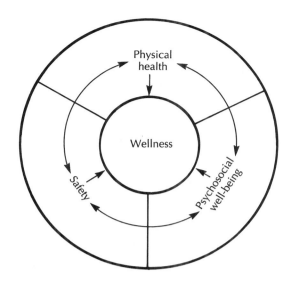

FIG. 10.1. The interrelationship of physical health, psychosocial well-being, and safety.

▶ PHYSICAL ASSESSMENT

The techniques for physical examination included in this chapter are not all-inclusive of the techniques used to conduct a total examination. However, this assessment outline assists you in completing a head-to-toe physical examination of an older adult. It is important to remember to report any abnormal findings to the registered nurse or the physician.

▶ HISTORY

When taking a history on any system, there is information you need in order to have an accurate record of the person's overall health. You need to know the person's:

- Exercise plan
- Eating pattern including recent weight loss or gain
- Consumption of alcoholic beverages, caffeine, and water
- Sleep pattern
- Smoking habits, or lack of them
- Stress management techniques
- Sexual activity
- Medication record, both prescription and over the counter

Once you have the holistic information listed above, you need to take a history and do an examination of the person's physiological systems. The following information will serve as a guide. If you identify aspects of the assessment or history that you do not understand or know how to do, discuss your concerns in class or privately with the faculty person. I am sure you have been taught how to do a history and physical on middle-aged adults. What you are learning in this chapter is not extremely different, yet it does include the aspects of a history and physical that are related to people who are growing older. It is important that you learn to adapt from one age group to another as you do your work of nursing.

You will find the following information written and presented in a very didactic manner. That is for ease and efficiency in your study of the material. It is specific and straightforward. So, please read on; I have tried to not deter you along the way with stories or casual information. Get into this material and master it. The nurse who can do an excellent history and assessment of a specialty group of people, such as older adults, is very desirable as an employee. An even more important point is that you will have the skills and knowledge to "pick up" on a subtle symptom, such as most older adults have "painless" heart attacks. That is important to know because it may save a life.

The material in this chapter is divided into three basic skills for doing an assessment.

They are history, inspection, and palpation, if it is appropriate.

HEAD, NECK, AND FACE

History

Evaluate the older adult's medical history for head injury, increased level of stress, thyroid dysfunction, neck injury, or infection.

Physical Examination

The assessment of the head and neck is the same for older adults as for younger people.

Inspection

Observe the older individual's head position. Note the size, shape, symmetry, and proportion of the head. If it appears abnormally large or small, measure the circumference or distance around the head. Evaluate hair distribution, pattern of baldness, and dryness of the scalp. Note if lice are found in the hair. The presence of lice demands immediate intervention. Assess the face for color, symmetry, and distribution of facial hair. Evaluate facial muscles by having the older adult demonstrate different facial expressions: raise eyebrows, close eyes, puff out cheeks, smile, show teeth, and frown. Note any wrinkles or dryness of the skin. Note the size of the neck. The trachea should be aligned with the midline of the suprasternal notch. Observe for symmetry of the neck muscles. Are they equal in size? Note venous distention, involuntary muscle tension, or swelling in the neck. Assess the active range of motion (ROM) of the neck by having the older adult tilt the head backward, forward, from side to side, and in a circular motion. ROM of the neck should be completed without limitation or pain.

Palpation

Palpate the alignment of the trachea. Palpate the cervical muscles, and note any tenderness. Palpate the carotid pulses one at a time. What does the pulse feel like? Is it bounding? Weak? Or does it have a vibration-type movement? As the older adult moves the neck, palpate over the spinal area for crepitus. Crepitus is a slight grating sensation that occurs when you palpate and is not normal.

Abnormal findings include edema of the face (especially around eyes), involuntary facial movements (tic, tremor, droop), lack of symmetry, unusual size and contour, and tenderness.

NOSE AND SINUSES

History

Ask the older adult to describe any problems with the nose or sinuses. Note that epistaxis (nosebleed) is more common in older adults than in younger adults.

Physical Examination

Inspection

Observe the size, shape, and color of the nose. Note any flaring of the nostrils during breathing and any nasal drainage. Ask the older person to tilt the head so you can examine the nasal cavity for swelling, drainage, polyps, and bleeding. The nasal mucosa should be moist and dark pink. Frequently, men have an increased amount of nasal hair. Assess the movement of air through each nostril by occluding the nostril not being examined and asking the older adult to inhale and exhale through the nose. Assess the older adult's ability to smell by asking the person to identify different common smells (almond, vanilla, cinnamon, coffee). It is abnormal for the smell to be perceived differently in each nostril.

Palpation

Palpate the nose for tenderness or masses. Abnormal findings include swelling of mucosa, bleeding, discharge, perforation, polyps, deviation of nasal septum. It is common to find nasal blockage, infection, crusting, and dryness.

Eyes

History

The nurse needs to discuss the following: vision changes, pain, excessive tearing or discharge, diplopia, infection, and cataracts. Ask whether the person wears glasses. When are the glasses worn? When was the last ophthalmic examination?

Physical Examination

Inspection

Assess both the external eye and visual acuity. Examine the eyes for position and alignment. Note the symmetry of the eyebrows, eyelashes, pupils, and irises. Changes in the appearance of the eyelids can be due to systemic diseases such as hyperthyroidism, myasthenia gravis, or palsy. The eyes should be evaluated for redness, swelling, and discharge. Pupils should be equal in size unless they have been unequal throughout life or have become unequal as a result of surgery or trauma. They may react more slowly to light than they did in the person's youth. Normally, the pupils are black, equal in size, round, and smooth. If the older adult has cataracts, the pupils may appear cloudy. Before testing visual acuity, you, as the nurse need to make sure that adequate light is available. If the older adult wears glasses, the lenses should be checked for cleanliness and alignment because those two factors can affect visual acuity. The line of the bifocals may cause double vision if the glasses are misaligned. Evaluate distant vision with a Snellen's eye chart. Test each eye separately, with and without glasses. After testing separately, test the eyes together with and without glasses. Any person with 20/40 vision or less should be referred to a physician or nurse practitioner. To test near vision, use a newspaper or other conventional reading material; measure the distance from the face to the reading material. Have an alternate plan if the person cannot read. A possibility is to have the person look at an artistic picture and describe the details to you.

Ears

History
The nurse needs to help determine the effect of hearing loss on the older person's life. Does the older adult use any corrective devices, such as amplifiers or hearing aids? The following are some questions that can be used to elicit a history: Have you experienced pain from your ears? Have you had dizziness? In what situations? How long did it last? What relieved the dizziness? Have you had any discharge from your ears? What color? What consistency? Did it have an odor? Have you experienced a sudden or rapid change in your hearing? What were you doing when it occurred? Does it come and go?

Physical Examination
Inspection
Observe the older individual in conversation. Does the person lean forward or cup a hand to the ear to hear? Is a loud speaking voice used?

Does the person request repetition of what has been said? If hearing loss is identified, speak to the person in a normal tone of voice and speak toward the better ear, if there is one. Assess the ear for size, shape, symmetry, redness, inflammation, swelling, discharge, and lesions.

Palpation
The surface of the skin of the ear should have a smooth texture. Palpate around the ear and ask the older adult whether any pain or tenderness is present.

Mouth and Throat

History
The first aspect of history taking related to the mouth is to establish whether the older adult has any dental complaints. The following questions can be used to elicit a history:

Do you have any pain or discomfort? Are any of your teeth especially sensitive to hot or cold temperatures? Have you noticed any swelling in your mouth or throat? Do you have any difficulty chewing or swallowing? How does food taste? Is your mouth dry?

Do your dentures fit properly? Do you have any sores or lesions in your mouth or throat? How often do you brush your teeth, dentures, or tongue? Do you use dental floss? If so, how often? When was your the last dental examination? What was the result? Do you clean your dentures at night in a cleaning solution?

Physical Examination
Inspection and Palpation
Inspection and palpation are used concurrently during the oral cavity examination. Use a gloved hand and a gauze pad to perform this part of the examination. If the older adult wears dentures, remove them before starting the examination. Evaluate both the fit of the dentures to the gums or alveolar surfaces and the dentures themselves. Dentures are considered to fit improperly if there is inflammation and ulceration of the palate, mucosa, and alveolar ridges. Examine the dentures for cracks, missing pieces, and rough edges. Dentures should be stable and remain securely fixed during chewing. Underlying tissues should be pink and adhere tightly to the bone. There should not be food, debris, or excessive denture adhesive on the inside of the denture. If the older adult does not have

dentures, examine the teeth. Note the number and position of teeth. Are they in good repair or can you see cavities and broken teeth? The gums should be pink, moist, and smooth. Inspect for signs of inflammation and lesions. The hard palate should be pale. The soft palate should be pink. Inspect for inflammation, lesions, pallor, and any purulent drainage or a white coating on the tongue. The uvula should be midline and red. It should move up as the older adult says, "Ah." Tonsils, if present, should be small, pink, and symmetrical. Check the gag reflex with a tongue blade. Both the top and bottom of the tongue should be examined. A smooth, painful tongue may indicate vitamin B_{12} deficiency. The tongue and mucous membranes should be pink, moist, and free of swelling and lesions. The tongue should relax on the floor of the mouth. Varicose veins on bottom surfaces of the tongue are common. To examine the tongue, ask the older adult to stick out the tongue. While you hold it out with a piece of gauze, inspect all sides of the tongue and the floor of the mouth. Report any white, scaly patches. The lips should be moist, smooth, and pink. Check the corners of the mouth for cracks.

Pedal edema should improve during the night while the older adult is asleep.

These cracks are a prime spot for *Candida* (yeast) infections.

NEUROLOGICAL SYSTEM

History
Does the older adult have any problems with headaches? Shaking or trembling? Confusion or memory loss? In assessing the neurological system, the nurse also should ask if the older adult has experienced seizures. Is there an existing seizure disorder? What type of treatment has been received? What were the circumstances occurring before, during, and after the seizure?

Physical Examination
Inspection
Initially, examine the older adult's level of orientation. Is the person alert, lethargic, or nonresponsive? Oriented to place, time, and person? As the older adult answers questions, observe the face for symmetry of movement when smiling, talking, grimacing, or frowning. Evaluate the older adult's appearance throughout the examination. Is the person dressed appropriately? Is the person wearing multiple layers of clothing? If so, are they appropriate for the weather outdoors? Is there body odor? Does the person appear well groomed? Is the older adult's behavior appropriate? Evaluate the strength and symmetry of the older adult's upper and lower extremities. This is commonly done by asking the person to squeeze your hands. Ask the person to walk across the room and observe the gait for symmetry, balance, and coordination during ambulation. Note any weakness.

PERIPHERAL VASCULAR SYSTEM

History
Some key history questions related to peripheral vascular functioning are listed below: Do you have diabetes? Do you wear garters or girdles? Do you wear ankle-, knee-, or thigh-high hosiery? When you take off your hosiery, is there an indentation in your leg that does not go away for several minutes? Do your shoes fit tightly? Do you have pain in your calves after walking? Do you ever experience pains, aches, numbness, or tingling in your calves, feet, buttocks, or legs? Are there any activities that you cannot do because of pains and aches in your extremities? What aggra-

vates your pain? What relieves the pain? Does walking or climbing stairs cause pain? Do you ever notice change in the color of your extremities, that is, red, blue, or pale? Have you noticed any hair loss over any part of your legs? Does your family have a history of problems with the legs? Do you sit for long periods of time with your legs crossed? Do you experience swelling of your legs at the end of the day? Does swelling return to normal in the morning?

Physical Examination

The physical examination of the peripheral vascular system includes inspection, palpation, and auscultation. The nurse should always compare one side of the body with the other when using these assessment methods.

Inspection

Skin color should be evaluated with the older adult lying down. Inspect the upper and lower extremities. Venous insufficiency is indicated if the legs are cyanotic when they are dependent (hanging down) or when petechiae or broken pigmentation is present on the skin over the legs. Chronic venous insufficiency is common in the elderly population. If the legs become pale when they are elevated and turn dark red when they dangle, arterial insufficiency is indicated. The signs of chronic venous insufficiency are as follows: distended tortuous veins, hair loss, hyperpigmentation, cool or normal skin temperature, pretibial edema/pedal edema that is worse during the day but improves at night when the older adult lies down to sleep. The signs of chronic arterial insufficiency include thin, shiny, atrophic skin; hair loss over feet and toes; thick and rigid toenails; and cool skin. Edema of the legs and feet should be noted. The nurse may choose to record the width of the edematous area by using a measuring tape. When measuring the legs to assess edema, be sure to measure at the same place on each leg. If you wish to monitor changes in edema, lightly mark the location on the leg you are measuring with a felt-tipped marker and measure in the same place each day. Stasis ulcers are rare with varicose veins but commonly occur with deep vein insufficiency. Venous stasis ulcers are located on the sides of the ankles. Arterial ulcers may involve toes or places where the skin has been bumped or bruised.

Palpation

Check the skin temperature of the older adults arms and legs by using the back of your hand. Increased temperature can be caused by a localized response to inflammation. Cool temperature Indicates decreased blood flow. Peripheral pulses should be evaluated by using the pads of the index and middle fingers. The pulse is evaluated for rate, rhythm, amplitude, and symmetry. Normal vessels feel smooth and resilient. In most older adults, increased resistance to compression may be palpated because of rigid and tortuous artery walls. The nurse should practice palpating the pulses of both a young person and an older person to be able to differentiate the changes associated with aging. Pulses should be evaluated one at a time (carotid, brachial, radial, femoral, popliteal, and dorsalis pedis). They should be regular, strong, and equal bilaterally. Lack of symmetry between extremities indicates possible impaired circulation. If you have difficulty finding a pulse, feel throughout the area where it is expected to be and vary the pressure of your finger. Be sure you are not feeling your own pulse. The rate you feel should be different from your own heart rate. If you had difficulty finding a pulse, you can mark its location with a felt-tipped pen once it is found.

CARDIAC SYSTEM

History

Older adults should be asked questions for assessment of cardiac disease risk factors, that is, smoking and exercise. Do you have any problems with dyspnea (explain this means shortness of breath)? Does your shortness of breath increase with activity (dyspnea on exertion)? Do you have chest pain? When does it occur? What are you doing when it occurs? Is the chest pain relieved by rest?

Physical Examination

Inspection

A cardiac physical examination procedure is the same for both older and younger persons. The older adult should be evaluated while lying down, sitting up, and standing. Observe the neck and chest to detect any visible pulsations, lifts, or heaves. The heartbeat is usually not visible, but it may be if the individual is emaciated. It is abnormal to observe the heart beating on the chest wall of an older adult who is obese or of normal weight. Note any cough, shortness of breath, venous or abdominal distention, or cyanosis of mucous membranes and nailbeds. The legs, ankles, and feet should be observed for edema.

Palpation
Feel the front of the chest over the heart for any thrills, heaves, or lifts. A thrill is palpable vibration. A lift or heave is a pulsation that is more forceful than anticipated. There should be minimal changes in the pulse when the older adult changes positions between lying, sitting, and standing. Press on the nailbeds and observe for the return of a pink color. This should occur quickly and is called capillary refill. It is abnormal for a refill to take longer than 2 seconds. Skin temperature should be palpated for unusual coolness or heat. The blood pressure should be checked using the orthostatic technique you learned in the last chapter. Orthostatic hypotension is a common problem with older adults.

Auscultation
Older adults have more rapid and less distinct heartbeats. Many older persons live normal, everyday lives with chronic atrial fibrillation. Any irregularity of the heartbeat noted while listening to the heart should be reported to the RN or physician. Infrequent extra beats (ectopic) are fairly common. Another common abnormal finding is a heart murmur. A heart murmur is caused by thickened and rigid heart valves and decreased strength of myocardial contractions. It sounds like a hum or click and results from turbulent or backward flow of blood through the heart. If detected, it should be reported.

RESPIRATORY SYSTEM

History
Questions that are used to assess an older adult's respiratory status include: Do you have any difficulty breathing? Do you get short of breath with exercise or exertion? Do you have a cough? Is your cough dry or productive? What color and consistency is the mucous that you cough up? Is there any blood in the mucus? Dyspnea or difficulty breathing is not a part of normal aging. It is often related to congestive heart failure (CHF), pneumonia, anemia, and other lung diseases. It is present in only one half of older persons with pneumonia. The first signs of pneumonia often

include a nonspecific deterioration in health, for instance, slight cough, altered mental status, and tachycardia.

Ask the older adult if there is any history of lung disease. If so, what effect does it have on activities of daily living (ADLs)? Is oxygen used? Ask questions to determine if the older adult is using oxygen safely in the home. Other questions that can be used to elicit history of lung disease follow:

Do you live in an area that has air pollution? Have you or any member of your family ever had tuberculosis? What is the date of your last chest x-ray study? Have you had the pneumonia vaccine (Pneumovax)? If so, when did you receive the Pneumovax? Have you had an influenza shot this year? Have you received one within the last year? Have you had a tuberculosis skin test? When?

Physical Examination
Inspection
In the older adult population, barrel chest, slight use of intercostal muscles, and slightly prolonged respirations may occur normally. If these signs and symptoms occur suddenly, they should be considered abnormal. The respiratory rate for normal older adults is 12 to 24 respirations per minute. A rate of 24 or greater is considered tachypnea. Observe for the use of accessory muscles and nasal flaring. A rate of less than 12 respirations per minute is considered bradypnea. Overt signs of the lower oxygen levels resulting from bradypnea include decreased consciousness, confusion, and lethargy. The character of respirations also should be evaluated. A normal respiratory rate is even and unlabored. The older adult's skin, lips, and nail color should be inspected for cyanosis and pallor. Posture while sitting and standing should be noted. Posture affects the ability to breathe.

Palpation
The anterior and posterior chest should be palpated for masses and tenderness of the ribs. The tracheal area should be palpated for any deviation.

Auscultation
Remember that an older adult can become dizzy from hyperventilation if asked to take deep breaths for a long time. Allow the person periods of normal breathing between deep breaths. Listen fully to inspiration and expira-

tion. Softer vesicular sounds and diminished breath sounds in the bases of the lungs are normal. Listen for abnormal (adventitious) sounds. These sounds are superimposed on the normal breath sounds. Crackles are often heard when the older adult has CHF or pulmonary edema. Crackles result from air passing through moisture and sound like hair being rubbed between the fingers. Scattered crackles in dependent lung segments of some older adults should not be mistaken for bronchitis or CHF. If the crackles disappear after coughing, they are not pathological. If they are present after coughing, pathology may be present. Wheezes are a whistling noise caused by air passing through a narrowed airway. This happens with bronchospasm and swelling of the bronchioles. It is commonly heard in chronic obstructive pulmonary disease (COPD) and in older adults with asthma. Pleural friction rub is due to inflammation between the membranes lining the chest cavity. It sounds like leather rubbing together.

GASTROINTESTINAL SYSTEM

History

In taking a gastrointestinal (GI) history, the nurse needs to focus on nutritional status, bowel habits, and medications. Ask the older adult or family member to give a 24-hour recall of the older person's diet. Evaluate the reported intake for nutritional balance. Is it full of fatty foods? Is it low fiber? Does it have a high starch content? Calculate the amount of fluids the older adult drinks in a 24-hour period. The older adult needs 2000 to 3000 mL of fluids per day. Continue with more health history questions:

How do you tolerate eating and drinking? Do you have problems with swallowing? Do you have the sensation of food stuck in your throat? What is your bowel routine? Do you have abdominal pain? Do you use laxatives? Have you used laxatives in the past? How long did you use them? What kind of laxatives? How often were they used? Have you experienced any recent injury or infection?

Physical Examination
Inspection
Inspect the skin of the abdomen and note any lesions caused by rubbing of belts or corsets over the years. Check for fungal rashes in skin folds of those who are obese or inca-

pacitated. Does the abdomen look rigid? If so, refer the individual to the RN or physician. Abdominal rigidity can indicate bowel obstruction.

Auscultation
Listen to the abdomen with your stethoscope. Mentally divide the abdomen into quadrants that intersect through the umbilicus. Auscultate each quadrant until you hear bowel sounds or if there are no bowel sounds, listen continuously for 5 minutes. Bowel sounds are decreased in the older adult because of decreased gastric motility that accompanies normal aging. While the history was being taken, did the older adult complain of pain in the abdomen? Ask the older adult to point to the area of pain. Right lower quadrant pain may indicate appendicitis. Left lower quadrant pain may indicate diverticulitis. Tenderness at the base of the xiphoid process may indicate stomach pain, hiatal hernia, or referred pain from the aorta. Palpation will provide further information.

Palpation
Relaxation of the abdominal muscles enhances palpation. If the older adult is obese, palpation may be difficult. If you palpate a mass in the abdomen, it could indicate diverticulitis, fecal impaction, mesenteric thrombosis, or cancer.

INTEGUMENTARY SYSTEM

History

History taking is the most important aspect of the skin assessment. The most common skin complaints are pain, pruritus (itching), paresthesia (numbness), and dermatitis. The nurse needs to find out as much as possible about any skin problem mentioned. Questions to ask include:

Do you have any skin problems? What kind? How were they treated? Are you allergic to any drugs or environmental allergens? What are they? How long have you had the allergy? Have you been exposed to an infectious disease? What is your history of sun exposure? What is your skin care regimen? Evaluate all medications the older adult is taking. Anything that can cause an allergic reaction, no matter how long the product has been used, should be discussed. Common allergens are soaps and topical medications.

Physical Examination
Inspection

Look at the older person's skin in a well-lit room. Skin folds should be evaluated for dampness, irritation, and fissures. Common skin folds are under the breasts and inguinal areas. Observe the scalp, behind the ears, the fingernails and toenails, genitalia, buttocks, and face. How clean is the older adult's skin? Is there an odor present? Assess skin color for variations that are not uniform and have changed since the previous examination. Note any pallor, jaundice, cyanosis, erythema, petechiae, and ecchymosis. Older adults with deeply pigmented skin tones should be evaluated for changes in color such as duskiness, graying, and blackish areas. Jaundice in a person of color should be evaluated on the hard palate and the soles of the hands and feet. Check pressure points over bony prominences, especially on individuals who are debilitated or immobilized. Pay particular attention to the areas over the scapulae, back of the head, ear lobes, hips, heels, coccyx, and elbows.

The Braden scale is one common assessment tool used to evaluate the risk of pressure ulcer formation. This is a helpful assessment to complete on every older individual who enters a health-care setting. It will provide baseline information on the older person's risk for pressure ulcer formation. Individuals at high risk should have preventive measures implemented from the start. The Braden scale (Fig. 10.2) also can be used for periodic assessment of the older person. If the older adult's risk for pressure ulcer development increases over time, new and more aggressive interventions for prevention should be implemented.

Evaluate the skin for lesions. Some lesions are normal. Table 10.1 describes normal and abnormal skin lesions. Note the consistency of the lesions. If there has been a change in color, consistency, edges or growth, the lesion may have changed from normal to abnormal.

Palpation

Check the skin for turgor. Gently pinch the skin on the forehead or anterior chest to see how quickly it returns to place. Poor turgor may be a normal aging change. It also could indicate dehydration and/or malnutrition. Palpate skin texture and note the temperature. Notice if the skin has become rough, dry, or coarse.

Normally, the skin is smooth with some dryness. Check the skin temperature with the back of your hand. During this evaluation, note the symmetry of temperature and texture.

MUSCULOSKELETAL SYSTEM

History

The most common musculoskeletal complaints are related to the joints. Complaints include pain, stiffness, redness, limitation in movement, and joint deformity. If the older person complains of pain, determine where the pain originates and where it radiates. The most common soft tissue problem is pain in and around the shoulder joint. If the older adult has a sudden onset of low back pain, report it to the registered nurse (RN) or physician. This could mean a compression fracture of the spine.

Physical Examination
Inspection

If possible, observe the older adult while the person is participating in ADLs and instrumental activities of daily living (IADLs). (See Functional Assessment section in this chapter.) This allows the nurse to assess ROM, muscle mass, and level of independence in self-care. Some decline in ROM is expected. There is a general rigidity of the lower extremities.

Observe the older adult's ability to walk. Have the person ambulate a specified distance to determine endurance. It is normal for older men to have a slight anterior-flexion of the upper body while the arms and knees are slightly flexed. Note the kind of shoes worn by the older adult. Intervention is necessary if the person has an unstable gait yet wears high-heeled shoes. Have the older adult transfer in and out of the bed and chair, on and off the commode, and from the commode to the bathtub. Observe for symmetry of movement. Determine if the person needs assistance. Some older people may be independently mobile with the use of a wheelchair. Assess their ability to maneuver the wheelchair in the environment. Check the older adult's feet for lesions and deformity because these can interfere with gait and mobility. As with physical examination of all of the systems, report all abnormal findings of the musculoskeletal system to the RN or physician.

Braden Scale
FOR PREDICTING PRESSURE SORE RISK

Patient's Name _____   Evaluator's Name _____   Date of Assessment

SENSORY PERCEPTION Ability to respond meaningfully to pressure-related discomfort	**1. Completely Limited:** Unresponsive to painful stimuli (does not moan, flinch, or grasp), due to diminished level of consciousness or sedation. OR Limited ability to feel pain over most of body surface.	**2. Very Limited:** Responds only to painful stimuli. Cannot communicate discomfort except by moaning or restlessness. OR Has a sensory impairment which limits the ability to feel pain or discomfort over ½ of body.	**3. Slightly Limited:** Responds to verbal commands, but cannot always communicate discomfort or need to be turned. OR Has some sensory impairment that limits ability to feel pain or discomfort in 1 or 2 extremities.	**4. No Impairment:** Responds to verbal commands. Has no sensory deficit that would limit ability to feel or voice pain or discomfort.
MOISTURE Degree to which skin is exposed to moisture	**1. Constantly Moist:** Skin is kept moist almost constantly by perspiration, urine, and so on. Dampness is detected every time patient is moved or turned.	**2. Very Moist:** Skin is often but not always moist. Linen must be changed at least once a shift.	**3. Occasionally Moist:** Skin is occasionally moist, requiring an extra linen change approximately once a day.	**4. Rarely Moist:** Skin is usually dry, linen requires changing only at routine intervals.
ACTIVITY Degree of physical activity	**1. Bedfast:** Confined to bed	**2. Chairfast:** Ability to walk severely limited or nonexistent. Cannot bear own weight and/or must be assisted into chair or wheelchair.	**3. Walks Occasionally:** Walks occasionally during day, but for very short distances, with or without assistance. Spends majority of each shift in bed or chair.	**4. Walks Frequently:** Walks outside the room at least twice a day and inside room at least once every 2 hours during waking hours.

FIG. 10.2. Braden scale for predicting pressure sore risk. (From Braden, B. J. & Bergstrom, N. [1992]. Pressure reduction. In G. Bulechek & J. McCloskey [Eds.], *Nursing interventions* [2nd ed., p. 63]. Philadelphia: W. B. Saunders, with permission.)

	1. Completely Immobile:	2. Very Limited:	3. Slightly Limited:	4. No Limitations:
MOBILITY Ability to change and control body position	Does not make even slight changes in body or extremity position without assistance.	Makes occasional slight changes in body or extremity position but unable to make frequent or significant changes independently.	Makes frequent though slight changes in body or extremity position independently.	Makes major and frequent changes in position without assistance.

	1. Very Poor:	2. Probably Inadequate:	3. Adequate:	4. Excellent:
NUTRITION *Usual* food intake pattern	Never eats a complete meal. Rarely eats more than ⅓ of any food offered. Eats 2 servings or less of protein (meat or dairy products) per day. Takes fluids poorly. Does not take a liquid dietary supplement. OR is NPO and/or maintained on clear liquids or IVs for more than 5 days.	Rarely eats a complete meal and generally eats only about ½ of any food offered. Protein intake includes only 3 servings of meat or dairy products per day. Occasionally will take a dietary supplement. OR receives less than optimum amount of liquid diet or tube feeding.	Eats over ½ of most meals. Eats a total of 4 servings of protein (meat, dairy products) each day. Occasionally will refuse a meal, but will usually take a supplement if offered. OR is on tube feeding or TPN regimen, which probably meets most of nutritional needs.	Eats most of every meal. Never refuses a meal. Usually eats a total of 4 or more servings of meat and dairy products. Occasionally eats between meals. Does not require supplementation.

	1. Problem:	2. Potential Problem:	3. No Apparent Problem:	
FRICTION AND SHEAR	Requires moderate to maximum assistance in moving. Complete lifting without sliding against sheets is impossible. Frequently slides down in bed or chair, requiring frequent repositioning with maximum assistance. Spasticity, contractures, or agitation leads to almost constant friction.	Moves feebly or requires minimum assistance. During a move, skin probably slides to some extent against sheets, chair, restraints, or other devices. Maintains relatively good position in chair or bed most of the time but occasionally slides down.	Moves in bed and in chair independently and has sufficient muscle strength to lift up completely during move. Maintains good position in bed or chair at all times.	

FIG. 10.2. (*Continued*)

TABLE 10.1. NORMAL AND ABNORMAL SKIN LESIONS

Normal Skin Lesions

Lesion	Description
Seborrheic keratosis	Raised; vary in size; tan to black in color; appear warty or greasy; frequently appear on trunk.
Senile purpura	Vivid purple patch; well demarcated; eventually fades.
Senile lentigines	Brown; irregularly shaped patches; age or liver spots; occur most frequently on back of hands, forearms, and face.
Cherry angioma	Bright; ruby red elevated area; frequently found on trunk; common; insignificant; increase in size and number with age.
Sebaceous hyperplasia	Yellowish, flat, solid elevations with central depression; looks like a small doughnut; common on face, forehead and nose; more common in men.

Abnormal Lesions

Lesion	Description
Senile or actinic keratosis	Precancerous; superficial patch covered by a persistent scale; common on sun-exposed areas.
Squamous cell carcinoma	Firm, red-brown nodule; may arise from senile keratosis; common on sun-exposed areas and in fair-skinned clients.
Basal cell epithelioma	Starts as pearly colored solid elevation on face or ear; ulcerates leaving a crater with an elevated border and depressed center.
Malignant melanoma	Brown, black lesion; may have flecks of red, white, or blue irregular border, irregular surface; arise from moles or appear as new pigmented, irregular lesion.
Lentigo maligna melanoma	Less aggressive form of malignant melanoma specific to the elderly; arise from lentigens that enlarge laterally.

Source: McGovern, M., & Kuhn, J. K. (1992). Skin assessment of the elderly client, *Journal of Gerontological Nursing, 18*(8), 40–41, with permission.

REPRODUCTIVE SYSTEM

History: the Female Patient

Although questions about sexual functioning and the reproductive organs may be uncomfortable for both the nurse and the older adult, it is important to ask them. Ask the older woman if she knows about breast self-examination (Fig. 10.3). If not, there is a need for education on the subject. Do not be surprised if she is familiar with breast self-examination and does it regularly. Many older women are more compliant than younger women in performing this examination. Inquire about symptoms of breast cancer. Does the person have any pain, nipple discharge, lumps, skin discoloration, or change in breast shape? Is there any family history of breast cancer or other cancerous conditions? Determine if the older woman has used estrogen or other medications that affect the breasts, such as digitalis, thyroid drugs, and antihypertensives. Has the older woman ever had an abnormal Papanicolaou (Pap) smear? If so, was she treated? Did she receive any medications for menopausal symptoms? Was there any unusual bleeding since menopause? Some common physical complaints that older women experience with intercourse include vaginal dryness, pain, and limited mobility from arthritis. These complaints should be addressed and ways to deal with them should be suggested. Lubricants and using different positions during intercourse, such as the side-lying position, can help the older woman manage these concerns. Note discussion in chapter 8 on sexually transmitted diseases.

History: the Male Patient

The older man should be evaluated for symptoms of benign prostatic hyperplasia (BPH). Is there any change in the urinary stream? Any dribbling of urine? A sense that the bladder is not completely empty after urinating? Is there urinary frequency? Urgency? Burning on urination? Does the older man experience nocturia? How often? Review his medications and note whether he takes diuretics or an anticholinergic that might worsen BPH. Does he realize the importance of checking his breasts periodically? It is possible for males to develop breast cancer but not as often as women.

OBSERVE FOR SYMMETRY, LUMPS, DIMPLING, NIPPLE RETRACTION, OR FAILURE OF NIPPLE ERECTION

GENTLY SQUEEZE NIPPLE AND OBSERVE FOR SECRETION, AND NIPPLE ERECTION AFTER EACH NIPPLE IS GENTLY STIMULATED

WHILE LEANING FORWARD, OBSERVE BREASTS AS THEY ARE REFLECTED IN MIRROR TO DETECT IRREGULARITY, RETRACTED AREAS, NIPPLE RETRACTION ESPECIALLY ON ONE SIDE ONLY

FEEL FOR NODES, IRREGULARITY, AND TENDERNESS BOTH IN BREASTS AND AXILLARY AREAS

FIG. 10.3. Breast self-examination. (From Venes, D. J. [Ed.]. [2001]. *Taber's cyclopedic medical dictionary* [19th ed.]. Philadelphia: F. A. Davis.)

Physical Examination

Inspection

During the examination process, you should inspect the external genitalia on both the male and female older adult. Assess for skin or mucous membrane lesions, rashes, discoloration, hair loss, inflammation, discharge, asymmetry, and circumcision.

URINARY SYSTEM

History

In gathering information about the urinary tract, the nurse needs to discover the chief complaint, and the nature and extent of the older adult's underlying problem. The most common complaints are urgency to void, leakage when changing position, pain on urination, frequency of urination, voiding small amounts, and incontinence caused by coughing, sneezing, and laughing. The subject of urinary incontinence frequently causes the older adult to feel embarrassed. Incontinence may cause the older person to withdraw from usual social contact for fear of having an accident. It is also a major risk factor for pressure ulcer formation and urinary tract infections. Thus, despite the difficulties and embarrassment that may be associated with discussing incontinence, it is a serious problem that can have multiple untoward effects. If the older adult reports any complaints related to the urinary tract, determine the person's normal urinary and bowel habits before the symptoms began. Assess the past medical history for childbirths, previous surgeries involving the lower abdomen and pelvic floor, renal disease, and bladder cancer. Evaluate the older adult's medications. Diuretics and antiparkinsonian drugs can affect the urinary system. Periods of prolonged rest or immobility can cause urinary stasis. Urine that is allowed to pool in the bladder creates a favorable environment for the development of infection. To empty the bladder fully, it is important for the older adult to be able to use the sitting-with-legs-dependent position. Full bladder emptying may not be possible on a bedpan. Decreased fluid intake results in low urine volume and infrequent urination. This can create pooling of the urine and increase the risk for infection. It also can lead to dehydration, elevated blood sugar levels, and electrolyte imbalance. These conditions may manifest themselves in the older adult through alterations in mental status.

Physical Examination

Inspection
Assess urine amount and color for the presence of any sediment.

Palpation
Palpate the abdomen for distention of the bladder and signs of pelvic discomfort or masses.

▶ FUNCTIONAL ASSESSMENT

For an older adult, a functional assessment is as important as a physical assessment. Very often, the older person demonstrates changes in function as the first or only sign indicating the onset of illness. Although the older person has many chronic illnesses, these typically are not problematic until function is affected.

Functional assessment includes a holistic approach to evaluating the older adult that includes physical, cognitive and social function. Physical function is comprised of the individual's current health status in addition to how well the person performs ADLs and

IADLs. Cognitive function includes the individual's memory, judgment, and thinking abilities. Cognitive function is discussed in Chapter 12 and is not included in this section on functional assessment. Social function involves a psychosocial approach to determine how the individual interacts with the environment and with others.

Functional assessment involves evaluating the older adult to determine what the person can do (strengths) and cannot do (deficits). What the health-care team members see as a deficit may not correlate with what the older adult views as a problem. Both the older adult's true abilities, as assessed by the nurse, and the older adult's perception of these abilities must be considered.

Functional assessment assists in setting realistic goals. Cure, as a goal, is not appropriate for an older individual with chronic, irreversible conditions. The goal, for this person, would be to maximize functional strengths and compensate for deficits to achieve and maintain optimal independence in function.

In almost any health-care setting, the nurse is the health-care professional who spends the most time with the older adult. This affords the nurse many opportunities to observe the client's physical functioning. A decline in functional ability may represent a change in an underlying chronic disease or the onset of a new acute illness. Monitoring functional status helps track improvements and setbacks. It also indicates when additional services are needed. Use of a formal tool to evaluate functional status allows the nurse to validate, monitor, and clearly communicate clinical impressions to other members of the interdisciplinary health-care team (IDT).

ACTIVITIES OF DAILY LIVING

The Katz ADL scale (Fig. 10.4) is widely used to assess ADLs. It is a well-rounded tool that is appropriate for use in most settings, including home, hospital, and nursing home. ADLs are those performed in taking care of oneself. The following areas are considered ADLs: bathing, dressing, toileting, feeding, ambulating or transferring, and continence. Direct observation is the most valid indicator in assessing ADLs. Watch the older adult perform ADLs and check for abnormal body movements. Rate the older adult on each

Activities of Daily Living (ADL) Scale
Evaluation Form

Name _____ Day of evaluation _____

For each area of functioning listed below, check description that applies. (The word "assistance" means supervision, direction, or personal assistance.)

Bathing—either sponge bath, tub bath, or shower

☐ | ☐ | ☐

Receives no assistance (gets in and out of tub by self, if tub is usual means of bathing) | Receives assistance in bathing only one part of the body (such as back or a leg) | Receives assistance in bathing more than one part of the body (or not bathed)

Dressing—gets clothes from closets and drawers, including underclothes, outer garments, and using fasteners (including braces, if worn)

☐ | ☐ | ☐

Gets clothes and gets completely dressed without assistance | Gets clothes and gets dressed without assistance, except for assistance in tying shoes | Receives assistance in getting clothes or in getting dressed, or stays partly or completely undressed

Toileting—going to the "toilet room" for bowel and urine elimination; cleaning self after elimination and arranging clothes

☐ | ☐ | ☐

Goes to "toilet room," cleans self, and arranges clothes without assistance (may use object for support such as cane, walker, or wheelchair and may manage night bedpan or commode, emptying same in morning) | Receives assistance in going to "toilet room" or in cleansing self or in arranging clothes after elimination or in use of night bedpan or commode | Doesn't go to room termed "toilet" for the elimination process

Transfer

☐ | ☐ | ☐

Moves in and out of bed as well as in and out of chair without assistance (may be using object for support, such as cane or walker) | Moves in and out of bed or chair with assistance | Doesn't get out of bed

Continence

☐ | ☐ | ☐

Controls urination and bowel movement completely by self | Has occasional "accidents" | Supervision helps keep urine or bowel control; catheter is used or person is incontinent

Feeding

☐ | ☐ | ☐

Feeds self without assistance | Feeds self except for getting assistance in cutting meat or buttering bread | Receives assistance in feeding or is fed partly or completely by using tubes or intravenous fluids

SOURCE: Courtesy of Sidney Katz, MD. Reprinted with permission.

For additional information on administration and scoring refer to the following references:
1. Katz S. Assessing self-maintenance: activities of daily living, mobility, and instrumental activities of daily living. *J Am Geriatr Soc.* 1983;31:721–727.
2. Katz S, Akpom CA. A measure of primary sociobiologic functions. *Int J Health Services.* 1976;6:493–508.
3. Katz S, Downs TD, Cash HR, et al. Progress in development of the index of ADL. *J Gerontol.* 1970;10(1):20–30.

FIG. 10.4. The Katz Activities of Daily Living Scale. (From Katz, S., Ford, A., & Moskowitz, R. [1963]. The index of ADL: A standardized measure of biological and psychosocial function. *Journal of the American Medical Association 185*, 914. Copyright 1963, American Medical Association, with permission.)

Instrumental Activities of Daily Living (IADL) Scale

Self-Rated Version Extracted from the Multilevel Assessment Instrument (MAI)

1. Can you use the telephone:
   without help, — 3
   with some help, or — 2
   are you completely unable to use the telephone? — 1

2. Can you get to places out of walking distance:
   without help, — 3
   with some help, or — 2
   are you completely unable to travel unless special arrangements are made? — 1

3. Can you go shopping for groceries:
   without help, — 3
   with some help, or — 2
   are you completely unable to do any shopping? — 1

4. Can you prepare your own meals:
   without help, — 3
   with some help, or — 2
   are you completely unable to prepare any meals? — 1

5. Can you do your own housework:
   without help, — 3
   with some help, or — 2
   are you completely unable to do any housework? — 1

6. Can you do your own handyman work:
   without help, — 3
   with some help, or — 2
   are you completely unable to do any handyman work? — 1

7. Can you do your own laundry:
   without help, — 3
   with some help, or — 2
   are you completely unable to do any laundry at all? — 1

8a. Do you take medicines or use any medications?
   (If yes, answer Question 8b) Yes — 1
   (If no, answer Question 8c) No — 2

8b. Do you take your own medicine
   without help (in the right doses at the right time), — 3
   with some help (take medicine if someone prepares it for you and/or reminds you to take it), or — 2
   (are you/would you be) completely unable to take your own medicine? — 1

8c. If you had to take medicine, can you do it
   without help (in the right doses at the right time), — 3
   with some help (take medicine if someone prepares it for you and/or reminds you to take it), or — 2
   (are you/would you be) completely unable to take your own medicine? — 1

9. Can you manage your own money:
   without help, — 3
   with some help, or — 2
   are you completely unable to handle money? — 1

SOURCE: Lawton MP, Brody EM. Assessment of older people: self-maintaining and instrumental activities of daily living. *Gerontologist.* 1969;9:179–185. Reprinted with permission.

For additional information on administration and scoring refer to the following references:
1. Lawton MP. Scales to measure competence in everyday activities. *Psychopharm Bull.* 1988;24(4):609–614.
2. Lawton MP, Moss M, Fulcomer M, et al. A research and service-oriented Multilevel Assessment Instrument. *J Gerontol.* 1982;37:91–99.

FIG. 10.5. Instrumental Activities of Daily Living Scale. (From Lawton, M. P., & Brody, E. M. [1969]. Assessment of older people: Self maintaining and instrumental activities of daily living. *Gerontologist, 9,* 179–185. Copyright © The Gerontological Society of America, with permission.)

of the ADL items of the Katz scale. Using the scale supplies specific information on how the older adult performs in each of the ADL areas, and the composite score can give you and others on the IDT an overall view of the person's level of ability. The score also gives an objective means to monitor progress over time. Goals in each of the ADL areas can be set on the basis of scores on the scale.

INSTRUMENTAL ACTIVITIES OF DAILY LIVING

Instrumental activities of daily living include the ability to use the telephone, cook, shop, do laundry, manage finances, take medications, and prepare meals. These activities are needed to support independent living. Lawton's scale for IADLs is used widely (Fig. 10.5).

If possible, observe the older adult while the person is performing IADLs. Look for abnormal body movements such as tremors or twitching, for lack of balance, or for poor vision. In addition to checking the person's ability to complete the IADL, it is important to assess the older adult with regard to safety. The older person may be able to cook a meal, but, if the burner is left on, a serious safety concern exists.

Many times, in completing an IADL assessment, the nurse must rely on reports from the older adult or family members. Keep in mind that individuals tend to overrate their abilities and family members tend to underrate them.

Tools for assessing ADLs and IADLs are used to measure the older person's ability to do self-care and home-care tasks. They can be used to help identify needed services and to monitor the progress or deterioration of the older individual.

SOCIAL FUNCTION

Social function is how the older adult interacts with self, the environment, and others. It is the degree to which a person functions as a member of the community. Cultural and socioeconomic background and the older adult's environment define and limit social activities and relationships. Self-concept affects the older adult's ability to perform self-care activities. Psychological interventions may be necessary to enhance the older person's self-esteem before achieving independent functioning.

▶ CONCLUSION

This chapter contains a great deal of information about performing a holistic physical assessment as well as a functional assessment. In order to be an effective gerontological nurse, you need to be very good at both of these skills. There is a great deal of information in this chapter. They only way you will learn it is to go over it several times, practice asking the questions, and practice the skills. Have the courage to use the skills (even with a cheat sheet) whenever you go to your student clinical assignments. This is not a chapter to read and then move on to the next one. This is the one you need to internalize through rereading and practice. Best wishes!

CASE STUDY

Miss S. is an 85-year-old woman who is has been admitted to the medical unit where you work. She has been there for 2 days while being treated for CHF. You are assigned her care for the next 12 hours. In report you are told Miss S. is uncooperative and incontinent. Miss S. is responding well to her medication regimen for the CHF and will be discharged tomorrow.

Discussion

1. What is your priority in terms of assessing Miss S. today?
2. How will you meet the requirements of the priority assessment items?
3. What other points of concern should you address in your assessment?
4. How will you do that?

Solutions

In doing a holistic assessment, it is important that you determine the underlying cause of "little" problems as well as the big ones. The big problem for Miss S. is the management of her CHF. According to the report, that is going well. Of course, you need to verify that her medical treatment is still managing her symptoms. This is the priority concern because it is life threatening as well as the reason she was admitted to the hospital. How will you assess the CHF? Here are some suggestions:

1. Assess for edema by checking her ankles, abdomen, lumbosacral area and hands for swelling, and listening to her lungs for adventitious breath sounds.
2. Is she able to perform her ADLs without dyspnea?
3. Does she understand her medication administration?

Now let's consider her incontinence and lack of cooperation. Some nurses would not be concerned about these items, but because you are committed to holistic nursing care, these concerns are important to you. One idea should come to your mind right away. Assume Miss S. is on furosemide (Lasix) for the CHF. Lasix is associated with increased urination. At age 85, this probably is a major inconvenience for this person. Has she cut down on her fluid intake in order to decrease the stress urination and incontinence, which has resulted in an electrolyte imbalance and confusion? This is what I would investigate as I did my assessment. It will be a very serious problem if it is not resolved before Miss S. goes home.

STUDY QUESTIONS

Please select the one best answer.

1. The following are normal aging changes except:
   a. Presbyopia, presbycusis
   b. Presbyopia, urinary incontinence
   c. Kyphosis, ptosis
   d. Osteoporosis, arteriosclerosis
2. Activities of daily living include:
   a. Shopping
   b. Managing finances
   c. Bathing
   d. Using the telephone
3. A common tool used for evaluating ADLs is:
   a. Lawton's scale
   b. The mini-mental status examination

   c. The Katz scale
   d. a and c
4. A common symptom of myocardial infarction with the older adult is:
   a. Chest pain
   b. Lethargy
   c. Confusion
   d. b and c
5. An important health problem the nurse should help the older adult prevent is:
   a. Fecal impaction
   b. Dehydration
   c. Malnutrition
   d. All of the above

Vivian J. Koroknay

chapter **11**

Common Clinical Problems: Physiological

▶ INTRODUCTION

With aging, every body system undergoes some changes. These changes, although not necessarily resulting in illness or disease, cause health problems that are more prevalent in the older age group. As you learned in a previous chapter, most people who are older than 65 years of age have multiple chronic diseases. The combination of normal aging changes along with underlying chronic diseases means that the older person has less physical reserve than a younger person has to respond to the increased demand of an illness. With diminished physical reserve, the older adult is less capable of adapting to physical stressors and is at increased risk for suffering such clinical problems as immobility, falls, incontinence, pressure ulcers, and alteration in nutrition and sleep. This chapter reviews the clinical problems that are common to older adults. In addition, effective management approaches, based on the nursing diagnoses, are discussed.

▶ ALTERATION IN MOBILITY

The process of aging, combined with the presence of chronic illness, places the older adult at risk for developing an alteration in mobility status. Immobility is a major medical disability for the aged, and one that is frequently overlooked by health-care providers. Immobility often leads to numerous complications for older people in long-term care facilities, as well as the hospital and the community. Nursing management is essential to maintaining and improving one's ability to be mobile.

THE MUSCULOSKELETAL SYSTEM

Normal aging changes that occur in the musculoskeletal system increase the risk of developing problems related to mobility. The bones of an older person are less dense and more brittle. This is due to changes in the formation of bone at the cellular level. As a result, older adults are likely to develop osteoporosis and to suffer the subsequent risk of bone fractures.

With a fracture, mobility is restricted still further. Mechanical stresses, such as walking and standing, tend to stimulate the process of bone formation. When the body is immobilized, there is bone dissolution. This process is called *disuse osteoporosis*, and it will make the bones of the older person still more brittle.

Generalized muscle weakness is also a normal aging process. There is a noticeable decrease in muscle strength with aging. The antigravity muscles are most affected by this change so that standing up can be a difficult movement. In time, if muscles are not used, walking, balancing, and turning become severely impaired. At complete rest, muscle strength can decline at a rate of 5% a day. The loss of muscle mass is not just a symptom of generalized deterioration but also a factor in the risk of falling.

The mobility of the joints is affected by the length and composition of the muscle fibers. When there is immobility, the muscles that bridge the joint shorten. With decreased muscle length, as well as thickening of the joint cartilage (the connective tissue that surrounds the moveable surfaces of the joint), the joints become stiff, which seriously impacts the ability of the person to move.

Osteoarthritis, or degenerative joint disease, occurs in 83% to 87% of people when they are between 55 and 64 years of age. It is marked by deterioration of the cartilage and formulation of new bone at the joint surfaces. With aging, the cartilage is less elastic, thicker, and more easily stretched. As a result, the joint is stiff and there is decreased range of motion to the joint. Over time, the older adult can lose the ability to mobilize efficiently as a result of stiffness in the joints. As joints are immobilized, contractures (a permanent contraction of the muscles that bridge the joint) can develop and further limit mobilization.

THE CARDIOVASCULAR SYSTEM

Many of the changes in the cardiovascular system that accompany aging are closely related to inactivity. Similarly, these aging changes can be exacerbated, or become more severe, when there are prolonged periods of immobility. One such aging change is that in oxygen consumption, which is referred to as $\dot{V}_{O_2}$. $\dot{V}_{O_2}$ measures the body's ability to transport oxygen from the atmosphere to the various tissues of the body. In aging, as well as during periods of immobilization, this ability decreases. $\dot{V}o_2$ is affected by cardiac output (the amount of blood pumped from the heart to the body), which is known to diminish in aging. Physical exercise causes the active tissue to use more oxygen and eliminate carbon dioxide, which increases cardiac output. With prolonged immobility, cardiac output during exercise does not increase as efficiently as in an active ambulatory person.

Oxygen consumption and cardiac output also are known to decrease with aging. This change is evident from the fact that the pulse rate of an older person does not increase in response to exercise as efficiently as in younger people. After physical exertion, the pulse takes longer to return to a normal level. The inefficient cardiac response to activity causes activity intolerance.

THE RESPIRATORY SYSTEM

As is true of all of the systems, aging changes to the respiratory system put the older person at risk for complications when immobility is present. Normal anatomical changes in the aging body compromise lung function. Increased rigidity of the rib cage, kyphosis, and osteoporosis reduce the compliance of the chest wall, making it more difficult to inflate the lungs fully. The reduced compliance of the chest wall makes it more challenging for the older adult to maintain activity, and it also increases the potential for complications caused by immobility. The lungs of most older adults have diminished vital capacity (the amount of air that can be expelled from the lungs following inspiration). Other changes include less efficient gas exchange by the alveoli and less stretchability of the lung tissue. The result is impaired ventilation and decreased blood supply to the lungs. Such changes may not only hinder the older person's ability to move, but more important, place the older patient at increased risk for developing atelectasis (collapsed lung) and pneumonia, when immobilized.

RESPONSE TO ILLNESS

Chronic health problems may cause older people to restrict their movement. For instance, poor eyesight may cause someone of any age to avoid activity because of fear of falling over an obstacle. Pain in the joints due to arthritis or pain in the lower extremities due to impaired circulation generally limit ambulation and cause older adults to become sedentary. Shortness of breath or angina secondary to chronic cardiopulmonary disease also may cause the individual to avoid activity.

Acute health problems can lead to immobility. The onset of an acute illness, whether or not it requires hospitalization, may lead to confinement in bed. Often well-meaning family and health-care providers actually encourage immobility. Bed rest often is ordered during hospitalization for an acute illness. Unfortunately, unlike a younger person, the older adult who is on bed rest deteriorates rapidly and may develop irreversible complications. Although rest can promote healing, immobility promotes deterioration. Prolonged immobility is detrimental to both the physical and mental health of a person of any age. When immobilized, the older person can develop complications such as contractures, pneumonia, pulmonary emboli, thrombophlebitis, pressure ulcers, incontinence, constipation, renal stones, dehydration, loss of appetite, and psychological problems related to sensory deprivation and depression.

▶ NURSING IMPLICATIONS

Nurses, as well as the older people to whom they give care, need to be aware that promoting physical activity not only prevents complications but also slows the rate of the aging process. In the hospital setting, the time for enforced bed rest needs to be limited as much

POINT OF INTEREST

Although immobility is a prevalent health problem, it is not often addressed in the care of the older adults. Identifying immobility as a patient-care problem and intervening to prevent it are central to nursing care of the older person. In addressing mobility needs, the licensed practical nurse (LPN) may prevent complications and shorten the length of time the older person is in the hospital or nursing home.

as possible. As soon as it is medically safe to do so, the nurse needs to ensure that the patient is up and out of bed. If orders for bed rest are in effect, it is the nurse's responsibility to inquire whether such orders can be changed. Even transferring the patient from a supine to a sitting position has beneficial effects. While on bed rest, older adults can be taught isometric and active range-of-motion exercises. If the patient is incapable of performing these exercises independently, then the nurse must assist the patient to meet this need through passive range-of-motion exercises.

As soon as it is medically indicated, the patient should be ambulated with assistance. This intervention is as important to the person's health as receiving the proper medication or a dressing change. Nursing staff should support physical therapy services by ensuring that appropriate, sturdy footwear, eyeglasses, and any assistive devices such as canes or walkers are available. Because of reimbursement issues, hospital stays are

The potential for falls is closely related to many of the bodily changes that are associated with falls. Older adults who need assistance to ambulate or require a wheelchair need monitoring to avoid falls.

becoming shorter. Therefore, as soon as the patient is physiologically able, attempts to restore functional ability should begin.

As in the hospital setting, promoting functional mobility is central to the care of the older person at home or in a nursing home. The nursing home environment offers different possibilities for fostering mobility. Unlike the hospital setting, where the presence of an acute state may impede the nurse's attempts to restore function, the nursing home environment allows the nurse to monitor and promote mobility over an extended period of time. All residents should be considered for assisted walking unless the underlying chronic illness absolutely precludes such an activity. The older person who does not walk deteriorates even further and eventually loses all ability to walk. Family members and other caregivers for the older adult who lives at home need to be taught the importance of mobility.

▶ POTENTIAL FOR INJURY FROM FALLS

As with alteration in mobility, the potential for falls is closely related to many of the bodily changes that occur with aging. The aging of the musculoskeletal system, which may cause a deterioration in mobility, also may increase the older person's risk for falling. One third of adults who are older than 65 years of age living in the community, and one half of those older than 80 years of age fall each year. In nursing homes, a fall rate of two per residents per year has been reported. Most falls do not result in serious injury; however, 230,000 falls per year result in hip fractures, and 9500 persons 65 years of age or older die each year as the result of a fall or fall-related injury. The presence of chronic illness accompanying the aging process places all older adults at increased risk for falls.

When an older person falls, the person often becomes fearful of falling again. This may cause the older adult to limit activities, to become more withdrawn and dependent on others, less mobile, and more at risk for future falls. Caregivers also may place restrictions on the older person's mobility to prevent another fall. At home, the family may admonish the older person to restrict activities so that a fall will not occur again. In the health-care setting, restraints may be used to prevent the risk of another fall. These options do not promote health for the person.

Factors that predispose to falling are typically divided into two categories: intrinsic and extrinsic. Intrinsic factors include factors inherent to the individual, such as normal aging changes, deficiencies in health status, changes in mental status, immobility, and changes in functional ability. Extrinsic factors refer to environmental conditions, which may include poor lighting, slippery floors, inappropriate or poorly placed furnishings, and inadequate footwear. Falls among older adults often stem from the presence of intrinsic factors that hinder the older person's ability to manage the environment or from environmental conditions (extrinsic factors).

INTRINSIC FACTORS

Age-related changes in posture, balance, gait, and vision predispose the older person to falls. Postural changes are common in older people and are due to a decline in strength and flexibility. In older adults, the head tends to be carried forward, the shoulders may be rounded, and the upper back may have a slight curvature, or kyphosis. Changes in posture and spinal alignment can affect balance and increase the risk of falls.

POSTURE AND BALANCE

The body's ability to maintain its coordination in a standing position and to react to prevent a fall is dependent on coordination among the musculoskeletal system, the neurological system, and the visual system. Postural sway occurs when one or more of these three systems is not functioning at an optimal level. Balance problems are associated with postural sway, which can cause falls. Prolonged bed rest, aging changes, medications, and the presence of some chronic diseases are contributors to postural sway.

Postural reflexes play a role in fall prevention by responding to disturbances in balance during standing or walking. With aging, these reflexes become slower; therefore, older people are less able to "catch" themselves when they trip or begin to fall. Inactivity may result in a slower response to disturbances in balance.

Gait

With aging, the gross motor movements necessary for maintaining posture and gait, or walking, are altered. The gait of older people often is marked by decreased speed and step height; small, hesitant steps; diminished arm swing; and stooped posture. These changes are almost universal in the population older than 80 years of age. The alterations in speed of movement and maintenance of upright posture adversely affect balance and often lead to a higher incidence of falls by the older person.

Vision

All older people experience changes in vision as part of the normal aging process. With aging, there is a decline in visual acuity, peripheral vision, depth perception, night vision, and tolerance for glare. The loss of vision that accompanies aging is a risk factor for falls because there is a decreased ability to focus on objects at a distance and to judge distances correctly. The result is that an older person may miss a step or trip over a curb. The decline in peripheral vision may cause an individual to trip over objects at the edge of the visual field. Visual deficits can compound a gait disability because vision is necessary to maintain stability while walking.

These normal, age-related changes in posture, gait, and vision, when compounded by the presence of an underlying chronic or acute illness, make falls the leading cause of death from injury in the group over 65 years of age. Because of the presence of these intrinsic factors, many older people are less capable of coping with the extrinsic factors that may be in the environment.

EXTRINSIC FACTORS

At least 50% of the falls affecting older adults result from environmental factors. Such factors may include clutter in the halls, inadequate lighting or glare, or unsafe furniture or equipment in the person's immediate area. Attempting to function in an area that is not designed to accommodate the aging person's needs can diminish the older person's confidence. The individual may begin to fear falling and eventually become more sedentary. Such behavior eventually leads to a loss of function and an increased need to depend on others for activities of daily living.

Nursing Implications. As health-care providers, it is important for nurses to understand the role that both intrinsic and extrinsic factors play in falls. The individual's ability to maneuver safely in the immediate environment is best monitored by the nurse. In both the home and the institution, most falls occur in the bedroom and the bathroom. Therefore, it is important to assess the older person walking about the bedroom, getting into and out of bed, and getting on and off the toilet. Only by assessing the individual's ability to manage these daily activities in their own environment, can you, the nurse, begin to anticipate needs and take steps to prevent a fall before it occurs.

Having assessed the older person's safety, the nurse, along with members of the interdisciplinary health-care team (IDT), should plan care according to the observed need. For instance, the nurse may observe that the older person cannot safely get on and off the toilet independently and may advise the individual not to attempt this maneuver unassisted. If the person is not cognitively intact, you may use a toileting schedule to discourage the individual from attempting self-toileting when you, the LPN, or other caregivers are not present to assist. If the older person cannot safely ambulate alone, the IDT may

decide that physical therapy is indicated or that a program of daily assisted ambulation should be initiated. Older adults who cannot safely stand or walk unassisted, but who may still attempt these actions, should not be left alone for extended periods of time. One idea is to bring the person out of the room so staff members can observe the older adult and in that way keep the individual safe. When someone who is not safe is left alone, mobility alarms would help the staff know when the individual is getting up unassisted. Certainly, all members of the team need to remember to remove clutter and maintain clear walking paths for older people, to adjust lighting to provide an optimum environment, and to wipe up spills from the floor as soon as they occur or are noticed.

▶ ALTERATION IN ELIMINATION

URINARY INCONTINENCE

Urinary incontinence, a problem that affects approximately 10 million Americans, is defined as an involuntary loss of urine that is sufficient to be a problem. It is a problem most often seen in the elderly population; 15% to 30% of noninstitutionalized people older than 60 years of age and half of all nursing home residents are affected. The cost of caring for individuals with urinary incontinence is approximately $7 billion annually for individuals living in the community and approximately $3.3 billion for nursing home residents.

Even greater than the economic cost are the psychological and social costs to the individual who is incontinent of urine. Incontinence is seen as a major reason older adults are placed in nursing homes. Furthermore, people who are incontinent may feel embarrassed and socially isolated. They may withdraw from participation in social activities and become depressed. Incontinence is associated with the development of other health problems such as skin breakdown, behavioral disturbances, and urinary tract infections.

AGE-RELATED CHANGES AFFECTING INCONTINENCE

Although incontinence is more prevalent in the older population, it is not a normal aspect of aging. There are, however, a number of age-

---

CRITICALLY EXAMINE THE FOLLOWING:

You have been asked to present the educational section at the next staff meeting. Your nurse manager has requested that you develop a teaching plan for your colleagues regarding the importance of mobility in older adults. You were asked to discuss two former patients who had mobility problems. As part of your lesson plan, write out the reasons an older person should be mobile. Identify ways mobility can be done successfully with the following former patients. They are as follows:

1. An 87-year-old man with a fractured hip. He is deconditioned (a word from a previous chapter, do you remember it?), yet insists he can walk "by himself."
2. A 72-year-old woman who is "pleasantly confused" while recovering from a fractured femur. She is experiencing a great deal of pain and thinks you are her son. Address the issue of restraint use with both patients as well as their ambulation plans. Bring your best lesson plan to class to share with others.

related changes that make the older person susceptible to developing incontinence. In older clients, the bladder capacity diminishes to about half that of young adults. The diminished ability of the kidneys to concentrate urine makes urinary frequency and nocturia (excessive urination at night) common problems for the older person. In addition, many older people experience sudden and unexpected contractions of the detrusor muscle (the smooth muscle that makes up the outside wall of the bladder), which cause an urgent need to void. Changes in the central and autonomic nervous systems of the older person cause a decreased ability to contract the external sphincter of the bladder, which further exacerbates urinary urgency. Many postmenopausal women experience thinning and weakening of the muscles of the pelvic floor and the urethra due to estrogen loss. In men, an enlarged prostate, often associated with aging, may lead to urinary retention, irritability of the detrusor muscle, and bladder spasms.

The urinary urgency that many older people experience often leads to incontinence in an institutional setting. When the older adult cannot go to the toilet independently or, as often as needed, incontinence is likely to result. This is further exacerbated by the immobility that results from being ill or from needing medical interventions such as intravenous therapy.

TYPES OF CAUSES OF INCONTINENCE

For the nurse to intervene in the management of incontinence, it is important to understand the underlying causes of incontinence. Incontinence can be a result of a chronic problem, or it can be the result of an acute situation.

Acute Incontinence

Acute or transient incontinence is incontinence that occurs because of the presence of another medical problem and often resolves when the underlying illness is treated. The following mnemonic demonstrates the possible causes of acute incontinence:

D: Delirium
R: Restricted mobility, retention (acute)
I: Infection, inflammation, impaction
P: Pharmaceutical, polyuria, psychological

Delirium is an acute confusional state that is brought on by an acute illness and that disrupts the physiological homeostasis in the older patient. In a delirious state, the patient is not aware of the need to void, nor does the person have the capability to get to the toilet.

Restricted mobility, as already discussed, is a common cause of incontinence in the elderly population. Acute urinary retention is often caused by anticholinergic and narcotic medications, and may result in overflow incontinence.

Urinary tract infections (UTI) cause frequency, urgency, and painful urination. This condition can lead to increased bladder contractions and incontinence. Many residents in long-term care have bacteria in their urine, a condition that is asymptomatic and does not require treatment. However, when bacteriuria is accompanied by urinary incontinence, the patient should be treated and the effect of the treatment on the incontinence noted.

It is important to remember that fecal impaction often obstructs the bladder outlet and may cause overflow urinary incontinence. In overflow urinary incontinence, the bladder retains urine, and when it reaches its capacity, the individual begins to drip or leak urine. In postmenopausal women, the changes that occur in the lining of the vagina and urethra because of lower levels of estrogen may cause inflammation and weakening of the pelvic floor, which can, in turn, cause incontinence.

Many drugs can cause urinary incontinence. The following is a list of drug groups that adversely affect the older person's ability to maintain continence:

- Sedatives/hypnotics
- Antipsychotics
- Narcotics
- Anticholinergics
- Alpha-adrenergic blockers
- Diuretics

Endocrine disorders that lead to hyperglycemia or hypercalcemia may cause urinary incontinence. Psychological causes that have been associated with urinary incontinence include depression and confusional states.

Nursing Implications. As nurses, it is important to understand that most instances of bladder incontinence are transient and, very often, reversible. In most cases, acute or transient incontinence can be resolved with treatment of the underlying illness or with discontinuation of a causative drug. Incontinence should never be accepted without first ascertaining that the older person has been assessed for underlying conditions and that treatment has been initiated.

Chronic Incontinence

There are four types of persistent or chronic incontinence. Incontinence is considered to be persistent if it continues after reversible causes have been ruled out or treated. Persistent or chronic incontinence usually has a gradual onset, worsens over time, and occurs when there is a failure to either empty or store urine.

Urge Incontinence. Urge incontinence is the most common form of incontinence in long-term care facilities. It is closely associated with stroke and Alzheimer's disease. In this type of incontinence, the patient or resident feels the urge to go but does not have enough time to get to the toilet before the urine is released.

Stress Incontinence. Stress incontinence occurs when a small amount of urine is released after there is a sudden increase in intra-abdominal pressure caused by coughing, sneezing, laughing, or lifting. This type of incontinence results when the bladder outlet sphincter is incompetent or weak. Stress incontinence is more common in women and is often a result of damage to the pelvic muscles during childbirth.

Overflow Incontinence. Overflow incontinence is present in approximately 15% of nursing home residents. It is caused by bladder outlet obstruction that results in impaired bladder emptying. When the bladder is not emptied sufficiently, the resident experiences frequent dribbling of urine.

Functional Incontinence. Functional incontinence results when the individual is unable or unwilling to attend to toileting needs. In this situation, the bladder and urethra function normally, but cognitive, physical, psychological, or environmental impairments make it difficult for the older person to get to the toilet. Inaccessible toilets, unavailable caregivers, depression, or inability to find the

toilet are all possible causes of functional incontinence.

Nursing Implications. Treatment of urinary incontinence is based on the underlying cause. Medication intervention may be used to treat infection, replace estrogen, or stop abnormal bladder muscle contractions and tighten sphincter muscles. Surgical intervention is used to correct anatomical anomalies and remove obstructions. Behavioral interventions require that the health-care professional provide education and positive reinforcement to the client. At times, behavioral interventions may be used in combination with medical or surgical interventions.

Behavioral Interventions. Behavioral interventions, which are most often provided by nursing personnel, are also called training procedures and include the following:

- Bladder training (retraining)
- Habit training (timed voiding)
- Prompted voiding
- Pelvic muscle exercises

These techniques are most helpful with stress and urge incontinence.

Bladder retraining is used to restore the normal pattern of voiding by inhibiting or stimulating voiding. The goal is to lengthen the period of time between voidings. This is best done by instructing and assisting the individual to learn to suppress the urge to void in an attempt to increase the amount of urine the bladder can hold. This technique is used with individuals who are capable of understanding and remembering the instructions. Most bladder-retraining schedules begin with a schedule of toileting every 2 hours and gradually increasing the amount of time between voidings.

Prompted voiding is different from bladder training in that the goal is not to increase bladder capacity but rather to teach the incontinent person to be aware of toileting needs and to request assistance from the caregiver. In this technique, the person is asked to try to use the toilet at regular intervals and is praised for maintaining continence and using the toilet. The schedule that is followed usually involves toileting on awakening, after meals, at bedtime, and, if awake, at night. More voiding times can be added if the individual's voiding schedule indicates that need.

This intervention works well with moderately confused people.

Habit training works best with cognitively impaired or confused people and requires the caregiver to take the patient to the toilet at regular intervals. The toileting schedule may be every 2 to 4 hours, or the caregiver may toilet the individual on awakening, after meals, at bedtime, and at night, if awake.

Kegel's exercises are used to alleviate stress incontinence. The goal of such exercises is to strengthen the pelvic floor muscles. Patients who are taught Kegel's exercises must be cognitively intact and willing to participate in this exercise regimen. The exercise consists of the person contracting the pelvic floor muscles and holding them for 3 to 4 seconds and then relaxing the muscle. This should be done 10 times in succession at least twice a day.

In dealing with incontinence, nurses play a key role in both education and treatment. Incontinence is not a normal part of aging but is more prevalent in the aging population. Many forms of incontinence are reversible, and all attempts should be made to assess, treat, and resolve incontinence when it is present.

CONSTIPATION

Bowel functioning and the avoidance of constipation are common concerns for the older adults. Many older people were raised during a time when anything but a daily bowel movement was considered abnormal. The concern regarding this problem is appropriate because numerous age-related changes in the gastrointestinal system make constipation more likely.

It is probable that an older person has an extended gastrointestinal transit time as a result of slower peristalsis. More water is removed from the stool when it is in the colon for longer periods of time. This causes the stool to become harder and more difficult to pass. Immobility, decreased exercise, and a lack of fiber and water in the diet are common problems in the older population, and these factors tend to exacerbate the tendency to become constipated. Certain drugs also may lead to constipation and include the following:

- Aluminum-containing antacids
- Anticholinergics
- Calcium carbonate
- Iron salts
- Laxatives (when abused)
- Opiates
- Phenothiazines
- Sedatives
- Tricyclic antidepressants
- Diuretics
- Calcium-channel blockers

Immobility is particularly problematic in the maintenance of regular bowel movements. Muscular atrophy, a loss of tone in the muscles of the intestine, and generalized weakness of the muscles necessary for the expulsive mechanism of evacuation occur during periods of immobilization. The overuse of laxatives also causes a loss of muscle tone in the bowel.

Immobility not only affects the physiological functioning of the gastrointestinal system, but it also prevents the individual from interacting efficiently with the environment to meet the needs of the body. Factors such as strange environments, disruption of the usual elimination patterns, being forced to defecate in an unnatural position in unnatural surroundings (as occurs with the use of a bedpan), and suppressing the urge to defecate because of the inability to get to the toilet will inhibit normal defecation.

Nursing Interventions

Nursing interventions aimed at prevention of constipation should be focused on establishing a regular pattern of bowel elimination that is not associated with straining or discomfort. It is important for the older person's overall health to attempt to correct constipation without resorting to the use of laxatives. These interventions should include increasing physical activity, increasing water intake, increasing dietary fiber, and establishing a regular bowel routine. Regular exercise stimulates motility in the gut.

The older adult should be encouraged to drink 1500 to 2000 mL of fluids daily unless this is contraindicated by other health problems. Dietary fiber also plays an important role in the avoidance of constipation. Fiber holds water, thus making the stool softer and bulkier, which speeds the passage of stool through the intestine. It can be difficult to increase fiber in the diet of the older person because of lifelong dietary preferences and poor dentition. It may be helpful to consult a dietician. Although prunes and prune juice are often used to combat constipation, they may not be the best choice. Prunes have only 2 g of fiber per prune, and prune juice has none. Furthermore, prunes mimic the action of cathartics, and there may be rebound constipation when the use of prunes is discontinued.

Assisting the patient to develop a regular bowel routine is an essential part of bowel maintenance, and one in which you, as the nurse, play a pivotal role. In facilitating regular bowel routines, the nurse must assess how much, if any, assistance the patient requires in getting safely to the toilet. The use of bedpans should be avoided if at all possible, but when they are used, the patient should be in an upright position unless this position is contraindicated. The nurse also needs to ensure that regular toileting times are maintained and that privacy is provided during toileting time.

▶ ALTERATION IN SKIN INTEGRITY: PRESSURE ULCERS

A pressure ulcer is defined as any lesion caused by unrelieved pressure that results in damage to the underlying tissue. Pressure ulcers are an extremely serious health problem that can lead to pain, extended hospital stays, and further complications from infection. In hospitals, the pressure ulcer rate has been estimated to be as high as 29.5%, and in nursing homes it is estimated to be 23%. Older persons are particularly at risk, with those older than 70 years of age accounting for 71% of all patients with pressure ulcers. A mortality rate of approximately 60,000 deaths per year is associated with pressure ulcers. In nursing homes, 66% of those residents who develop a pressure ulcer die. It is estimated that patients with pressure ulcers require 50% more nursing care than those without them. Because pressure ulcers are, for the most part, preventable, maintaining adequate skin integrity is a quality-of-care issue for all nurses. Even more important than knowing the various treatment modalities is knowing how pressure ulcers develop. You need to become an expert in prevention techniques.

RISK FACTORS

Mechanical Risk Factors

Four mechanical factors that contribute to the development of pressure ulcers are pressure, friction, shearing, and moisture.

Pressure. Pressure ulcers usually occur over bony prominences where normal tissue is squeezed between the internal pressure of the bone and an external source of pressure or friction, such as the chair or the bed. External pressure that lasts long enough and is sufficient to decrease blood flow results in inadequate oxygenation and nutrition to the area and the subsequent development of a pressure sore. Immobility is the most important risk factor in the development of pressure sores. Pressure of high intensity that is left unchecked for more than 2 hours can result in irreversible tissue damage.

Shearing. When the head of the bed is elevated more than 30 degrees and the person slides toward the foot of the bed, shearing occurs. In this situation, the skin over the sacrum does not move, whereas, the subcutaneous tissue and gluteal vessels are stretched. This results in rupture of the blood vessels. Subcutaneous fat, which lacks the ability to stretch, is particularly vulnerable to injury from shearing forces. Sores that develop on the sacrum, heels, and anterior tibial region are most probably a result of shearing. When shearing and pressure are both present, the amount of pressure necessary to cause tissue damage is half the amount that causes tissue damage when shearing is not present.

Friction and Moisture. Friction occurs when the skin is moved across the sheets, such as when the patient is being pulled up rather than lifted up in the bed. The result of this motion is damage to the epidermis, which can lead to ulceration or a break in the skin. Moisture caused by perspiration or incontinence can increase the friction between the surface and the skin. Moisture also can cause maceration (softening of the skin), which weakens the skin and increases the risk of infection. In the presence of moisture resulting from urinary or fecal incontinence, the risk of pressure ulcer development on the sacrum and buttocks increases fivefold. Incontinence is a strong predictor of skin breakdown.

Physiological Risk Factors

In addition to mechanical forces, there are also factors that are inherent to the individual that increase the risk of skin breakdown.

Aging Skin. Aging skin increases the likelihood of developing pressure ulcers because it is less resistant to the mechanical forces that can damage the skin. With advancing age, there is a decrease in the thickness of the cell layers of the epidermis, a flattening in the epidermal/dermal interface, and a loss of subcutaneous tissue. In turn, these changes cause impaired wound healing and decreased thermoregulation, causing the skin to become more fragile.

Immobility. Immobility, combined with the age-related changes of the skin, greatly increases the risk of pressure ulcer formation. Normally, spontaneous body movements that occur during sleep and throughout the day protect the skin from pressure. A number of situations, however, prevent the body from spontaneous movement. These include a physical disability, loss of sensation, the presence of pain, or the use of sedating drugs or anesthesia. The use of physical restraints also causes immobility.

Malnutrition. Another physiological factor that can lead to pressure ulcer formation is malnutrition. Deficiencies in zinc, iron, vitamin C, and protein adversely affect the health of the skin. The more severe the malnutrition, the more severe the pressure ulcer is. In patients who have had weight loss or who are underweight, it is important to check the albumin level of the blood. A serum albumin level below 3.5g/dL indicates that nutritional intervention is necessary to prevent skin breakdown. Malnutrition and the subsequent weight loss lead to loss of muscle mass and subcutaneous tissue. This diminishes the body's protective padding and increases the pressure over the bony prominences.

Staging

Pressure ulcers are graded according to the degree of tissue damage. The staging of a pressure ulcer dictates the type of treatment to be implemented. Staging provides a means of describing an ulcer that allows for the ulcer to be monitored over time. A commonly used

Aging skin increases the likelihood of developing complications because it is less resistant to the mechanical forces that can damage skin.

staging criteria is presented in the following list:

> Stage I: Nonblanchable erythema of intact skin. (The skin is reddened, even in the absence of direct pressure.)
>
> Stage II: Partial-thickness skin loss involving epidermis or dermis. The ulcer is superficial and presents clinically as an abrasion, blister, or shallow crater.
>
> Stage III: Full-thickness skin loss involving damage to or necrosis of subcutaneous tissue that may extend down to, but not through, the underlying fascia (the fibrous membrane covering the muscles). The ulcer presents clinically as a deep crater with or without undermining (connecting) of adjacent tissue.
>
> Stage IV: Full-thickness skin loss with extensive destruction, tissue necrosis, or damage to muscle, bone, or supporting structures (for example, tendon or joint capsule). Undermining and sinus tracts also may be associated with stage IV pressure ulcers.

Prevention

Assessment of risk is a vital first step in prevention of pressure ulcers. If a patient is found to be at risk for developing pressure ulcers, then interventions to prevent skin breakdown can be initiated before an ulcer develops. A number of assessment tools are available. If necessary, review the Braden Scale presented in the previous chapter.

Assessment should be done within the first 24 hours of admission to a hospital or nursing home and be repeated 24 to 48 hours following admission. Ongoing assessment is necessary to prevent new skin breakdown. This should be done every 24 to 48 hours in the hospital, monthly in the nursing home, and whenever there is a change in the patient's condition. Once the patient is found to be at risk for alteration in skin integrity, preventive measures should be aimed at reducing pressure on bony prominences, preventing shear or friction, keeping skin clean and dry, and providing adequate nutrition and hydration.

To reduce pressure, the patient should be repositioned at least every 2 hours. This decreases the amount of time that pressure is exerted on any one body part. The appearance of reddened areas indicates that more frequent turning or other interventions may be indicated. When placing a patient on either side, a wedge should be placed behind the patient to prevent the individual from lying directly on the trochanter (the bony prominence located below the neck of the femur). Although at one time it was common practice to massage reddened areas over bony prominences, this is no longer the practice. To do so may exert pressure on the area and may cause further breakdown of the small capillaries in the area. In some cases, it may be necessary to use pressure-relieving devices, such as air-, water-, or gel-filled chair pads or mattresses, as well as foam heel protectors and mattresses. The use of egg-crate mattresses, although common, does not provide sufficient pressure relief to prevent pressure ulcers. Walking programs and passive and active range-of-motion exercises not only improve muscle strength and joint flexibility but are important in the prevention of skin breakdown as well.

To reduce friction, patients should be lifted and not pulled when repositioned. The use of a lift sheet or a turn sheet is essential to distribute the patient's weight evenly and avoid undue friction and stress on the skin. Shear can be reduced by decreasing the amount of time and frequency that the patient's head is elevated in the bed. When out of bed and in a chair, the patient should be repositioned at least every 2 hours, and long-term sitting should be discouraged. While in the chair, the individual needs to be examined for appropriate posture and alignment because an inappropriate sitting posture can lead to pressure ulcers and increased shearing forces.

Although skin should be kept clean and dry to prevent pressure ulcers, older adults do not need to be bathed daily. Excessive bathing and rubbing can be drying and damaging to the skin. Using a mild cleansing agent that does not promote dryness and patting the skin dry are essentials of good skin care for the older person. A diet that provides adequate nutrition and hydration and that meets the protein and vitamin requirements of the individual promotes skin integrity. A dietary consultation is needed in a patient who has skin breakdown or has an albumin level below 3.5 g/dL.

Treatment

Sometimes, despite vigilant nursing care, a pressure ulcer does develop. Often an underlying disease state can defeat attempts to prevent skin breakdown. The treatment of

CRITICALLY EXAMINE THE FOLLOWING:

You are a home health nurse for an 79-year-old woman who is cared for by her husband with drop-in visits from three daughters. Sarah, the patient, is home bound because of general fatigue and post-operative bilateral total knees. She can ambulate with a cane, but is fearful and will not leave the house except on rare occasions. She says she is happy to be at home with her husband and not to have the arthritic knee pain. The problem? She is in bed and a recliner chair most of the day and night. Her husband lifts her to and from the chair and bed when Sarah is "too tired to move herself."

You have noticed that Sarah's buttocks are reddened, as are her heels. What should you do about your assessment.? Focus on a teaching plan for this couple. (I know this is the second teaching plan you have been asked to do in this chapter. My hope is that after doing the first one, and sharing it with your fellow students, this one will be easier to write).What do they need to know about pressure ulcers? What is the best way for you to share the hazards of Immobility with Sarah? What can you do to prevent the stage I pressure ulcers from developing into something worse? Do your best thinking and be prepared to share it with the class.

pressure ulcers is extremely individualized, and there is much controversy as to which treatments and skin care products to use. The technology and products for treatment of pressure ulcers are changing every day. Treatment is aimed at promoting a healing environment by providing adequate circulation and oxygenation to the impaired tissue, and maintaining a clean and dry wound area. Exudate should be removed as much as possible and infection should be treated with the appropriate antibiotic. Any necrotic tissue needs to be débrided or removed before treatment of the ulcer can proceed. This should be done only under the supervision of a registered nurse.

▶ ALTERED NUTRITIONAL STATUS

Adequate nutrition is essential to the maintenance of health, prevention of disease, treatment of chronic illness, and recovery from acute illness. When the body is inadequately nourished, the individual is more likely to develop an illness and is less able to recover from illness. Caloric or protein malnutrition is present in 12% to 50% of the older population.

To be adequately nourished, the body must have a sufficient intake of carbohydrates, fat, protein, vitamins, minerals, and water. Difficulty obtaining appropriate nutrition can be a result of lack of knowledge about good nutrition, inadequate income or means of obtaining the appropriate foods, lack of socialization (which may lead to disinterest or overindulgence in food), or housing that is not adequate for storing and preparing nutritionally sound meals. The older person's diet is often lacking in calcium, vitamin C, riboflavin, niacin, and iron. A deficiency of any essential nutrient can cause changes to the body that, if left unchecked, can lead to illness.

RISK FACTORS

Anorexia (loss of appetite) is a major cause of inadequate nutritional intake in the older population. Poor dentition, poorly fitting dentures, or the lack of dentures may make it difficult for the individual to chew; and a soft or puree diet may be unappetizing. Not only may diminished mobility make it difficult for the older person to obtain and prepare food, but a sedentary lifestyle may lead to a decreased appetite. Polypharmacy, a situation not uncommon to the elderly patient, can adversely affect appetite by altering taste sensation, impairing cognition and mood, or interfering with the absorption of nutrients. Other causes of anorexia in older adults may include the increased incidence of chronic illness, social isolation, depression, and unappetizing institutional foods.

Changes in the metabolism of older people translates into changes in nutritional requirements of the body. With aging, there is a decreased metabolic rate. This means that the body requires fewer calories for maintenance. Decreased mobility and the loss of muscle mass associated with aging also suggest that older people may need to decrease their caloric consumption. However, older adults use more energy than a younger person to do the same activities. Therefore, if the individual is active, there may actually be a need to increase the caloric intake. Furthermore, with aging, the body does not metabolize protein as efficiently, so older people may need more protein in their diet.

Maintaining adequate nutrition in older persons who have a disease process poses a particular challenge to the nurse. People with advanced dementia may have weight loss even when there is an adequate intake of nutritional requirements. It is suspected that this weight loss may be due, in part, to the increased use of antibiotics in a population that tends to have a higher rate of infection. Neuroleptics, another commonly used class of drugs in the demented patient, also may cause a loss of appetite. It has been postulated that there may be a disturbance in the metabolism of patients with advanced Alzheimer's disease, and this, too, may account for the unexplained weight loss in this population. The term, "failure to thrive," has been used to describe another entity associated with weight loss. Failure to thrive occurs when some elderly nursing home residents experience a gradual decline in physical and cognitive functioning associated with weight loss, withdrawing from food, withdrawing from human contact, and exhibiting signs of depression.

Assessment

Assessing the nutritional status of the older person can be a difficult task for the nurse. The recommended daily allowance (RDA) that is established by the National Academy of Science Research Council is one way of monitoring how well an individual is meeting nutritional requirements. It is important to realize, however, that the RDA does not consider the specific needs of the population older than 65 years of age. Furthermore, additional nutrients that may be needed as a result of infection or chronic illness are not addressed by the RDA.

Further complicating the assessment for malnutrition are the changes of the aging body itself. Many of the physical manifestations of malnutrition are similar to changes that are associated with aging. These changes include dry, thin hair; dry, flaky skin; sunken eyes; dry oral mucosa; weight loss; and muscle weakness. Using skinfold measures to estimate percentage of body fat may not yield accurate information because mean body mass (muscle tissue) decreases with age. Probably the most reliable indicator of adequate nutritional intake is a normal serum albumin level (3.5 to 5.5 g/dL). Monitoring an individual's weight over time is also an appropriate means of recognizing alteration in nutritional status.

Nursing Implications. To re-establish adequate nutritional intake, health-care providers should strive to maintain oral feedings, possibly with appropriate modifications. This may mean making the diet more palatable with foods that have different textures and flavors. Providing the individual's food favorites whenever possible is also a good approach. Asking the help of family to provide favorite foods for the patient may be necessary. Making sure that the older person has dentures and that they fit well, and then providing a diet that is appropriate for the individual's dental status, is imperative. Everyone responds well to meals that are served in an attractive manner and in an environment that is relaxed and pleasant. Nursing staff should strive for this kind of atmosphere during mealtime by not raising their voices and trying to keep noisy dietary carts out of the eating area. Eyeglasses help the resident to see the food on the tray, and hearing aids allow the resident to socialize with table-mates during mealtime. It is important that the nurse make sure that the individual has whatever assistive devices are needed to make the eating experience a more pleasant one.

If, despite these efforts, the patient's nutritional status does not improve, the nurse needs to consider other interventions. It may be necessary to offer more assistance with meals. The individual may need to be fed, to have containers opened, or may just need ongoing gentle encouragement throughout the meal to continue eating. Often, gently touching the arm or shoulder while encouraging feeding helps the older adult to attend to the task of eating. Touch is a caring behavior that indicates both value and respect for the person being touched. Older people often are not touched or hugged frequently and generally respond positively to the act of being touched. A nutritional supplement also may be needed.

The dietician should assist in deciding what, if any, supplements are needed. Liquid dietary supplements are best offered between meals so that the supplement is not substituted for the meal itself. The supplement can provide a large percentage of the RDA requirements but does not completely meet all dietary requirements.

Tube feedings and parenteral feedings can be used when all other attempts at oral feedings have failed. However, these methods have numerous complications. Striving to maintain adequate oral intake should be the goal of all nursing personnel. Adequate nutrition affects every aspect of the individual's health and well-being.

▶ SLEEP PATTERN DISTURBANCES

Older people often complain of not getting enough sleep or not feeling well rested after sleeping. Indeed, sleep disturbances do increase with age. It is estimated that sleep pattern disturbances affect half of those older 65 years of age who live at home, and two thirds of those living in institutions.

NORMAL SLEEP PATTERNS

A review of normal sleep patterns is necessary to understand the changes in sleep patterns that tend to occur with aging. There are five stages to normal sleep. During stage I, the individual is just nodding off, can be easily awakened, and may still have some fleeting thoughts. During stage II, a deeper stage of relaxation occurs: some eye movement is noted through the lids, there may be some brief fragmented thoughts, and the individual can still be easily awakened. Stage III is the early stage of deep sleep. Temperature and heart rate are reduced and muscles are relaxed. The individual is more difficult to arouse. This leads to stage IV, the period of deep sleep and relaxation. This is the restorative stage of sleep, where all body functions are reduced and considerable stimulation is needed for the individual to wake up. About 45 minutes into the stage IV, the period of rapid eye movement (REM) begins. During this phase, vital signs increase and may be irregular, and the body is in an arousal state, with bursts of central nervous system activity. Dreams occur during REM sleep. It is a stage of sleep important for learning, memory, adaptation, and problem solving. It is considered the mentally restorative stage of sleep. Insufficient REM sleep can cause emotional dysfunction that may progress to psychoses. REM sleep occurs approximately every 90 minutes during the stage IV sleep.

AGE-RELATED CHANGES IN SLEEP PATTERNS

In the course of aging, people tend to sleep less than 8 hours per night. Older people have an impaired capacity to maintain sleep; therefore, sleep tends to be marked by more frequent and prolonged awakenings during the night. In addition, stage IV and REM sleep diminish. In extreme old age, changes in cerebral blood flow and organic brain syndrome also are associated with a shortening of the REM stage of sleep.

The sleep patterns of older people can be disturbed by such factors as needing to void frequently during the night (nocturia) and changes in vision and hearing that cause incorrect perceptions of their immediate environment. These changes can lead to ineffective sleep or sleep deprivation. Sleep deprivation is marked by fatigue, tiredness, eye problems, muscle tremor, muscle weakness, diminished coordination and attention span, apathy, and depression.

SLEEP DISORDERS

In addition to age-related changes in sleep patterns, there are sleep disorders that are common to older adults. Sleep apnea affects 20% of the older population. This is a medical condition in which breathing stops for 10 seconds or more, numerous times throughout the night. Sleep apnea is associated with high blood pressure, obesity, heart disease, and stroke. Death can result because of the effect on the cardiovascular and respiratory systems. The affected patient complains of excessive daytime sleepiness and constant interruption of sleep. Cessation of breathing for 10 or more seconds, followed by very loud snoring or choking, is the primary objective symptom of sleep apnea. It often is discovered first by night-shift personnel when the patient is admitted to the hospital or nursing home. The treatment for sleep apnea is usually weight reduction, continuous positive airway pressure (CPAP), oxygen, and occasionally, surgery. CPAP is a technique that forces air down the nose, through the throat, and into the lungs; it is used during sleep for those who have been diagnosed with sleep apnea.

SUNDOWN SYNDROME

Sundown syndrome is another disorder that affects many older people. Sundown syndrome is defined as the appearance or exacerbation of symptoms of confusion associated with the late afternoon or evening hours. This syndrome is marked by behaviors such as agitation, restlessness, confusion, wandering, and screaming that occur usually in the evening hours (sundown). Little is known about this disorder, which is a tremendous management problem for caregivers. Risk factors for sundown syndrome seem to be impaired mental status, dehydration, being awakened frequently during the night for nursing care, and recent relocation either to a new room or to the institution.

NURSING INTERVENTIONS

Sleeping medications, tranquilizers, and sedatives are commonly used to promote sleep but should be avoided at all costs in older persons. Sedatives and barbiturates that depress the central nervous system may lead to other problems by depressing vital body functions, lowering basal metabolic rate, decreasing blood pressure, and causing mental confusion. Sleeping medications decrease spontaneous body movements that may lead to skin breakdown. Most of the medications used to promote sleep are not efficiently metabolized by the aging body, and thus the patient may experience a hangover effect the next day. In addition, these drugs tend to cause blurred vision, dry mouth, and urinary retention. Because it is known that the aging person cannot sleep as long as younger individuals, it is unreasonable to put an individual to bed at 8 P.M. and expect that person to stay in bed until 7 A.M. the next day.

There is much the nurse can do to promote sleep without resorting to the use of medications. Meeting the individual's comfort needs by offering back rubs, snacks such as warm milk, assisting with toileting needs, providing socks or an extra blanket to increase body temperature (which may be diminished in the older person), repositioning, and alleviating pain are just a few of the nursing interventions that may reduce insomnia. If these interventions do not promote sleep, it is prudent to allow the patient to come out of the bed and perhaps sit for a while in a comfortable chair near the nurses' station. This may reassure the patient of the surroundings and prevent the individual from attempting to get out of bed unassisted, perhaps risking a fall. During the daytime, increased motor activities and time out of doors, if possible, have been found to promote sleep.

▶ IATROGENESIS

Iatrogenic disorders can be defined as those disorders that the patient acquires as a result of receiving treatment by a physician, nurse, or other member of the IDT. Iatrogenesis also can occur if the patient does not receive treatment when it is indicated, or receives incorrect treatment. The older person often presents with numerous chronic conditions that require complex interventions, numerous medications, and increased exposure to the health-care system. This puts older adults at increased risk of suffering untoward effects of medical treatment. Iatrogenic disorders include those previously discussed in this chapter: immobility, falls, incontinence, malnutrition, pressure ulcers, and disturbances in the sleep-wake cycle.

Studies have found that 30% to 40% of people older than 65 years of age suffer from iatrogenic complications. Common causes of iatrogenesis in the hospital are misuse or overuse of drugs, prolonged immobilization, nosocomial (hospital-acquired) infections, and malnutrition and dehydration secondary to preparation for diagnostic tests. In the nursing home, common iatrogenic disorders include immobilization, adverse drug reactions, falls, pressure ulcers, and nosocomial infections.

Iatrogenic disorders often cause a vicious circle in which one disorder quickly leads to another. For instance, consider the older person who is admitted to the hospital for abdominal discomfort. This person is unable to sleep and is prescribed a sleeping pill. Having taken this medication, the person is groggy when getting out of bed and sustains a fall. The staff, not wanting the patient to be hurt again, apply a restraint. The patient is now unable to get up and suffers from some of the adverse sequelae of immobility, such as incontinence, disorientation, and pressure ulcer formation. In time, the patient's muscles become deconditioned, and the next time the patient is assisted out of bed, there is another fall, the person suffers a hip fracture, and the cycle continues. One can see what a high price is paid for the negative effects of medical and nursing interventions.

▶ CONCLUSION

The health-care needs of older adults are multiple and complex. Health-care providers often are not educated in the normal aging process or the older person's response to illness and health-care interventions. As a result, the layperson as well as the health-care provider may believe that there is little that can be done to improve the health status of older adults. Not only is this not true, but this attitude can lead to a self-fulfilling prophecy in which older people are expected to be ill and to experience functional decline. In turn, assessment and interventions aimed at correcting the illness, promoting function, and averting a subsequent decline may not be initiated, and the older person is likely to become more ill and more dependent on others. Licensed practical nurses can and should play a pivotal role in ensuring that the health-care needs of the older person are being met. They also need to be aware of the problems that besiege the older person as a result of medical interventions. It is important to know that iatrogenesis can be prevented. Many of the clinical problems that the older person faces, both in health and in illness, can be averted or alleviated with nursing interventions that are focused on improving and maintaining wellness and promoting function.

CASE STUDY

Mrs. S. is an 84-year-old widow who was admitted to the hospital following a right cerebrovascular accident (CVA). Her medical history includes hypertension, atrial fibrillation, and bilateral total hip replacements due to degenerative joint disease. Before the CVA and this hospitalization, she was living in her own apartment, where she was social and able to meet her own needs except for shopping and heavy housecleaning. Her family did those things for her. When admitted to the hospital, she was found to have left-sided weakness and some speech problems, although she could be understood.

The family is planning to admit her to the nursing home; they do not know if she will be able to return to her apartment, but they are hopeful that she will be able to go to an assisted living apartment. The report given to the nursing home from the hospital includes the following facts:

- During her hospitalization she became incontinent. A Foley catheter was placed to control the urinary incontinence, but she subsequently developed a urinary tract infection, so the catheter was removed.
- She developed aspiration pneumonia, which the physician assumed was due to aspirating food because of a swallowing deficit from her stroke. Her diet was changed to puree, and she has had no further episodes of aspiration, although she is taking only about 30% of her diet.
- She has started physical therapy and has progressed from the parallel bars to short distances with a walker. She does not own a walker, so she has not walked on the unit, only in the therapy department.
- Mrs. S. has not spoken much during her hospitalization, although she follows simple directions. The nurse thinks that she "might be a little confused at times."
- Her blood pressure is well controlled with diuretics.
- The family is very concerned that if she falls, she may damage the hip replacements, and they have requested that she be restrained.

Discussion

Examine the list of facts in the case study for iatrogenic problems. How would you prevent such problems? How would you deal with them?

Solution

In this case study, there are a number of iatrogenic problems that the nursing staff should address. The report from the hospital notes that Mrs. S. had a Foley catheter inserted because she was incontinent. The question the nurse should be asking here is "Why is Mrs. S. incontinent?" True, the incontinence can be a result of damage from the stroke, but until attempts are made to take the patient to the bathroom, one cannot be certain. It may be that Mrs. S., having had a stroke that affected her speech, could not tell the staff that she needed to go. She may have to go to the bathroom as soon as the urge presents itself. A prompted voiding schedule would be helpful in beginning to assess whether this incontinence is reversible. A Foley catheter should not be the first intervention used in the presence of incontinence. In this case, the use of the catheter prolonged the hospitalization by causing a urinary tract infection.

Another possible iatrogenic problem may be aspiration pneumonia. In this case, iatrogenesis may be a result of something that should have been done that was not done. In a patient who has had a stroke and who has difficulty talking, one should consider the possibility of a swallowing deficit. Therefore, a patient, such as Mrs. S., should never be left alone to eat. In addition, the nursing staff should be assessing her during mealtime for any difficulty swallowing. If a difficulty is noted, a speech and swallowing consultation is warranted. Once the diet was changed to puree, Mrs. S. apparently had no further problems with swallowing but had a decreased nutritional intake. Again, the nurse needs to assess the patient to understand why the diet is not being taken. There may be a number of reasons: The patient may not like her diet, she may still be having difficulty swallowing and is afraid of choking again, or she may be depressed and without an appetite.

It is indeed a positive step that Mrs. S. has been started on physical therapy and is walking, but there is more that the nursing and therapy staffs can do to promote functional ambulation. Walking does not have to be done just in the therapy department. The therapist needs to lend a walker to Mrs. S. or to instruct the family to buy one for her so that ambulation can be done on the nursing unit. Therapy takes place for only about 1 hour a day. Walking the patient on the unit augments therapy, improves the patient's gait, helps her to regain her confidence in her functional ability, and prevents the negative effects of immobility.

The nurse reports that Mrs. S. might be confused; however, there is little evidence here to support that conclusion or to suggest that confusion should be expected. From the report, Mrs. S. was not confused before her hospitalization. If she is confused, it may be related to the urinary tract infection, the pneumonia, the relocation to the hospital, or the depression from the stroke. The possibility of confusion should not deter the nurse in any way from pursuing a plan of care that focuses on promoting the highest level of functional ability for this patient.

The family requests that Mrs. S. be restrained to prevent injury to her hip replacements. Instead of a restraint, the staff needs to consider ways of preventing a fall so that the family will not believe that a restraint is needed. Some possible fall prevention interventions might include helping the patient to understand her limitations, toileting the patient at regular intervals, promoting lower extremity strengthening through exercise, keeping the patient out of her room and within sight of the staff, and perhaps using an alarm if the patient is unpredictable in her attempts to get up. Because Mrs. S. is on diuretics, one would want to assess her for orthostatic hypotension as a possible fall risk factor. Honoring the family's request for a restraint may serve only to cause contractures, skin breakdown, a worsening of her urinary incontinence, depression, and general deconditioning related to immobility. The family needs to be educated to the dangers of using restraints. The use of restraints will not promote a positive outcome for this patient.

STUDY QUESTIONS

Please select the one best answer.

1. An example of an intrinsic risk factor for falls in the older person is:
   a. The use of diuretics
   b. Weakened muscles in the lower extremities
   c. Glaring lights in the hallway
   d. The use of a cane

2. To promote mobility in the older adult, the nurse would:
   a. Turn the patient every 2 hours
   b. Encourage the patient to cough and take deep breaths
   c. Ask the family to bring in the patient's walker from home
   d. Assume that the physical therapist is helping the patient to walk

3. The best way to promote urinary continence in the older person is to:
   a. Stop giving the diuretic because it causes the patient to have urinary urgency
   b. Obtain a urine specimen for culture and sensitivity
   c. Offer the bedpan every 2 hours
   d. Assist the patient to the toilet in the morning, after meals, and at bedtime

4. When seeing a reddened area on the patient's coccyx, the nurse would do all but one of the following interventions:
   a. Turn the patient every 2 hours
   b. Ask the doctor to order a medication to treat the skin
   c. Help the patient to the toilet more frequently
   d. Measure how much of the diet the patient is taking every day

5. Which of the following is not an example of an iatrogenic disorder?
   a. Falling because of dizziness after receiving mediation for pain relief
   b. Depression because of a stroke
   c. Incontinence because the patient could not find the bathroom
   d. Loss of weight because the patient cannot chew the food that is provided

Jeanne Robertson Samter

chapter **12**

Psychological Assessment

Learning Objectives

After completing this chapter, the student will be able to:

1. Identify three cognitive functions.
2. Describe two benefits of using a standardized examination to screen for cognitive functioning.
3. Identify four uses of psychological assessments.
4. Describe the impact of depression on the mental status score.

▶ INTRODUCTION

Psychological assessments are essential tools in identifying the mental health of older adults in all health-care settings. Such assessments provide the basis for determining how much of a return to normal an individual can expect to achieve. Psychological assessments are important in any health-care setting, but especially when the focus is restorative care.

Restorative care, in its truest application, requires a body-mind-spirit connection. Relate this concept to Jean Watson's theory of caring—the two theories are conceptually the same, and it is hoped that they are beginning to have meaning for you in your practice. Nurses practicing within this framework are concerned with the physical indications that a person is declining such as falls, incontinence, and immobility. Behavioral, or psychological, indicators have received less prominence in terms of restorative care. Some examples are failure to eat and a decline in functional level, such as severe memory loss or confusion without a physiological basis.

Although one can expect a certain amount of decline in older people who have vascular and central nervous system (CNS) disease, it is important to identify the psychological areas of decline and recognize when interventions are essential. Maintenance of mental health and cognitive functioning is as important to restorative care as is maintenance of physiological processes. Nurses working with elderly people need to understand basic concepts of mental health and cognitive function so they can participate in the older adult's care more effectively. Assessment tools provide a brief, methodical approach to noting changes commonly found in individuals with cerebrovascular diseases, delirium, and dementia disorders.

▶ MENTAL HEALTH

Over the years, clinicians in the field of mental health have tried to diagnose symptoms, traits, and patterns of behavior that identify disease. The view that identification and treatment of disease establishes health is known as the medical model. The simplest definition of mental health, then, would be the absence of identifiable disease. A more positive approach is to define the traits of the mentally healthy personality.

Practitioners use terms that have been formulated by theorists to describe and discuss psychological problems. Words such as *id*, *ego*, and *superego* are used by therapists who base their practice on Sigmund Freud's theory. *Enmeshment* is a term used by some family therapists to describe interactions among family members that keep them dependent on each other. A therapist practicing within a Gestalt framework may focus on the feeling experiences of an individual.

The current trend is to identify wellness in mental health. Although it is difficult to define wellness, some of its characteristics have been described by psychologists, nurses, and physicians. Some of these characteristics are given in the following list:

- A clear meaning and purpose in life
- A strong reality orientation
- An ability to cope creatively with life's situations
- A capability for open, creative relationships

Mental health is not necessarily a product of good nurturing or of a life of positive experiences. There are individuals who function well in life, for example, they maintain a satisfying job and career, have a family, and make a contribution to their community, despite poor nurturing and environmental handicaps. Most views of mental health now embody a continuum of health and illness. This continuum is dynamic rather than static. There are a number of situations that have an impact on the functioning of an individual. These situations include the following:

- The death of someone close
- Unemployment
- The birth of a child
- Relocation

Any individual, if sufficiently stressed, can demonstrate some signs of impairment. One concept refers to the continuum of functioning as a scale of the differences in people. Individuals higher on this scale require more stressors to impair their functioning than individuals lower on this scale. These individuals choose a life course based on thought and conviction rather than on impulse, and they show an ability to stand by a belief that is different from that of their peer group.

It is important for nurses working in the field of gerontology to identify and promote positive mental health traits. Nurses can then reinforce healthy traits and interactions in older persons. This is nursing care being given in the nursing model (Watson's theory) rather than the medical model. Because it is nursing model care, it is both caring and holistic, which are strong traits of the profession of nursing, and characteristics you want to work to develop as a licensed practical nurse (LPN).

COGNITION

Cognition is a mental activity concerned with processing information. It refers to a broad range of mental behaviors, including awareness, thinking, reasoning, and judgment. This process is very complex and involves a number of abilities or functions. Because it cannot be directly observed, many psychologists define cognition in terms of cognitive functions. There are a number of ways of conceptualizing the cognitive functions. One scientist's definition is perceiving, thinking, remembering, communicating, orienting, calculating, and problem solving.

Memory

In general, the more active people have been, the better their overall memory is as they age. A dysfunction in memory occurs in almost all of the cognitive disorders common in the older adults. Generally, psychologists refer to two categories of memory, short-term memory (STM) and long-term memory (LTM). The time interval for measuring STM is seconds, whereas for LTM it is minutes and beyond. Recently, there has been an interest in the study of very remote memory. Many elderly persons demonstrate excellent long-term recall, although this recall may be rooted more in a belief than in fact. This means that the stories they tell of their childhood or young adulthood are stories based on their belief systems rather than on what actually happened. This skill may be enchanting to staff and can be used effectively as a tool for reminiscence to strengthen a person's self-esteem.

Memory functions are extremely important to a person's ability to think. A deficit in STM means that a person is unable to recall some of today's events. An older adult with severe impairment of STM experiences the routine of each day as a new experience. Such a person is trapped in an endless cycle of requesting basic information about the environment from strangers, such as "Where is my room?"; "When do we eat?"

Memory impairment limits the ability of a person to form a new idea or relate one fact with another. It is nearly impossible for memory-impaired individuals to organize new information into categories. A place where one can put something (a pair of glasses) for safe keeping may change several times a day. This makes a never-ending search for an important item an everyday event.

Screening for memory impairment is the most important part of any assessment for the elderly. The loss of STM is the first symptom of Alzheimer's disease. A stroke also may impair memory function, but in this case, the type and extent of impairment depend on the loca-

Reminiscence is an excellent tool to use to strengthen the resident's self-esteem.

tion of the damage. Other STM deficits may be due to depression. Individuals suffering from depression are inattentive to their environment. They often are preoccupied or self-absorbed. A decline in STM, then, is an important finding on assessment and should prompt further investigation.

Perception

Psychologists believe that all behavior depends on how one sees one's self, the situation one is in, and the interaction between the two. Behavior changes as individuals become aware of details in their surroundings. Learning, problem solving, remembering, and forgetting are all part of one's awareness of the environment. Effective communication with an older person depends on the nurse's ability to understand the perceptual world of that person. With such an understanding, the most bizarre behavior often becomes comprehensible.

The first phase of forming a perception is the ability to use the five senses to collect information about the environment. Frequently, in older adults, there are real impairments in the sense organs. In the previous chapter, you learned about the deficits in vision, hearing, touch, taste, and smell in older persons.

There is an emotional or feeling component to perception as well. Individuals take in information from the environment and form opinions about such information. Perceptions are normally evaluated against past experiences. An older adult may compare a meal eaten within the institutional setting with recollections of meals eaten with the person's own family. These recollections of past experiences are a part of forming perceptions.

Perceptual distortions also are known as hallucinations and delusional thinking. Although both may indicate a psychiatric illness in younger individuals, perceptual distortions are common in dementing illnesses. Impaired memory and a natural distrust of a strange environment exaggerate this tendency in the institutionalized older person.

Orientation

Orientation refers to a person's awareness of self in the context of a particular time and place. Tests for orientation determine whether

the persons being tested know their names, where they are, and the approximate time of day. Sometimes the expression "oriented times three" is used to indicate that an individual's orientation to time, place, and person is correct. Assessment of orientation is covered on every mental status examination. This is important information because a disturbance in orientation is one of the most frequent symptoms of brain disease. Awareness of time and place requires that individuals know where they are and can remember it. In this way, individuals keep in touch with ongoing history. Orientation depends on a person's ability to link each minute with the previous minute. Disorientation with respect to time is the first major confusion to occur as a result of dementia. Loss of a sense of place is likely to follow. Last, the person loses the ability to recognize other people and eventually cannot remember who he or she is.

Thinking

Every area of the brain is involved in the mental operation of thinking. The ancient Greeks believed there were "higher" levels and "lower" levels of thinking, a distinction that is still relevant. Higher-level thinking includes the ability to form concepts and think in an abstract manner. Asking a patient to interpret a proverb tests the patient's ability to think abstractly. If a person interprets the proverb "a stitch in time saves nine" in a way that conveys that prompt attention to a problem prevents trouble in the future, the person's ability to abstract think is considered intact. A concrete interpretation adheres closely to the exact meaning of the phrase. Concrete thinking is a "lower" mental ability. Someone with concrete thinking may answer the question about the proverb with something like, "If I make nine stitches, the cloth will hold."

Thinking processes have a hierarchical order. The lower mental abilities are more enduring and less affected by brain injuries and disease processes. The higher levels of thinking tend to be more fragile. At first glance, interpreting proverbs may seem a bit removed from a person's ability to function in the real world. The use of good judgment, the ability to think abstractly, and the capacity to reason, however, are higher-level abilities that indicate the difference between independent and supervised living. To some extent, these abilities can be determined by proverb interpretation. In general, tests for abstract thinking are not included as part of the short tests of mental function.

Communicating

The only vehicle for viewing thinking processes in an individual is communication. People understand human thought when it is reflected in language. It is important to assess language problems because they are common in cerebrovascular and dementing disorders. Assessment of communication patterns, word order, and the general sense of a sentence provide a window into the dementia process. This is especially true with the patient who has experienced a stroke. Sometimes, patients who have had a stroke will have severe problems with communication. Small connecting words such as "if," "and," and "but," are missing. There are also several types of aphasia that impair an individual's ability to communicate.

Calculating

Calculating is a cognitive function that must be assessed carefully in terms of the person's intelligence and educational level. Poor performance may indicate dementia or delirium, anxiety, or depression. Serial 7s is one test that can determine a person's ability to calculate. The person is asked to subtract 7 from 100 and then to subtract 7 from that remainder, continuing five times. A nurse interviewed a moderately to severely impaired patient with Alzheimer's disease. Although the patient was completely disoriented with regard to time and place and could not recall the names of three objects even seconds after they were told to him, he performed magnificently with the serial 7 calculations. In seconds he completed the operation, then turned to the nurse, announcing proudly that mathematics was always his favorite subject. The patient had been a judge.

CRITICALLY EXAMINE THE FOLLOWING:

Whenever you are asked to complete this type of exercise, you are asked to think on a higher level. Has it seemed that way to you? Think back to your reactions in doing the critical thinking assignments. Did you avoid doing some? Were you irritated or upset at any of the assignments? Did you enjoy the challenge of doing them? Were you bored with them, and saw them as not being a challenge? Take some time and consider your reactions to these assignments. Consider how you felt when certain items were discussed in class. Did you benefit from the thinking of your classmates? Were your ideas and thinking valued by others? Take the time to write your reactions regarding the higher-level thinking experiences. Be prepared to share them in class.

Problem Solving

Problem-solving skills are essential to an individual's ability to function in any environment. Even some very demented people can demonstrate aspects of problem-solving ability. Individuals in the early stages of Alzheimer's disease frequently make lists. Lists are coping devices that enable the recall of event sequences. When asked questions of orientation, some elders search for familiar cues in the environment. Examples of this behavior include the patient who was asked the date, spied a newspaper, then winked, and smiling broadly gave the correct answer. Another patient called to a nursing assistant passing by the door. When the nursing assistant entered the room, the patient asked her for the date and promptly relayed this information to the nurse interviewer.

A individual's environment is filled with a multitude of clues that facilitate orientation, aid a failing memory, and maintain a stable perceptual field. Use of these clues enables older adults to maintain communication with nurses, other patients, and families. Because a patient's environment is rich with problem-solving clues, room changes and unit changes should be made infrequently and only after the most careful thought.

▶ ASSESSMENT TOOLS AND HOW TO USE THEM

Mental status examinations are the most frequently used psychological assessments. Mental status assessment includes probing of the cognitive functions as well as level of consciousness (LOC). In selecting a tool, it is important to remember that examinations with brief instruments are generally better tolerated by the elderly person. A short examination is much less tiring for an older person to sit through than a lengthy one. No brief instrument, however, is a perfect detector of cognitive impairment.

Screening tools initially may seem intimidating or cumbersome to use in clinical practice. Most tools are short and can be easily committed to memory after using them a few times. All of the following tests are easy to learn and administer: Pfeiffer's Short Portable Mental Status Questionnaire (SPMSQ; Pfeiffer, 1975), Folstein's Mini-Mental Status Exam (MMSE; Folstein, Folstein, & McHugh, 1975),

Kahn's Mental Status Questionnaire (MSQ; Kahn, Goldfarb, Pollak, & Peck, 1960), Jacobs' Cognitive Capacity Screening Exam (CCSE: Jacobs, Bernhard, Delgado, & Strain, 1977), and Kiernan's Neurobehavioral Cognitive Examination (NCSE; Kiernan, Mueller, Langston, & Vandyke, 1987). These scales are compared in Table 12.1 and are listed with a brief description in Box 12.1.

A very important factor to consider in the scoring of all tests is that test results are influenced by the educational level of the person being tested. An older adult with a lack of a formal education can score several points lower than an older person with greater deficits but more education. Some of the mental status tests have a method of scoring to correct for education.

There are some important reasons for an LPN to gain skills in using assessment tools. A standardized test allows you, as the caregiver, to collect pertinent information in a short period of time. The collection of this information is organized and methodical. The initial test establishes a baseline and allows for comparison of changes over time.

MEMORY

Assessing memory functions is the most important assessment in working with cognitively impaired older adults. There are three steps in the memory process. Each step needs accurate assessment. The first step is reception (encoding), followed by storage (retention), and finally, retrieval (recall). Folstein's MMSE tests memory by asking the older adult to repeat three words after the nurse for three times, for example, apple, ball, and lamp. The number of trials it takes for the older person to recall the three items is noted. Immediate repetition enables the nurse to determine whether the person has heard the three words correctly. Once the older adult repeats them accurately, the nurse requests that the person remember them. In 5 minutes, the nurse asks again for the older adult to recall the three objects. Each item recalled is given a score of 1.

ORIENTATION

All short mental status examinations include questions about orientation. Time orientation is tested by asking for the date (day, month, year, and day of the week) and the time of day. Because older adults often become quite skilled in using clues from the environment, it is important to remove newspapers or calendars that may help them find the answer. An older adult can sometimes have an accurate sense of time passing yet may not remember the exact date. The nurse may ask questions such as "How long has it been since you last saw me?" or "What was your last meal?"

Assessment of orientation in place generally begins with questions about the name or location of the place in which the person is being examined. You, as the LPN, need to determine whether patients know the kind of place they are in, for example, a nursing home or hospital. Short mental status examinations ask questions about the state, county, or country of residence. Many moderately to severely demented people are not able to recall places. It may be more functional to question an older adult regarding the location of the bedroom or the dining room, for example, "Can you tell me where your room is?"

LEVEL OF CONSCIOUSNESS

The determination of a person's LOC is an important assessment to make in the event of delirium or a head injury. Folstein's MMSE is one tool that screens for LOC. It is important for the nurse to know the four levels of consciousness and to be able to define each in behavioral terms. The first level is *alert*, which means that the person is awake and responding in an appropriate manner. The next level is *lethargic*. A person is lethargic when the individual can be aroused and, once aroused, responds in an appropriate manner and with an orientation that is consistent. The third LOC is *stuporous*. If a person can be aroused but responds inappropriately when aroused and then returns to sleep when the stimulus is stopped, the person is stuporous. This response may be the initial phase of a delirium. *Comatose* is the fourth level. A person who is comatose does not respond to any stimulus except deep pain.

BOX 12.1. BRIEF DESCRIPTION OF COMMON SCREENING TOOLS

The MMSE was developed by Folstein to be used with medical and psychiatric patients. Scores in the range of 9 to 12 indicate a high likelihood of dementia. Scores of 25 and higher are considered normal.

The SPMSQ was developed by Pfeiffer. This test is a little quicker to administer than Folstein's MMSE. Questions of orientation and memory are addressed and there is one question concerning calculation. LOC is not assessed. An advantage over the MMSE, however, is that there are specific directions for scoring this test so as to correct for education and race. A test score of 8 to 10 indicates severe intellectual impairment; 5 to 7, moderate impairment; 3 to 4, mild impairment; 0 to 2, intact status.

The MSQ was developed by Kahn. This questionnaire has two versions: one for the institutionalized elderly patients and the other for use with adults in the community. Five or more errors indicate severe impairment, 3 to 5 errors indicate some impairment, and fewer than 2 errors indicates no impairment.

The CCSE was developed by Jacobs. This mental status questionnaire was adapted specifically to diagnose diffuse organic mental syndromes on busy medical wards. A score of less than 20 indicates diminished cognitive capacity.

The NCSE was developed by Kiernan for use with behaviorally disturbed adults in acute diagnostic units. This test differs from the others in that it has two separate scores. One score is given for LOC, orientation, and attention. Another score is given for language, construction, memory, calculations, and reasoning. The two separate scores enable clinicians to differentiate areas of impairment more clearly. This examination is two pages long, with directions to the clinician on how to administer it. It can be completed in 5 minutes by nonimpaired patients and by most patients with impairments in 20 minutes.

	NCSE	KAHN	SPMSQ	MMSE	CCSE
Level of consciousness (LOC)	X			X	X
Cognitive functions					
Remembering	X	X	X	X	X
Communicating	X			X	
Problem solving					
Perceiving					
Thinking	X				X
Orienting	X	X	X	X	X
Calculating	X	X	X	X	X
Corrects for education and culture		X	X		X
Number of questions	2 PG	10	10	30	30
Time required (minutes)	5–20	5	5	10	10

Source: Gurland B. J. (1987). The assessment of cognitive function in the elderly. *Clinical Geriatric Medicine, 3,* 53–63. CCSE = Cognitive Capacity Screening Exam; MMSE = Mini–Mental Status Exam; NCSE = Neurobehavioral Cognitive Status Exam; SPMSQ = Short Portable Mental Status Questionnaire; SQ = Mental Status Questionnaire.

DELIRIUM AND THE MENTAL STATUS EXAMINATION

Nurses sometimes have a difficult time recognizing delirium. Sudden onset is the most significant feature described by experts. Older individuals, however, may develop a delirium gradually, over the course of 2 or 3 days. One sign is a fluctuating LOC. This can vary from mild confusion to stupor in an active delirium, which is frequently characterized by visual hallucinations. A nursing home resident was being assessed for delirium by the nurse. The resident, who was talking about snakes in her bed, suddenly stopped and turned to the nurse. "Your hands are very chapped, she said. "You should use gloves to do your housework. I always did." Then the resident returned to her delirious state.

Another feature of delirium is disorientation. One person may be mistaken for another. Sometimes an older adult imagines being at home or in another location. Other cognitive functions may become impaired. There also may be a disturbance in the sleep cycle. Many delirious elders are awake all night and then sleep during the day.

VALIDITY AND RELIABILITY OF ASSESSMENT SCALES

Whenever a questionnaire is used in any clinical setting, psychologists are concerned about two questions: validity and reliability. Is the test question a valid question? For example, does the question really measure memory, or orientation, or thinking? Validity is determined by the agreement reached by a panel of individuals who are experts in the content of the particular test questions used. The more experts are involved in designing the process, the greater the validity of the test questions. Reliability is concerned with consistency. Will two nurses, each asking the same person the same questions, get the same answers? When the answer to this question is "yes," the test questions are reliable. All standard mental status questionnaires considered in this chapter are valid and reliable instruments. They have been used by a variety of experts for a number of years with consistent results.

Because rating scales are designed to collect standard information about older persons in a methodical way, nurses should review the methods of using the rating scales together. This practice ensures that information is gathered in the same way. One nurse can interview an older adult while another nurse observes. Then they can reverse roles and compare the answers they received. Some experts recommend continuing this technique with 10 patients or until 80% of the ratings are the same.

► WHEN TO ASSESS

Many hospitals and nursing homes use some sort of standard mental status examination to screen for gross impairments on admission. This is an excellent practice. Although some initial confusion, agitation, or depression is often seen in older adults who are newly admitted because of transitional stress, this practice, if consistently done, helps staff to get a baseline of the person's overall cognitive function. The assessment can be repeated if the older adult demonstrates acute changes in behavior, mental status, or functional level, for example, if there is a decline in activities of daily living (ADLs). Although screening tools are not diagnostic, that is, they do not point out the exact nature of the problem, they do show, in a factual way, specific areas that have changed.

▶ ASSESSMENT TECHNIQUES

Older adults generally remain cooperative unless they perceive the questions asked as challenging their mental competence. Catastrophic reactions such as screaming or leaving the room angry can be precipitated when a person is pushed to perform beyond the person's competency. An older adult's refusal to answer questions should be accepted. This information in itself is significant. Older person's, aware of their cognitive impairments, may become defensive when their vulnerabilities are exposed. Attention to the following factors promotes the success of the psychological assessment.

TIMING

The timing of an interview is an important factor in determining success. Regular staff, especially primary nursing assistants in the nursing home setting, are especially skilled in knowing the best time to interview a resident. Allowing an older person to select a time may be the most effective way to gain cooperation.

PRIVACY

Privacy is very important. Questions, which to caregivers may seem routine, are often considered deeply revealing and very personal to older persons. All interviews should be conducted in the person's room or a location that ensures confidentiality.

ELIMINATION OF INTERRUPTIONS

Interruptions undermine the importance of psychological assessments. They negatively affect a person's attention span, and they distract the nurse from focusing on the person being interviewed. Some interruptions are beyond your control as the nurse and occur regardless of the precautions taken. Reasonable efforts should be made to eliminate as many interruptions as possible, because they have an impact on the reliability and validity of the assessment.

POSITIVE INTRODUCTION OF THE ASSESSMENT

Introducing the psychological assessment in a positive and respectful manner is useful. Describing the test as "a lot of silly questions" may prompt the response that "If they are so silly, why should I answer them?" Let the older adult know that the information gained from this assessment will help the nurses in planning and giving care.

▶ WHAT TO DO WITH THE ASSESSMENT INFORMATION

All information obtained from the older person must be used on the individual's behalf. This information should be dated and appear in an accessible place on the chart with a notation that this document must remain on the chart. In general, assessment information is not updated unless a client demonstrates a behavioral problem or has a marked decline in functional level.

APPLICATIONS IN CLINICAL PRACTICE

In the hospital or nursing home, psychological assessments may be used as one of the factors determining the unit assignment of a new patient/resident on admission. They contribute to the identification of the person's strengths and potentials. When used in conjunction with the person's ability to perform ADLs, psychological assessments may point out the need for psychiatric evaluation. When a person's mental functioning appears much lower than the score of a psychological assessment might indicate, a mental illness is suspected.

Psychological assessments can be used as a basis for care planning. This is especially important when an older adult's social graces lead staff to the conclusion that the person is functioning at a higher level than is the case. Many individuals with a dementing process learn strategies to cover for losses in cognition. They may rely on list making, props in the environment, and social cues from others. Staff sometimes can make excessive demands on older persons if they are unaware of cognitive deficits.

Psychological assessments can allow a broad determination of the effects of an intervention. For example, a person with sadness, who wishes to die, may be treated with an antidepressant. Effective treatment may enhance the abilities of depressed older persons to attend to their environment, thereby improving memory and perception. On the mental status examination, such people may achieve higher scores in the area of recall. This information is useful to a consultant when a more extensive evaluation is considered necessary. It is helpful to be able to tell a consultant that an older adult has dropped four points on Folstein's MMSE because the examination was conducted 6 months earlier. It also is useful to note the specific area of decline, for instance, the area of decline is in orientation to time and place or in immediate recall.

Older adults vary greatly in symptom severity and the rate of progression. Although in the later stages of dementia, older persons present very much the same regardless of disease process, the initial symptoms may clearly demonstrate one disease over another. For example, the initial symptom of Alzheimer's disease is the gradual progressive decline in the ability to learn new information. The most significant early symptom of Pick's disease is a change in personality. This is an important distinction.

Therefore, symptoms of dementia are a moving target that must be tracked. The tracking is done by frequent, well-recorded assessments. If an assessment tool has been used to establish a baseline in the early stages of the disease process, it may contribute to the diagnostic process.

▶ OTHER ASSESSMENTS

ASSESSING DEPRESSION

Although recent research indicates that depression is no more prevalent in older people than it is in younger people, its manifestation is different and, therefore, difficult to identify. It is important for you, as the nurse, to gain skill in the assessment of depression because of your focus on the quality of life for all people. There is a heavy emotional cost to depression that ultimately affects the immune system. This can lead to cancer and other physical illnesses as well as infections.

Depression, therefore, predicts the onset of disability almost as powerfully as disability predicts depression. Older individuals who are depressed are in a high-risk category for institutionalization because they are less motivated to care for their personal hygiene and nutrition. This increases their vulnerability to disease. Depressed individuals are frequently withdrawn and socially isolated, so they have weak support systems. The path to a nursing home for these individuals is apt to be very short and direct.

It is a fact that people older than 65 years of age are beginning to face some significant losses: economic, vocational, family supports, and friendships. Physical disabilities, however, are frequently viewed as the beginning of the end. "If you have your health, you have everything," one grandmother reports. The loss of health signals a life of dependency for most older adults.

Generally, the most impressive feature of depression is an unpleasant mood. To psychiatrists, the term *clinical depression* refers to a cluster of specific symptoms. These symptoms are clearly defined in a diagnostic manual called the *Diagnostic and Statistical Manual* (DSM-IV) (1994) and must be present for a specified duration. Depression may be chronic or acute, and the symptoms may vary in intensity as well. Severe depression is thought to impair cognitive functioning at any age. Memory seems to be the function most influenced by a depressed mood, but there are many ways that memory can be affected. For example, information committed to memory when a person is depressed is likely to be biased. Other clinicians focus on the ability or lack of ability of older adults to attend to their environment as the indicator of a depression. Methods for the identification of depression in the elderly population are controversial. Use your own skills and life experience to process the responses of the older adult you are interviewing to try to identify expressions or behaviors of depression. Report your results to the registered nurse (RN).

ASSESSING PAIN

Chronic pain may leave a person totally fatigued and unable to participate properly in a restorative care program. In addition, some behavioral problems in institutionalized older adults stem from ineffective pain management. A psychiatric evaluation may be

Pain assessment in the elderly population is a demanding and necessary skill.

requested for screaming or abusive behavior on the part of a resident of a nursing home who, in fact is simply experiencing pain. A failure to identify pain as a factor affecting behavior and function may result in poor medical management.

Pain in older people is frequently either over- or undertreated simply because it is difficult to assess. Some older adults want every ache treated with a drug, whereas others maintain a stoic attitude: "Why bother? There is nothing that can be done, anyway." Often, older people perceive pain differently. In fact, some pain receptors may not be as acute as they were in the past. Medical journals document clinical cases describing "silent" myocardial infarctions or "painless" intra-abdominal emergencies. These cases may not, in fact, be silent or painless but may reflect an older person's normal aging situation.

Some barriers to pain assessment are cognitive impairments, delirium, and dementia. People who have a dementia process or a stroke and became aphasic may be unable to give an accurate pain history. They may not be able to describe when the pain started or at what point in the day the pain becomes most severe. Most people describe the pain in the here and now.

A person in pain is often self-absorbed and inattentive to activities in the environment. Because pain frequently leads to depression, the mental status examination score may demonstrate a decline in recall.

Delirium may be one manifestation of an attempt to treat a person's pain. An assessment for delirium should be made whenever there is a change in the LOC after the start of any new drug, particularly a pain medication. A sensitivity to medications that results in delirium makes pain management difficult.

Multiple chronic disease processes as well as acute diagnoses compound the difficulty. There even may be an acute exacerbation of a chronic problem. These multiple sources of pain make diagnosis difficult, and pain management becomes a challenge.

MYTHS OF PAIN

One of the myths regarding pain in older adults is that pain is normal. As body systems begin to wear out, one might expect an increase in pain. Pain, at any age, however, is the most common symptom of a disease process and should be investigated and treated.

Another myth is that pain and sleep are incompatible. Nurses often disbelieve a patient's complaint of pain when they bring a pain pill and find the person asleep. The wrong conclusion is drawn. It is believed that an individual really in pain could not possibly sleep. The exhaustive feature of pain, however, is seldom considered in the assessment process.

The last myth is that narcotic drugs are not safe for older people. Narcotics provide effective pain relief for some chronic conditions and terminal illnesses. These drugs should be used on a scheduled basis, for example, every 4 hours or every 6 hours. Use of a narcotic on an "as needed" basis does not provide effective pain management. Some nurses believe that narcotics dull an older person's LOC. They fear that an older adult will not be able to benefit from the support of family or friends in the time remaining before death. Effective relief of pain actually promotes interaction, and the initial drowsiness soon wears off.

Methods of Assessment

Although pain is a highly subjective experience, there are two methods for assessing it. Simple observation from a nurse, who knows the person well, can be very effective. A grimace or clutch of the chest provides a vivid picture of pain. Assessment questions may follow these observations. There are clinical practice guidelines for acute pain management that identify the quantifiable measures of pain that should be considered in an assessment. These measures include the intensity of the pain, the duration of the pain, the quality of the pain, and the personal meaning this pain has to the older adult. Also included is the impact on the person's functioning.

Assessment tools are available. A good tool addresses the older person's pain history and coping strategies for dealing with pain, as well as medications in the past that have been effective. It is important to ask questions that help to describe or define the pain. Noting the intensity and duration assists in providing an objective measure to a highly subjective experience. Simply asking "How is your pain today?" may prompt the response "Well, it is there."

The simplest method of pain assessment is the use of a pain intensity scale. You, as the nurse, can draw a line indicating that the far left (L) end of the line defines no pain and the right (R) end represents the most pain the person has ever experienced. The person can point to the place on the line that reflects current pain level.

▶ SUMMARY

Observations of a person's behavior and functional status are subjective and often inconsistently reported. It is difficult to get a clear idea of decline or progress over time without some objective measures. Psychological assessments and other assessment tools provide the means for collecting factual information about older adults.

Brief mental status examinations universally identify assessments of memory and orientation as the two features that provide the most information about an individual's cognitive functions. Assessments help establish a person's baseline functioning. They can be used to establish a diagnosis, plan care, and evaluate treatment efforts. Psychological assessments also enable the nurse to define problem areas in a more specific manner to consultants. Older adults cooperate well with assessments if the nurse is sensitive to timing, respects the person's privacy, limits interruptions, and presents the assessment tool in a positive manner. Other assessments that can provide important information in planning care are those that assess depression and pain.

▶ CONCLUSION

Many institutionalized elderly patients are all too aware of their declining abilities. These losses have a dynamic impact on their self-concept. A life once vital and central to a young family now does not seem worth the effort to maintain. A lowered self-concept and diminished self-esteem complete the picture of physical decline. The process can become circular without the intervention of a caring and knowledgeable staff.

The performance level of most individuals improves in a supportive environment. Therefore, recognition and reinforcement, both of cognitive skills and abilities, and of attributes of mental health can positively affect restorative care efforts. Nurses who consistently identify strengths in a factual way are instrumental in improving the quality of life for older adults In their care.

CASE STUDY

Ms. F. is 81 years old. She had a long career with the government that involved traveling all over the world. Although she never married, she is a devoted aunt and a vital member of her extended family. She is the youngest of three siblings. Her two older brothers live in New York and California. Despite the distance, the three communicate regularly through letters and telephone calls. Nieces and nephews are always attentive to Ms. F. She never spends a holiday alone.

The retirement years for Ms. F. became the highlight of her life. She continued her travels, sometimes with friends and at other times with a niece or nephew.

Only one problem seemed to dampen Ms. F.'s life. In her middle years, every once in a while (3–5 years), she became depressed, or "blue" as she describes it. Two episodes she "toughed out" on her own. Although she continued to function in her job, her appetite diminished. She woke up at 3:00 A.M. on most days and had no energy to do much of anything. In a couple of months, the blueness lifted, and she returned to the good life. These periods seemed to have no precipitating event. She saw a psychiatrist for the first time when she was 54 years old. He prescribed an antidepressant, nortriptyline (Pamelor). This medication was successful in treating the depression. After 6 months, the medication and brief therapy were stopped. She did quite well in the following years.

When she was 78 years old, Ms. F. made the decision to come to a nursing home. Her family thought she was having some minor problems with memory. Although she denied feeling depressed, she noticed a real decline in her energy level and ability to do for herself. She was placed on a unit with other residents who functioned independently. A niece came to help her decorate her room. Whatnots displayed unique treasures from a life of travel.

Based on this information, answer the following question:

1. With respect to the administration of the mental status examination, the charge nurse decided:
   a. Not to give the examination. It would be insulting to Ms. F. to be questioned in such a way.
   b. To check with Ms. F. regarding a good time to conduct some routine admission assessments, which would include the MMSE.
   c. That Ms. F. was doing so well there was no need for such a test.
   d. To ask the social worker to conduct this examination in a few weeks after the resident had adjusted better.

Ms. F. was a trim woman and her clothing was exquisite. From the start, the other residents seemed to respect her. Although she did not become a member of one of the unit cliques, there was no one who did not accept her and welcome her company when she sat down. Her admission MMSE score was 29/30. She was unable to recall one object after 5 minutes.

A few months after admission, some of the residents began to remark to the staff that Ms. F. was ignoring some of their efforts to engage her in a conversation. She started retreating to her room a little more. In general, she seemed more withdrawn. She favored a chair off to herself rather than an available seat in a group of other residents.

Based on this information, answer the following question:

2. The charge nurse was concerned. She went to visit Ms. F. in her room. The two problems the charge nurse was assessing in this interview were:
   a. Delirium and dementia
   b. Depression and dementia
   c. Depression and hearing loss
   d. Depression and possible delirium

Ms. F. was a little vain and disclosed to the charge nurse during this interview that her hearing was not what it used to be. "I don't want to wear a hearing aid," she said. The charge nurse convinced Ms. F. that a routine audiology appointment might be useful.

She was scheduled for a clinic appointment the following week. She had a great deal of wax buildup that was interfering with her hearing. When the wax was removed, her hearing improved, but the audiologist convinced her that a hearing aid would be most beneficial and told her," It's an attractive device and can be made to fit your glasses." The persuading force was Ms. F.'s love for classical music. Clearly, she had not been able to enjoy her music with the hearing loss. She ordered a hearing aid.

The bad weather set in, holidays came and went, and Ms. F. holed up in her room "reading the paper." As spring approached and there were a few days of good weather, Ms. F. could not be dissuaded from staying in her room. When Ms. F. was weighed routinely, staff were horrified to note a 10-lb weight loss. In reviewing the minimum data set (MDS), the staff noted that she had lost a total of 15 lb in 3 months.

Based on this information, answer the following question:

3. The charge nurse decided to conduct a mental status examination. Ms. F. agreed to being tested. The nurse noted that it took four repetitions of the objects for her to recall them. In 5 minutes she could not recall a single object. Because Ms. F. was well oriented, the nurses believed that:
   a. There was some dementia.
   b. She needed a battery for her hearing aid.
   c. She was depressed.
   d. A combination of a, b, and c.

The psychiatrist was called to assess Ms. F. He determined that she was depressed and recommended nortriptyline (Pamelor), an antidepressant. The primary physician prescribed Pamelor 25 mg every evening. After 3 weeks, the nurses reported that Ms. F. was smiling and seemed to be out of her room more. Her appetite was a little better; at least she ate a good breakfast. The primary physician conferred with the psychiatrist and increased the Pamelor to 50 mg daily. Six weeks later Ms. F. was on the porch enjoying lovely June days. She had been in the facility for a year. The charge nurse decided to repeat the mental status examination to determine whether there was marked improvement in her depression. Ms. F. was able to recall two out of the three objects. Her recall had improved. She was a little vague about the date; however, she knew the season, month, and year.

Based on this information, answer the following question:

4. The charge nurse wondered if:
   a. Ms. F. was just a little confused
   b. Ms. F. might have a disturbance in orientation related to a dementia process
   c. An adjustment in the antidepressant might be appropriate
   d. She should discourage Ms. F. from subscribing to a daily newspaper because it might be too tiring for her declining abilities

Toward the end of November Ms. F. slipped. Although she did not fall, she injured her back when she grabbed onto the support rail in her bathroom. The nurses noticed that she held on to the furniture and walls as she walked. She had radiographs, which revealed osteoporosis. The staff and primary physician discussed with her the idea of using a walker to get around. She agreed to try this and went to physical therapy (PT) for an evaluation and a walker. Two weeks later, the resident was still complaining of pain. She stayed in her bed more and did not come out for meals. Aspirin was ordered for her pain. Staff came by to visit. A few more weeks passed. Answer the following questions about this situation:

5. Some of the staff believed that:
   a. The resident was exaggerating her problem to get more attention
   b. The resident was depressed because of the pain and decline in function
   c. The resident had more extensive physical problems than they realized
   d. That further assessment was needed to determine the factors behind the resident's decline

6. The charge nurse decided that the following assessment(s) would help staff understand the resident's decline:
   a. Pain history and physical assessment per physician
   b. Nurse Interaction focused on Identifying depression, if it existed
   c. MMSE
   d. All of the above

The resident described the pain as severe, the worst she had ever experienced. The physician decided to hospitalize her for more tests. Hospital laboratory work showed dehydration. Magnetic resonance imaging (MRI) revealed that there was a disc pushing in on the spinal cord. The doctor ordered intravenous fluids and meperidine (Demerol) to manage the pain. When the charge nurse stopped by the hospital to see Ms. F. on the way home from work, she was shocked to find that Ms. F. did not remember her and believed it was nighttime. She had no idea where she was and had no recall from one moment to the next. It was January, and she believed it was June.

Answer the following question regarding this situation:

7. The charge nurse realized that her resident:
   a. Was depressed

b. Was in extensive pain
c. Had not heard a word she had said
d. Was delirious

During her hospital stay, Ms. F. was treated for gastrointestinal problems related to aspirin use and had back surgery that resulted in some postoperative complications. When Ms. F. returned to the nursing home, it was spring. She had a marked decline in her functional ability. She was now in a wheelchair and had been assigned to another unit. The staff from her original unit visited her to help her get adjusted. They focused on her abilities and her life of travel. They invited her to visit them and attend groups on the first floor. Ms. F. seemed very vague to them. The nurses felt sad and wondered whether Ms. F. would ever again be as bright and interested in her surroundings as she had been on their floor.

The MMSE was repeated. The nurses on the third floor realized from the MMSE that Ms. F.'s cognitive status had changed significantly. There were deficits in orientation and memory. Her ability to perform calculations, however, had not declined.

In a postadmission care conference, the staff identified Ms. F.'s resident care needs. Answer the following question about this determination:

8. They believed that they must implement all the following except:

a. To assist the resident to accept her decline
b. To assess her ability to move about and participate in a walking program
c. To request a psychiatric evaluation
d. To encourage her to participate in all unit activities

The resident slowly began to respond to the staff's plan of care. She was restarted on an antidepressant that had been stopped while she was in the hospital. She responded well to a walking program. Although she had lost some of her agility, she achieved some independence with a walker. Her dementia had advanced slightly, but she could and did participate in activities. It was decided that staff would continue to do an MMSE annually to monitor her progress.

Solutions

1. b
2. c
3. c
4. b
5. d
6. d
7. d
8. a

STUDY QUESTIONS

Please select the one best answer.

1. The health-care providers who are best qualified to conduct psychological assessments, such as Folstein's MMSE, are:
   a. Psychologists
   b. Nurses
   c. Social workers
   d. Psychiatrists

2. The social worker of a unit annually conducts an MMSE on all the residents. She informs you that Mrs. H.'s score in the area of orientation has dropped 2 points from last year. You suspect that the drop is due to:
   a. Delirium
   b. Arthritis
   c. Progression of dementia
   d. Depression

3. The activities department has alerted you to the fact that, recently, Mr. J. has not been interested in attending programs sponsored by their department. This morning, he complained to you that he believes that he is having problems with his memory. He did not eat breakfast and only picked at his lunch. He denies feeling depressed. You conduct an MMSE. There is a change in score from the admission MMSE conducted 3 months ago. His immediate recall of three objects on Folstein's MMSE has declined. You suspect:

   a. Delirium
   b. Progression of dementia
   c. A urinary tract infection
   d. Depression

4. Mrs. C. does not come out of her room for breakfast. The night shift staff report that the resident was up all night and that she has a fever. You go to Mrs. C. to determine whether you can assist her. She seems to be asleep. When you touch her arm, she opens her eyes. She does not quite recognize you, her favorite nurse. She believes that it is bedtime and her main concern is that her husband (who has been dead for 20 years) is late coming home from work. When you leave the room she returns to "sleep." Yesterday her MMSE score was 30/30. You know immediately that she is:
   a. Depressed
   b. Having a massive stroke
   c. Delirious
   d. Confused, due to dementia

5. Important considerations when conducting psychological assessments are:
   a. Timing
   b. Privacy and elimination of interruptions
   c. Positive introduction of the assessment
   d. All of the above

Colleen Brill and Mary Ann Anderson

chapter **13**

Common Clinical Problems: Psychological

Learning Objectives

After completing this chapter, the student will be able to:

1. Recognize three behaviors that may signal the presence of a psychological problem in an older adult.
2. Explain how to use nursing interventions for older adults with common psychological problems.
3. Discuss how to manage difficult behaviors of older adults.
4. Compare reality orientation, reminiscence, remotivation, resocialization, and validation techniques.
5. Select important information about psychological medications to include in teaching.

▶ INTRODUCTION

Psychological problems are disturbances in mental or emotional health that occur as a result of external or internal stimuli. These problems are usually assessed by examining thought patterns, behaviors, and emotions. Because psychological difficulties are not as obvious as some physical problems that can be diagnosed by laboratory tests, it may be difficult to diagnose and correctly treat older adults with these problems.

Almost any psychological problem that can occur with other age groups, also can occur with older adults. A few of the more common psychological problems found in clinical situations are described in this chapter. A glossary of terms used in this chapter is presented in Box 13.1.

▶ GENERAL GUIDELINES FOR COMMUNICATING WITH OLDER ADULTS

It is helpful to review some basic principles for good communication, particularly as they relate to communicating with the older person with psychological disorders. It is important to practice the skills outlined throughout this chapter in order to develop your own style for working in an individualized way with each person in your care.

BOX 13.1. GLOSSARY OF PSYCHOLOGICAL TERMS

Anxiety: generalized unpleasant feeling of apprehension.
Behavior modification: treatment method of changing behavior.
Bipolar affective disorder: psychological disease involving mood swings from mania to depression.
Delirium: sudden, reversible state of confusion.
Delusion: false, fixed idea or belief.
Disorientation: state of not knowing what day or time it is, or not knowing where one is.
Hallucination: false sensory impression, often seeing or hearing something that is not there.
Illusion: misperception of a real event or object.
Neurolinguistic programming: a way of communicating using neurological, behavioral, and speech patterns.
Neurotransmitter: chemical in the brain that carries electrical impulses to neurons.
Paranoia: way of thinking that systematically interprets others as being intentionally harmful.
Phobia: exaggerated fear of a particular object or group of objects.
Schizophrenia: psychological disease involving severe thought and perception disturbances.
Sensory deprivation: condition of decreased stimulation that can cause hallucinations, illusions, and disorientation.
Social support: emotional and physical assistance given by loved ones.
Somatization: extreme preoccupation with physical problems.

FORMING RELATIONSHIPS WITH PEOPLE WHO HAVE PSYCHOLOGICAL PROBLEMS

Generally, relationships have three stages. During each stage, there are concepts with which you should be familiar. At the beginning of a relationship, people sometimes are uncomfortable. After all, they are sick and you are new to them. As time goes on and trust is established, people enter a stage of the relationship that allows for more open communication that can be therapeutic in its purpose. The last stage of a relationship involves termination or saying good-bye. Problems in relationship building can be prevented by understanding these normal stages.

Beginning a Relationship

People who have psychological problems may not be easy to get to know initially. They may have had problems starting relationships all their lives, and forming a relationship with a new nurse might be difficult. Some people with mental illnesses have trouble trusting others and find it difficult to trust a new nurse or a new roommate in a hospital or long-term care facility. There are some things that can be done to help make the beginning of a relationship more comfortable.

If the person with a psychological problem does not talk or becomes upset at first, do not take it personally. Remember that the person may be feeling uncomfortable and unsure of how you will react. You, as the nurse, can be creative in dealing with problems like this and need to respond in a natural way. Some approaches to consider are using humor to diffuse tension or finding an interest of the person's, such as fly tying or crocheting, and asking him or her about it.

Important points to keep in mind are the need to establish trust and not to reject the person. You may need to try saying to the individual, "It seems like you'd rather not talk right now. I'll come back in an hour and sit here (or at the desk, or at a table) just in case you want to talk to me then."

Developing a Relationship

Once you have developed a trusting relationship with an older adult, you are ready to be an instrument in the work of healing for a person with psychological problems. With the development of trust, the older person is able to share with you such emotions as fear, anger, and the symptoms of more serious illnesses such as delusions or hallucinations. Your responsibility is to listen and guide the discussion.

If the older person has a serious disease, most of the verbal therapy is done in group or private sessions with nurse practitioners or psychologists. Then your responsibility is to listen, be genuine, and report anything unusual to the registered nurse (RN).

Ending a Relationship

Nurses begin and end relationships with many people every day. Sometimes this happens in small ways, like taking a weekend off or going away for a conference or vacation. Sometimes it is more permanent, like discharging a person to another facility or to the home, changing jobs, or saying good-bye to a person who is dying. During this phase of a relationship, people in general try to avoid the termination process. This often is done when the patient ignores you and other staff members, or by acting out.

If a nurse is going away for a short period of time, the older adult may start demanding more attention by ringing the call light more frequently, by becoming angry or irritated by small things, or by not responding or talking. To prevent this from happening, it is best if the person knows as soon as possible when to expect the separation. Provide opportunities to talk about it openly with you. If a permanent separation is approaching, some kind of formal farewell, like a good-bye party, might be helpful. Taking pictures with patients and staff also can help ease the difficulty of a separation. If an older person is being discharged home, do not always assume it is a joyous occasion. Sometimes the situation at home is worse than being in the nursing home or hospital. Even if a person is looking forward to going home, mixed feelings may exist about having to adjust to another new situation. Remember the difficulty of transitional stress.

It is not unusual for someone who is about ready to go home to suddenly become worse. If this happens, it may be a clue to you that the person is having problems with ending his or her present relationships. If you, as the nurse, talk about this openly by sharing feelings like "Things just aren't going to be the same around here without you, Mr. M.," the person may be more willing to discuss personal feelings.

VERBAL COMMUNICATION

Communication skills described in general nursing books also can be used successfully with older adults. There are some skills that are important to emphasize when working with elderly people who have psychological problems. The following discussion includes validation techniques, which are especially useful with the disoriented. There will be more information about validation therapy (VT) later in the chapter.

OPEN QUESTIONS

Verbal communication can be helpful by using open questions instead of closed questions. A closed question is a question that can be answered with a simple "yes" or "no." An open question tends to encourage the person to talk more. Open questions are asked using such words as "who," "what," "where," "when," and "how." "Why" questions usually are not very helpful, especially with someone who is disoriented. Some people with psychological problems may not be able to logically or rationally answer a "why" question. If a resident in a nursing home says she is looking for her mother, you may validate her by asking open questions like "What does your mother look like? What did you like to talk about with your mother? What did you and your mother do together?" If you were to ask "why" do you want your mother, the resident often would not be able to tell you.

GIVING INSTRUCTIONS

When giving directions, it is best to do so slowly, one step at a time. Individuals who are disoriented may not be able to perform any self-care activities unless they are prompted by very simple cues. Telling people who are disoriented to brush their teeth may not get any results. But if you tell them to pick up the toothbrush, then pick up the toothpaste, then put the toothpaste on the brush, then put the brush in the mouth, and then brush up and down, they may be able to do more than you originally thought.

GUIDED CHOICES

Some people may not respond to open questions as well as they do to guided choices.

When asked "What would you like to do today?" someone with a psychological problem may not know how to respond. However, when given a choice between two activities, with choices given one at a time, the person may be able to make a choice. An example of guided choices is: "Would you like to go to singing time today? Would you rather go for a walk outside?"

EMPATHY AND GENUINENESS

When a nurse shows the desire to understand someone, it promotes more meaningful communication. Empathy can be expressed by maintaining eye contact, using a caring tone of voice, listening closely to what someone says, and making statements such as "This must be difficult for you," or "It sounds like you are having a rough time right now."

The opposite of empathy is patronizing a person. Using a tone of voice as if talking to a child is an example of being patronizing. This type of communication keeps the nurse from using empathy and is not helpful in communicating with older adults. Referring to an older person as "honey" or "dearie" is also patronizing and, therefore, a hindrance to effective communication. Another example of patronizing behavior is referring to an older person in a report to another nurse as a "real cutie" or a "sweetheart."

It is important that the nurse be genuine when showing empathy. Being genuine means that nurses must truly represent themselves. Finding things you sincerely want to say to a person is more important than saying the right thing from a book.

LISTENING

Listening to someone includes listening to feelings, words, and behaviors. Sometimes people with emotional problems may forget or confuse the facts or use words that do not make sense. When this happens, it is especially important to listen to feelings instead of trying to get the facts straight. If a resident is incomprehensible but is speaking loudly and has tearful eyes, you might respond by saying, "This is extremely frustrating for you."

Another aspect of listening is to make sure the older adult can hear you. A review of the basic principles may help you. Start by being directly in front of the person. Stand so there is not a bright light (a window on a sunny day) behind you so the person can read your lips as well as listen to you. Speak in a normal tone; do not shout even if the person cannot hear you. If you suspect the person is having difficulty hearing you, move closer to the person. Ask permission to move close to one of the person's ears and repeat what you were saying, in a normal tone. If the person seems comfortable with touch, place your hand on a shoulder and express nonverbal acceptance and caring with touch. Remember to smile and do not act rushed even if you are. You may find other successful methods for promoting the older adult's way of listening. If so, use them and share them with others.

VALUES AND CULTURE

There are many different motivations for behavior during a conversation. Two that can enhance or Interfere with effective communication are the values and culture of the nurse and the older adult. What one person sees as normal may be seen as unacceptable or offensive by a person who has different values or comes from a different cultural background.. For example, the nurse who has been educated to value touch as a way of communicating concern, and an older adult who

Do you recognize the cultural background of this woman by looking at her clothes? It is important to gather information quickly on cultures unfamiliar to you so you can give complete, holistic health care. This woman is Guatemalan.

perceives touch, without permission, as an invasion of privacy will have problems with the communication process.

Nurses know that older adults, as with other age groups, come from a wide variety of backgrounds. A Hispanic resident may stand very close while talking to staff members. A staff member who is not aware of this cultural difference may interpret such behavior as being intrusive. An older Japanese person who values modesty may have difficulty talking openly about bowel and bladder problems. Some Native Americans want their Shaman, or medicine man, to perform a sacred "sing" to help them heal. This ritual involves music, dance, and numerous family members and friends. In order to have meaningful communication with older adults, all caregivers need to understand and respect the variety of differences that can occur because of personal values and cultural behaviors. If you recognize that you need more information about the cultural diversity of the people to whom you give care, there are excellent textbooks available for independent study. It would benefit you to locate one and review the information you need. Some people with emotional problems have trouble trusting others. It is important to develop trust with such people.

Being patient also is very important. Some nurses have to be available to their patient for several days before seeing a positive response. When the results do come, and the nurse is able to communicate successfully with the older person, it is a very rewarding experience.

NONVERBAL COMMUNICATION

Psychologists say that nonverbal communication, such as tears or the inability to smile, is the most honest communication a person can make. In order to be an effective listener, you need to both watch and listen to what is being said. Using direct eye contact and a caring tone of voice can help the communication process. Positioning the body at eye level also helps.

Touch

Touching is an important part of communicating with people. Many older people miss human contact and enjoy being touched. However, a person with psychological problems may become frightened, withdrawn, or

Remind Client of	Touch Technique
Mother	Palm of hand in a light circular motion on the upper cheek
Father	Finger tips, in a circular motion, medium pressure, on the back of the head
Spouse/lover	Hand under the ear lobe, curving along the chin, with both hands, a soft stroking motion downward along the jaw
Child	Cupped fingers on the back of the neck, with both hands, in a small circular motion
Brother/sister or good friend	Full hand on the shoulders and upper back by the shoulder blades; use full pressure in a rubbing movement
Animals/pets	Finger tips on the inside of the calf

Source: Feil, N. (1989). *Validation: The Feil method.* Cleveland, OH: Edward Feil Productions, pp. 47–48, with permission

POINT OF INTEREST

In all likelihood, you will not eagerly want to use the touch techniques just described. This is a test of courage of sorts. These touch techniques have a powerful impact on people with dementing illnesses. You need to have the courage to step into the situation and give the techniques a try. What if you use the rooting reflex touch on a resident and the person reacts loudly and with fear or anger? Don't walk away and say that technique never works. Instead, critically examine what has happened and consider why the mother of the older person did to cause such a strongly negative reaction so many years later. You have learned something important about the person by using this technique. It is that the mother was not a positive influence in the older person's life and the issues surrounding the mother may need to be resolved for the older adult.

agitated if touched. When the nurse touches someone who has an emotional problem, it is a good idea to ask the person first if it would be all right. Saying, "Would it be okay if I gave you a hug?" might be a way of asking for permission. Carefully note the response of the person to both the question and the actual touch. Some people who are very withdrawn may respond only to touch.

Touch can be used to stimulate sensory memories as well. Different people respond to touch in different ways. A list of common responses to touch is found in Table 13.1. A person who talks about his mother or says, "Ma, ma, ma" repeatedly may respond well to stroking on the upper cheek. This stimulates the rooting reflex and can bring back memories of a loving mother. Stroking the upper arm from the shoulder to the elbow is perceived by many people as a universal symbol of friendship. It feels comforting and safe to have someone touch In that way. If a patient is agitated, you may want to try stroking their upper arm while you talk quietly and gently to the person. The results may surprise you.

Matching and Mirroring

Research has determined that it helps the communication process if a person can match or mirror another's behavior. Mirroring is doing exactly what the person is doing as if the person were looking into a mirror. Matching is using the same pattern or intensity of tone the person is using. This must be done in a respectful way and not as a way of making fun of the individual. If the nurse feels uncomfortable doing this, it is not genuine and does not help communication.

Matching and mirroring are nonverbal ways of helping someone know that you hear what he or she is saying. Matching of emotions can be done by labeling the emotion out loud and using the same intensity used by the older person. Mrs. C. may pound her fist on the arm of her wheelchair and say "I hate them, I hate them, I hate them." Using matching and mirroring, the nurse would pound on the table with the same rhythm she is using and say "You're angry, you're angry, you're angry," using the same intensity of emotion.

Symbol	Possible Meaning
Jewelry, clothing	Worth, identity
Shoe	Container, womb, male or female sex symbol
Purse	Female sex symbol, vagina, identity
Cane or fist	Penis, potency, power
Soft furniture	Safety, mother, home
Hard furniture	Father, God
Napkin, tissue	Earth, belonging, baby
Flat object	Identity
Food	Love, mother
Drink from a glass	Male power, potency
Any receptacle	Womb
Picking the nose	Sexual pleasure
Playing with feces	Early childhood pleasures

Source: Feil, N. (1989). *Validation: The Feil method.* Cleveland, OH: Edward Feil Productions, p. 73, with permission.

Universal Symbols

A universal symbol is an object in the present that represents something important from the past. Sometimes these symbols increase in importance for people who develop disorientation as they grow older. The symbols can be something that has meaning to the older person, such as a reminder of a hobby or life's work, or it can be a different type of symbol. A few typical symbols are listed in Table 13.2. An apron can be made with a large pocket in the front that can contain significant symbols. A farmer may fondle farm tools placed in the pocket of apron and by doing this revive a memory of a time in life he enjoyed. As he touches the tools, the nurse can encourage communication using these symbols of the person's previous life.

PROBLEM BEHAVIORS

If a person with a psychological problem begins to display any unusual behaviors, it may be due to a number of different causes. Recent changes in relationships may contribute to increased wandering, shouting, and aggressive or withdrawn behaviors. These behaviors are not uncommon after a room or roommate change, or when the person is becoming accustomed to new staff members. These behavioral changes may also indicate that a medication change needs close monitoring, or symptoms of the person's illness are becoming more acute.

When you are caring for a person exhibiting difficult behavior, you need to take special precautions. Be alert to any situation that would place you, the older adult, or other patients in danger. Report anything suspicious to the RN, and stay calm.

All persons with psychological problems do not act in a dangerous way. Some sit quietly and never talk or move. This person needs your attention and expertise as well. Talk gently and kindly to the person. Sit with this quiet individual even if there is no conversation. Touch the person if it seems acceptable. All of these simple acts indicate acceptance of the person and are important for healing.

What should you do if an older adult is "yelling" at you? First, do not respond with anger. Stay calm. Be empathetic and kind. Listen to what is being said in order to identify what the problem really is. Get help if you need it. Be alert to what is going on throughout the unit as well as with the individuals in your care.

Some older adults with psychological disorders suffer from hallucinations, delusions, and illusions. These are symptoms of serious mental illness. People exhibiting these symptoms may think that they are Jesus Christ, or they may see bugs crawling all over their arms, or they may think you are a princess and want to wait on you. When dealing with such problems, the first rule is to stay calm. The next most important thing is to tell the truth. Do not play into the symptom by saying "Yes, I am princess Laura," or something of that nature. Be caring, honest, and genuine with the person. Remember, it never is wrong to get help if you feel uncomfortable or in danger.

▶ AGITATION

Agitation can occur as a result of physiological or psychological problems. Some people become agitated owing to physical causes that result in delirium. Common psychological problems that can cause agitation are the manic phase of bipolar affective disorder, stress or anxiety, flashbacks from traumatic experiences, post abuse reactions, or dementia. When people become agitated, they also may become violent. Such violence can be directed toward themselves or others. Preventing agitation, and managing it once it occurs, can be accomplished by following a few simple principles. For example:

- Watch for signs of agitation. Some people show signs of increasing irritability before a severe problem occurs. Others may have sudden, explosive outbursts. Notice if someone is talking very loudly, pacing more or faster, or making threatening comments to staff or others. Before an actual outburst occurs, try to keep the person talking to you by using some of the communication skills discussed in this chapter. With many people who are agitated, simply matching their breathing patterns or tone of voice is calming. With most people who are agitated, it is best to step back about 4 to 6 feet while talking with them. With disoriented elderly people, the reverse may be true, especially if a sensory deficit is present. It may be more calming to move closer to maintain sustained eye contact and touch. This must be done cautiously to protect your own safety and that of others. If there is the possibility that other patients or visitors may be harmed, move them out of the way.
- If a person becomes physically aggressive,

it is important to remember that the thumb is the weakest point of the hand. If a person has a hold on you, the way to remove yourself is by rotating away from the thumb of the person's hand. For further information on intervention techniques, most psychiatric facilities provide training sessions that allow you to practice dealing with these behaviors in a way that minimizes harm to yourself and protects the agitated person.

DEALING WITH PSYCHOLOGICAL PROBLEMS CAUSED BY STRESS

Here are some general guidelines for dealing with older adults with psychological problems who are experiencing stressful situations. Making an extra effort to assign the same staff members to an older person may help to prevent emotional distress. This is true both in the hospital and in the nursing home. A hospitalized person may be assigned nine different nurses during a 3-day stay. The sheer number of names to remember is difficult, but it is especially challenging for the older adult with emotional problems.

In addition to the "normal" stress of being admitted to a hospital or nursing home, the person with psychological problems has to deal with whatever illness caused his or her admission and the symptoms of their psychological Illness. An example is a person who has hallucinations. Hallucinations are real to

Some people with emotional problems have trouble trusting others. It is important to develop trust with such people.

the person experiencing the event, and they add a tremendous level of confusion to the daily life of the person experiencing them. Hallucinations interfere with one's ability to accurately perceive information. Your instructions or even a greeting may be misinterpreted; medications may look like spiders; or walls and doorways may keep moving. The approach to such problems includes keeping the same caregiver with the person throughout his or her stay. The nurse will begin to understand the behaviors of the older adult and be able to work within the limitations of the mental illness of the person.

It also helps when the older person's familiar belongings can be kept in the room. This promotes self-worth and helps to prevent disorientation. Small objects and pictures can be placed near the older person during a hospitalization to prevent the disorientation that can accompany stressful changes during an illness. Playing taped music of familiar songs generally is better than television viewing in preventing sensory overload. These are just a few examples of simple nursing interventions that can be used to prevent psychological problems caused by stress in older adults.

VIOLENT BEHAVIOR

If older adults start to act violently, the nurse must remember to protect these persons from their own behavior at all times. The nurse needs to call for help and, as a member of a team, decide what the intervention should be. Do not raise your voice, stay calm. They are the basic rules for handling someone who is violent.

Some violent behavior can be life threatening. I remember the day I was on a psychiatric unit, and a former patient came to visit; he brought a gun with him. He started shouting and shooting at random. That was an extreme act of violent behavior. Fortunately, he was a poor shot. But, the absolute fear was overwhelming for the patients and almost so for the staff. The charge nurse began an interaction with the former patient, once he was through shooting, and the rest of us slowly gathered the other patients and took them to safety. There is no formula for what to do in every possible situation. Simply stay calm and safeguard the patients and yourself.

SEXUAL ACTING OUT

Acting out feelings of anxiety may take many forms. Sometimes older adults with dementia lose social controls and express sexual feelings openly. Some people, such as those in the early stages of Alzheimer's disease, have an increased desire for sexual activity. People with other types of psychological problems, such as bipolar affective disorder, demonstrate sexual feelings in ways that are not socially appropriate. Dealing with these behaviors is almost always difficult, no matter how experienced the nurse is. Always consider if the acting out is an expression of the need for affection and touch.

Notice any factors that seem to trigger the behavior in order to intervene before the behavior occurs.

CRITICALLY EXAMINE THE FOLLOWING:

Mrs. C. starts yelling and shouting, "Call the police, call the police." while she is throwing items at her roommate.
Possible Solutions:

1. Maintain eye contact, speak in a calm voice and call Mrs. C. by name.
2. Tell her to talk to you and ask, "Are you frightened of something?"
3. Have another employee remove the roommate to safety.

CRITICALLY EXAMINE THE FOLLOWING:

Mr. J. walks into the visitor's area, unzips his trousers, and begins to masturbate.
Possible Solutions:

1. Gently approach him and get his attention by moving in close and speaking to him. Say his name.
2. Quietly lead him to his room; make sure that he is safe and then give him privacy to do whatever he wishes sexually. Ask his roommate to go to the day room with you if necessary.
3. Give affection and attention when he is not sexually acting out.

► SPECIALIZED COMMUNICATING SKILLS

The hallmark of nursing care for persons with psychological problems is the ability to communicate effectively. In addition to the skills just described in this chapter, there are other communication skills that can be used to make it easier to talk to older people with psychological problems. Some standard communication skills, and concepts from neurolinguistic programming (Bandler, 1985) and validation (Feil, 1993) are described in this section.

Neurolinguistic programming uses observation of a person's words and behaviors to help establish the best way of relating to that person. Validation, a communication approach for relating to disoriented older adults, helps disoriented clients express themselves. Sometimes communication with someone who is disoriented is blocked by the listener's need to have the disoriented person think or talk in a "logical" way. When the listener is able to put away the need to communicate in a normal way, there is the possibility of communicating in other, more effective ways. When this happens, the listener is able to understand and validate the disoriented person's experiences.

PREFERRED SENSE WORDS

All people relate to their surroundings through their senses. Most people respond more through one sense than through others. How a person talks will give an idea of that person's preferred sense. If Mrs. J. says, "I see what you mean. Look at this," she probably is a person who responds best to sight or visual words. Some people respond best to hearing or auditory words, and others respond best to words about feelings or movement (kinesthetic words). A list of commonly used visual, auditory, and kinesthetic words is included in Table 13.3. The nurse can use the person's preferred sense to establish rapport. For example, if an older adult says, "No one listens to me anymore," a response like "What would you like for me to listen to, Mr. J.?" will receive a better response than "What would you like me to see, Mr. J.?"

VAGUE PRONOUNS

If a person is not able to fill in the details with enough facts to be understood, try using vague or ambiguous pronouns to help foster communication. Sometimes people refer to all women as "she" and all men as "he." If the nurse becomes too concerned about accurate details, the opportunity to communicate may be lost. Instead of worrying about the facts, such as who "he" or "she" is, try to focus on the feelings. If an older person says "She's all alone. She can't stay there," you can respond "You're worried about her. She's important to you." That type of sensitive response generally will elicit more communication.

SPEAKING SLOWLY

Many people who have emotional problems have slowed thought processes. When this problem is combined with normal aging changes, it is very important for the nurse to use slightly slower speech and wait a little longer for the person to respond. Asking questions one at a time, instead of running several questions together, can also make it easier to talk to an older person with an emotional problem.

ASKING THE EXTREME

When someone who is disoriented is upset about something he or she thinks happened, ask questions about the extremes of the situation. What is the worst? What is the best? Imagine the opposite. When is it better? When does it not happen? Suppose every night an elderly woman thinks some men are coming to attack her. The nurse might ask, "When do they usually come? When are they not there? What helps you feel safe? What doesn't help you very much?" Often by looking at the extreme of a situation, the person will recognize what is happening in the "here and now."

> **TABLE 13.3. COMMONLY USED PREFERRED SENSE WORDS**

Visual	Auditory	Kinesthetic
See	Listen	Feel
View	Hear	Grasp
Picture	Sound	Move
Look	Loud	Touch

▶ GRIEVING AND DEPRESSION

Surviving losses is part of the aging process. An older person may lose relationships with people through death, retirement, or relocation, or he or she losing the ability to maintain contacts with friends and family due to physical problems. An older adult also may suffer the loss of valued social roles, a home, financial security, vision, hearing, or other body functions. The grief process that occurs with the loss of a loved one is one of the most powerful losses a person can experience.

DEALING WITH GRIEF

It is helpful to keep in mind the stages of the grieving process—denial, anger, bargaining, depression, and acceptance—when dealing with losses (Refer to Chapter 6). These stages do not always occur with every person. Some people who experience losses may become angry but not go through the other stages. As a nurse, it is important to accept each person's response to grief and not have a preconceived idea of how a person should respond.

An older adult can be helped to talk about grief by asking open-ended questions such as, "What did you do on your former job? When did you start working there? How did you get started working there?" if the person is grieving over the loss of a job. Asking open-ended questions about feelings also can help another to express grief. Sometimes it can be uncomfortable to hear a person talk about negative emotions like anger and sadness. Encouraging someone to express feelings and allowing expressions of anger or crying can help that person deal with feelings effectively. Saying something like, "How did you feel about that?" or "What upset you the most about that?" can encourage someone to talk about feelings. Telling someone who is sad and grieving, "Don't cry now, it will be all right" only gives false reassurance and tells the person to keep such powerful emotions inside. If emotions are not expressed, they tend to be expressed later in dysfunctional ways such as extreme anger, agitation, or withdrawal.

DEPRESSION

Because depression is a part of grieving and loss, it is a serious problem among the elderly population. There may be other factors that contribute to depression as well. Most of the current theories about depression have a strong emphasis on neurobiological causes and take into account the fact that depression tends to run in families. Most researchers conclude that depression is linked to the amount of the neurotransmitters serotonin and norepinephrine present in the nerve synapses. Lower serotonin and norepinephrine levels seem to be associated with depression. Factors within the body can deplete these substances, but external factors such as stress or decreased exposure to light also can influence the amounts of neurotransmitters available to a person.

As health-care providers, nurses also know that regular exercise can help maintain a higher level of endorphins in a person's body. Endorphins are naturally produced morphine-like substances that help people feel better. If the ability to exercise is impaired, then the body and mind are affected, and depression may result. Getting exposure to sunlight also can affect some people by changing their mood. For the homebound elderly person, this may be a problem. A poor diet also may contribute to the development of depression. Many older people have poor nutritional intake due to a variety of psychological and physical factors such as poor denture fit, cost of nutritious foods, changes in taste sensations, and eating alone. When the effects of the losses of aging are combined with those from physical risk factors, it is clear why many elderly people are depressed. The good news is that most people who have depression can be helped by treatment. Medications that are used to treat depression are generally effective.

The tricyclic antidepressants were widely prescribed in the past and are still effective for many people. Major problems with using tricyclic agents are side effects related to the cardiovascular system and urinary retention. Many elderly persons have problems with heart disease and hypertension, and men may have prostatic hypertrophy. These problems can be contraindications for the use of tricyclic drugs. With the advent of serotonin-selective reuptake inhibitors (SSRIs) such as fluoxetine (Prozac), sertraline HCl (Zoloft), and paroxetine HCl (Paxil), safer treatment options are available for people who have depression and other physical problems. Another antidepressant used very effectively with many elderly patients is bupropion (Wellbutrin). Wellbutrin must be monitored

closely if there are any eating disturbances or
if there is a concern over weight loss.

Medications are an important part of treating depression but are most successful when
used in conjunction with other types of therapy. Individual therapy with a counselor
educated to work with older adults can help
the person develop coping skills for dealing
with depression.

DEPRESSION AND CONFUSION IN THE ELDERLY PATIENT

Assessing someone who is depressed is
complicated by factors that occur as a result of
normal aging. The previous chapter describes
how to assess someone with depression and
how to use standard measures of depression.
Some of the behaviors seen in those with
depression may be very similar to behaviors
seen with other problems common in older
people. Individuals who are depressed may
not care about their surroundings and begin
to be disoriented and confused as they draw
inward. It can be very difficult to know whether
the mental slowing and memory loss attributed to depression are actually caused by the
depression or represent changes commonly
found in the early stages of dementia. Many
elderly people who have depression are
thought to have dementia and are not treated
for their depression (Table 13.4).

DEPRESSION AND SUICIDE

Assessing for the risk of suicide is essential for
someone who is depressed. The suicide rate
among older adults is high. It may not seem
likely that an older person would have

thoughts about suicide, but it happens too
frequently. If an older person says something
like "I just don't want to live anymore," the
tendency may be to discount the person and
say "Oh, you don't mean that" or "You'll feel
better tomorrow, you're just having a bad day."
If a person expresses a wish to die, makes
funeral plans, has a major change in life, or
begins to give away cherished possessions, be
aware that these can be signs that the person
may be planning suicide.

Asking people whether they are having
thoughts about killing themselves is not
"putting the thought into their heads." Many
people are relieved to talk to someone about
suicide if asked in a calm, matter-of-fact
manner. Finding out whether the person has a
plan and what it is are essential pieces of information. If a homebound older adult describes
a hoard of potassium supplements or cardiac
medications that are readily available, and if
the person's conversation indicates a plan to
take the medication after the nurse leaves, that
is a situation requiring immediate action.
Persons who say they do not want to live, but
have not thought about how they would end
their lives, are at a much lower risk for an
immediate suicide attempt than those who
have a plan. Many incidents of so-called
noncompliance with medications are actually
intentional attempts to overdose. If an older
adult is having thoughts about suicide, listen
carefully, intervene immediately if necessary,
and refer the person for treatment.

FAILURE TO THRIVE

The term *failure to thrive* is most often applied to
young children who do not grow and develop
as expected. Some elders who are depressed
also may have a failure to thrive or a giving-up
complex. This may be the case when the older
person no longer makes an effort to continue
with life, for instance, by refusing to eat, refusing medications, or choosing to resist or
refuse treatment for health problems. If there
is not an intervention that involves the interdisciplinary team and the family, the older
adult may well die in this situation.

▶ DELIRIUM AND DEMENTIA

Because depression can cause some confusion and disorientation, it can be difficult to

determine whether the older person has a
problem with delirium, dementia, or depression (see Table 13.4). Many factors influence a
person's ability to think clearly.

Emotional stress and change can cause
anyone to have difficulty remembering scheduled appointments or to be distracted easily
from activities of daily living such as turning
off the burner when cooking. Sometimes physical factors such as illness, insufficient oxygen,
or high or low blood sugar levels may cause a
person to behave in a very bizarre way. The
person who has a problem with disorientation
can be found in any setting. When a person
becomes disoriented, the caregivers may
become resigned to the problem and consider
this to be a normal part of the aging process.
That is not a correct assumption. Clarification
of the differences between delirium and
dementia can provide guidance for effective
intervention in both situations.

DELIRIUM

The psychological problem of delirium refers
to a situation in which an older person has a
fairly rapid change in behavior and thinking
ability. Mental status changes that occur with
this acute problem usually affect individuals'
abilities to recall where they are, what day or
time it is, or even what their own names are.
Delirium may cause agitation or rapidly
changing moods. Someone who is delirious
commonly has an anxious facial expression.
Short-term memory may or may not be intact.
With delirium, the older adult pays little attention to surroundings or may respond slowly to
new surroundings.

The person with delirium usually talks in a
rambling way that does not make sense. The
individual may have difficulty staying awake or
have increased activity and be awake all the
time. Sensory and perceptual disorders such
as hallucinations and delusions may be present. For example, the perception that the
nurse holding a syringe or has a knife, or hearing a baby cry that is not there. Changes in
thought content and process also may be
present. Fixed ideas or beliefs may be evident,
as well as disjointed or flighty thoughts.

Delirium can result from a variety of physiological causes and can be reversed.
Malnutrition, electrolyte imbalance, infection,
acid-base imbalance, change in blood sugar,
hypoxia, drug reactions, dehydration, and
head trauma are a few of the common causes
of delirium. It is important to determine what
is causing the delirium because the sooner
the problem can be treated, the sooner the
delirium will resolve.

When an older adult has a period of delirium, it can be very upsetting for the family and
nursing staff. Explaining what is happening to

▶ TABLE 13.4. DIFFERENCES BETWEEN DELIRIUM, DEMENTIA, AND DEPRESSION

	Delirium	Dementia	Depression
Onset	Rapid	Slow	Rapid
Duration	Short	Long	Short or long
Night symptom	May worsen	Frequently worsen	Usually do not worsen
Cognitive functions	Variable	Stable	Variable
Physical causes	Common	None	Possible
Recent changes	Common	None or minimal	Common
Suicidal ideation	Rare	Rare	Common
Low self-esteem	Rare	Rare	Common
History of psychiatric symptoms	Not usually	Rare	Common
Mood	Labile	Labile	Depressed
Behavior	Labile	Labile	Slowed thought and motor processes

all of those involved can help reduce stress and make it easier for everyone to handle the problem behaviors that occur.

DEMENTIA

The symptom of dementia is usually defined as the loss of intellectual abilities to the extent that it interferes with normal activities of daily living. Dementia is characterized by problems with cognitive ability, personality changes, memory impairment, decreased intellectual functioning, and changed judgment and mood.

Dementia usually occurs gradually, over a period of months or years, and is the result of deterioration of the brain. This damage can be caused by neurological diseases such as Pick's or Huntington's disease, or can be the result of vascular problems such as multi-infarct dementia. Advanced AIDS also has an associated dementia. The most common type of dementia is associated with Alzheimer's disease (AD). It is estimated that, in the future, dementia will outweigh heart disease and cancer as a major health problem. This estimate is based on the growing number of elderly people in our society and the strong correlation between aging and AD.

Because dementia is such a significant concern, new approaches to dealing with this problem are being examined. Validation therapy (VT) is a way of communicating with people who have dementia (Feil, 1993). Validation means respecting the feelings of the person and confirming, that from the individual's perspective, the experience is true.

This therapy is being used in many countries for people who are disoriented to decrease stress, to promote self-esteem and communication, to reduce chemical and physical restraint usage, and to make it possible to sustain independent living for a longer period of time.

A brief introduction to VT follows. More information on communication strategies is given later in this chapter. For those with a special interest in validation, additional information is available by doing a topic search on the Internet.

Stages of Disorientation

Naomi Feil (1993) has described four stages of disorientation that occur with people who are "old-old" (older than 80 years of age). These changes occur in people who have had fairly normal lives until they reach their 80s, when they begin to show signs of disorientation.

Malorientation. Malorientation is the first stage of disorientation. People who are maloriented may initially appear as if nothing is wrong with them. These people may be oriented as to where they are and who the President of the United States is but are beginning to forget information important for maintaining normal activities of daily living. They may try to cover up their memory loss by making up excuses. They do not like to be around people who are disoriented because they are threatened by their own memory loss. They deny their feelings and blame other people for their problems.

People who are maloriented respond best to open questions about facts, not feelings. It is important to hold onto acceptable social roles and rules for people who are maloriented. Encouraging someone who has been a teacher to lead the Pledge of Allegiance may be a way of helping maintain dignity and promote self-esteem. Often, the technique of using commonly preferred sense words assists this person to relate to the caregiver. It is best to listen to the maloriented person until you identify what the person's preferred sense is, and then address the person with words that represent that sense. For example, someone who often says "Oh, yes, I see what you mean" probably is a visual person and may respond to visual words better than to other choices (see Table 13.3).

Time Confusion. As people become more disoriented, they withdraw more from the real world and retreat into their own inner world. During this stage, people lose a sense of real time and respond to an inner sense of time. Someone may think about the mother (who is dead) and, because past time has fused with present time, talks about her as if she was present.

Because the nurse feels a need to orient the time-confused person, he or she might say something like "Your mother is dead; you can't go to see her." This only agitates and distresses the individual, who has no real need to stay in a painful present reality. Using the validation approach, the nurse would move close, use touch, and say "You miss your mother. What color eyes did she have? Blue or brown?" This is an effort to stimulate pleasant thoughts and memories for the person. There are several different methods of touching a person with dementia that are designed to evoke feelings about a loved one. Refer to Table 13.1 to review common forms of touch.

Repetitive Motion. If people with dementia continue to retreat from present reality, they may enter the stage of repetitive motion. During this stage, movements or sounds are repeated constantly. Usually, speech is limited to single-syllable words, and eye contact is made only after someone touches and talks to the person. The use of touch with these people is very important. Individuals with repetitive motions are often ignored emotionally, with caregivers providing physical care only. Validation techniques of sustained eye contact, stroking, and touching can help reach people in this stage of disorientation and prevent the final stage, which is that of vegetation. When persons are in the repetitive motion stage, they often communicate through universal symbols. These people use objects to represent thoughts. A common example is carefully folding and holding or caressing a napkin, which could represent a baby. Other examples are given in Table 13.2.

Vegetation. The final stage of disorientation and withdrawal is vegetation. In this stage, very little movement or sound is noted. Eye contact is very rare. Using touch and familiar music can help reach a person in this stage.

Alzheimer's Disease

The most common type of dementia is AD. The disease was first described in 1906 by a neurologist, who observed neurofibrillary tangles in an autopsy of the brain. Although there have been many advances regarding AD over the years, the only way to conclusively diagnose AD is at an autopsy. This means that AD is usually diagnosed by first ruling out any other causes of delirium or dementia. When symptoms of dementia are present and no other organic disease causing behavioral and mental changes can be found, a diagnosis of AD can be made.

AD is commonly found in persons older than 80 years of age but can be found in persons as young as 30 years of age. Recent research findings indicate a strong correlation for increased incidence of AD as people age. There also seems to be a significant correlation between both Down's syndrome and head trauma in relation to AD.

At least half a dozen drugs are being investigated for use in the management of dementia. At present, the medication tacrine (Cognex) is being used with mixed success in the treatment of mild-to-moderate AD. Because of the effects of this drug on the liver, it is necessary to make frequent checks of liver enzymes.

▶ PARANOIA

Some people with emotional problems fear that other people are trying to hurt them. Such paranoid ideas are an indication of problems the person may have with trusting others. This can occur with dementia, schizophrenia, or other psychological problems. Many times, people who are paranoid seem very convincing and logical. Developing trust is the most important thing to accomplish with someone who is paranoid. This can be best done by being consistent and reliable in all you do with the person. Do not make promises you cannot keep. If you say you will do something, follow-up with the paranoid person is especially important. It is particularly important to avoid putting medicines in food or drink without the paranoid person's knowledge.

▶ DEVELOPMENTAL DISABILITIES

Historically, people who had developmental disabilities did not live to an old age. With advances in health care, more individuals who have developmental disabilities, such as Down's syndrome, are living longer. There is evidence that as individuals with Down's syndrome grow older, they are at high risk of developing AD.

Individuals with developmental disabilities may have some of the problem behaviors that have been identified in this chapter. Principles for setting limits on behavior include the following:

- Recognize the person's feelings and encourage expression of them.
- State the limit clearly.
- Point out ways that behavior can be expressed within the limits and what is outside the limits.
- Allow the person to express anger at having limits placed on him or her.

▶ SUBSTANCE ABUSE

Staff working with people who have chemical dependency problems recognize that there are a growing number of older adults with substance abuse problems. Because many older people are treated for a wide variety of physical problems, sometimes they receive prescription drugs from several different sources. The availability of prescription drugs contributes to problem of drug abuse among older persons.

Alcoholism is another problem for many elders. Many of the same reasons people use substances to self-medicate (depression, losses, loneliness) in other stages of life are even more of a problem for the elderly population. Because many of the memory lapses found with substance abuse are similar to those in the early stages of dementia, substance abuse may not be discovered until it is advanced. Sometimes, families have difficulty confronting older family members about substance abuse problems. The denial of a problem, which is characteristic of most substance abuse problems, is especially difficult to deal with when working with older adults. This then creates a problem with the treatment process. If a substance abuse problem is suspected, it is best to contact trained professionals to assist with interventions.

▶ EATING DISORDERS

Often, the reason for seeking health care is a problem with eating. Problems with eating can be due to physical factors, such as loss of taste sensation or poor denture fit, but many times, eating difficulties are due to psychological problems. Anorexia can be a symptom of a psychological problem, such as depression, or it can be a problem in itself.

Compulsive resistance to eating or anorexia historically has been most commonly found in young women. More and more clinicians are now describing similar symptoms in the elderly population. Eating or not eating can be used as a way of exhibiting controlling or resisting behaviors, especially in stressful situations. Compulsive overeating also can occur in the elderly population, as can the bingeing and purging found in bulimia. Some elderly patients with psychological problems have phobias related to certain foods. Others may become paranoid about food that they believed to be poisoned or contaminated.

Regardless of the specific problem, treating someone who has an eating disorder may require tremendous amounts of creativity. Sometimes, the only effective treatment is using a feeding tube until adequate weight gain is achieved. Behavior modification techniques, such as giving privileges for weight gain and withdrawing privileges for weight loss, may need to be planned by the health-care team or a psychiatric nurse specialist.

▶ GROUPS FOR THE ELDERLY

Many older adults with psychological problems can benefit from group interactions. Discussed below are some types of group therapy that have been used successfully with older persons.

REMINISCENCE

Based on memories of similar events or experiences, many older adults form bonds in groups. Stimulating memories of childhood or early adulthood can serve to improve feelings of self-worth and provide an opportunity to review their lives. Memories may stimulate laughter and happiness or other emotions and serve as a way of coping with present circumstances. Groups can be conducted around an

Many older adults with psychological problems can benefit from group interactions.

important event, such as Pearl Harbor Day. Common, shared experiences, such as early school days, can be recalled to promote socialization and provide mental stimulation. Reminiscence also can be used individually as a means of helping people wrap up any unfinished business in their lives.

A very structured form of reminiscence is the life review process. This process provides an opportunity for evaluation and integration of life experiences. People in the more advanced stages of disorientation are not able to benefit from this type of therapy.

REMOTIVATION

To improve interest in and quality of life, remotivation techniques can be used. The emphasis with remotivation is the use of real objects to stimulate senses and provide new motivation in life and the surrounding world. Pictures, plants, animals, or sounds can be used to encourage group interaction. Holidays, birthdays, or hobbies can be used to focus on remotivation for participating in the here and now. The focus is on factual information as opposed to exploration of feelings. These groups work best with those who have depression or early stages of disorientation.

RESOCIALIZATION

Encouraging residents to assume social roles can stimulate feelings of increased self-esteem. The focus for this group is on social roles and not on problem solving. Discussion may occur about previous social gatherings and how people behaved during these events. The emphasis is on the present and discussion of factual information.

Many older adults with psychological problems can benefit from group interactions. Group members are assigned roles, such as the greeter, or to serve each other refreshments. Feelings are not the focus of resocialization groups, which can be helpful for the mildly disoriented.

REALITY ORIENTATION

Helping residents become oriented to present reality is the goal of reality orientation. Constant reminders about the present, that is, where they are and what day it is, are given. Current events on the television or in the newspaper can be used as topics to stimulate discussions. The season of the year, holidays, and the weather are other topics to promote orientation to reality. These groups are focused on keeping people oriented to present reality and are not usually very effective with people who have more than mild disorientation.

VALIDATION

Validation groups combine some of the other types of techniques with group problem solving and a focus on support. Members are assigned roles, sing familiar songs, serve each other refreshments, and reminisce about the past. Movement is encouraged during group activities. The group is presented with a problem to solve. Resolving losses and expressing feelings are emphasized. Validation groups are most effective for people who have moderate disorientation.

▶ PSYCHOTROPIC MEDICATIONS

As with all medications, adaptation is necessary when using psychotropic medications with an older adult. Teaching the older person and his or her family about the reason for the medication, side effects, toxic effects, and what to do if a dose is missed are very important when psychotropic drugs are used with the elderly population.

Many psychotropic drugs require a period of time—sometimes several weeks—before a therapeutic effect is achieved. This waiting period may be longer for some older people. They may show more signs of toxicity at lower doses than usual because an impaired ability to excrete the drug results in a buildup in the bloodstream. Another possibility is that they may be more difficult to treat, because there are side effects due to the difference in distribution and excretion of drugs in the aging body.

Psychotropic medications work in the brain in a variety of ways. Most medications work by helping to change the level of neurotransmitters or chemicals in the brain. It is hoped that re-establishing a more normal balance will help the person have fewer psychological problems. Because these drugs work on the brain, it is important to use them only for psychological problems and not just because the resident has behaviors that irritate other people. Before any drugs are used to sedate a person with problem behaviors, all other types of nursing interventions must be used along with documentation of the interventions.

Because of physical health problems, some medications used to treat mental health problems may be contraindicated or may require careful administration in the older person. For example, an elderly man who has prostate disease may, if given a tricyclic antidepressant, have extreme difficulty voiding.

A common side effect of many psychotropic drugs is constipation. When combined with normal aging changes, the constipation resulting from psychotropic medications can become a troublesome problem for the elderly person.

Orthostatic hypotension is a problem that results from many psychotropic drugs. Simple teaching techniques can help manage some of the postural blood pressure changes; however, many times these changes are severe enough to require that the medication be discontinued.

▶ PHYSICAL AND MENTAL HEALTH

Because there is such a strong relationship between physical and mental health, many professionals believe that all diseases have both physical and emotional aspects. Some older people grew up in a time when it was frowned on to admit that mental illness existed, but it was more socially acceptable to have a physical problem. One grandmother described a time early in her marriage when she became so upset with her husband that she became "sick" and took to her bed for a week.

This expression of emotional problems through physical complaints is called somatization. Many times, if a stressful situation is encountered, the person who uses somatization may develop a backache, headache, or stomachache to avoid dealing with problems. This does not mean the ache is "all in the head," but it may mean the person finds it easier or more acceptable to have a physical pain than an emotional one. For someone who has done this for 80 or 90 years of life, it may be difficult if not impossible, to change their way of coping. The nurse can help the patient learn to meet needs more directly by encouraging the person to talk about feelings openly.

▶ PATIENT RIGHTS AND LEGAL RESPONSIBILITIES

The current standard of care in nursing homes and in mental health centers is that the older person has the right to the least restrictive form of treatment. Federal and state regulating agencies such as the Health Care Financing Administration (HCFA) have specific regulations protecting these rights. In most states, treatment can be administered involuntarily only if a danger exists to the individual or to others. The length of time allowed for this type of treatment varies from state to state but is usually only a few days. If a longer treatment schedule is required and the older person is unwilling to consent, then an application for guardianship may be made. This takes away the person's rights to make personal decisions and gives that to a guardian. This is a procedure that may be necessary for people with some types of mental illness, including dementia.

When agitated behaviors become severe, the nurse has to make a decision about how to handle the problem. Points that must be considered are the patient's right to the least restrictive treatment environment and the legal issues related to the use of chemical and physical restraints. If an older adult has an episode in which increased symptoms of bipolar affective disorder or schizophrenia are exhibited, an antipsychotic drug is likely to be more effective than for someone with dementia or delirium. Before giving a chemical restraint, it is necessary to try talking to the person as well as using behavioral interventions. When all else fails, physical restraints may be necessary on rare occasions.

▶ CONCLUSION

The care of elderly people in all arenas of nursing is an opportunity to practice the art of nursing on its highest level. The skills and understanding that are needed to give meaningful care to the elderly patient with psychological problems are complex and require a personal and professional commitment to the needs of people as they age.

CASE STUDY

Mr. A. is an 80-year-old retired farmer. He lived with his wife on the farm until 1 year ago, when he became too ill for his wife to manage his care alone. At that time, he became a resident of a nursing home in a nearby town. He has been forgetful for several years and now wanders the halls looking for his pickup truck. During the winter, he walked away from the nursing home and wandered for several hours. This resulted in frostbite on several fingers and toes. He becomes agitated when he is told that he can not go back to his home. What actions can be taken to assist Mr. A.?

Solution

Working with the entire nursing staff, a plan is developed for using validation therapy with Mr. A. When he asks about his truck or home, the staff ask him questions such as, "What color is your truck?"; "What did you do with your truck?"; "Where did you go?"; "With whom?" Coveralls with a front pocket are obtained, and a small hammer and screwdriver are placed in his pocket. His toolbox is brought into his room. The staff have put him in charge of a small garden outside the nursing home. Individual sessions of validation are scheduled 20 minutes a day, three times a week, by the activities staff.

Over a 6-week period, the staff notice that Mr. A. spends quiet, productive time in the garden area. He carries his tool box with him most of the time but does not use its contents. He no longer leaves the building except to work in his garden. He is still forgetful.

STUDY QUESTIONS

Please select the one best answer.

1. The best intervention for an elderly resident of a nursing home who suffers from paranoia is:
   a. To encourage him to lead a large group singing
   b. To plan one-on-one activities with staff and other residents
   c. To invite the resident to sit on the residents' council of the nursing home
   d. To have the resident join a weekly bingo group

2. An elderly homebound person taking medication for a psychological problem needs to know which of the following?
   a. If dizziness occurs, notify the nurse.
   b. It may take several weeks to get the desired effect.
   c. Report any changes in vision.
   d. All of the above.

3. Validation techniques are best described as:
   a. A way of helping someone resolve past experiences
   b. Helping someone find new meaning in growing older
   c. A reminder of a painful present reality

   d. Bringing someone from the past into the present world

4. When a hospitalized older adult suddenly becomes disoriented, the best intervention is which of the following?
   a. Ignore the person's feelings because they are a normal part of aging.
   b. Tell the person to cheer up because things are not so bad.
   c. Do not allow the person to talk about being sad because that makes it worse.
   d. Encourage the person to discuss feelings openly because it helps to talk about problems.

5. When teaching older adults or their families about the use of psychotropic drugs, one of the most important concepts to teach is:
   a. The meaning of the different colors of the medications
   b. The stress psychotropic drugs put on the kidneys
   c. To anticipate the chronic light-headedness that most people experience
   d. Not to expect the full effect of the drug for several weeks

Sister Rose Therese Bahr
Kathleen R. Culliton

chapter **14**

Restorative Care

Learning Objectives

After completing this chapter, the student will be able to:

1. Define rehabilitation and restorative nursing in a holistic framework.
2. Identify the clinical implications of restorative care in walking programs, continence training, and feeding and self-help programs.

▶ INTRODUCTION

Nurses strive to promote the health of older adults. Generally, nursing care involves assisting older adults in overcoming the symptoms of an acute health problem or the worsening of a chronic condition. Nurses use medications, treatments, and referrals to help the individual overcome physical, psychological, social, and spiritual illness. In the acute-care setting, nurses assist older adults through the crisis of illness and discharge them back into the community to their homes or a supportive living environment. The goal of nursing care is to assist older adults back to health and allow them to return to their homes. Assessment of their general health and ability to meet their personal needs are considerations during the discharge process. There are times an older adult is no longer physically or emotionally able to safely return to his or her home.

The purpose of this chapter is to present an overview of gerontological nursing concepts based on rehabilitative and restorative care. Both rehabilitative and restorative nursing care surpass the traditional custodial approach that has prevailed in the care of older adults before the initiation of the 1990 Omnibus Budget Reconciliation Act (OBRA) regulations. Data collection for residents in nursing homes is done on the minimum data set (MDS) (see Chapter 4) and emphasizes restorative care of older adults as a major priority of care.

Demographically, America is graying. Along with the aging process comes increased disability for many older persons. It has been statistically projected that 40% of all disabled persons in America presently are 65 years old or older. As the aging population increases, nurses are called on to provide rehabilitative and restorative care to more and more older people as they enter health-care facilities.

▶ UNDERSTANDING REHABILITATION AND RESTORATIVE CONCEPTS

Rehabilitation is the process of teaching and training individuals to achieve their highest level of independent function. People are most familiar with rehabilitation programs for spinal cord injuries. For older adults, the rehabilitation often is for treatment of a cerebral vascular accident (CVA) or deformity from arthritis and the surgery that often accompanies severe arthritis. Rehabilitative care is a multidisciplinary care model. Physical therapists, occupational therapists, speech therapists, dieticians, respiratory therapists, recreation therapists, social workers, psychologists, nurses, and rehabilitation physicians are members of rehabilitation care teams. Rehabilitation is initiated after an extensive assessment of an individual's physical, emotional, spiritual, and functional assets and liabilities. Assessment information is reviewed, along with the resources available to assist the individual to develop a rehabilitative plan. Often, an individual does not need all available services. Then the team is restructured to include the necessary health-care team members. This team works with individuals and their families to develop rehabilitative goals and to decide the best way to work toward the goals.

Selecting a short-term or long-term living environment is one of the first choices that a rehabilitation team must make. Every care environment has the potential to be a place for rehabilitation. The limiting factors often are not enough family support, environmental safety, insurance reimbursement, and access to the rehabilitation team. An older adult with a total hip replacement may want to go home, but home has an upstairs bathroom and there is no one available to prepare meals. These factors present a problem. A young man may be recovering well from knee surgery and want to have intensive inpatient therapy, but his insurance company does not approve the cost. An elderly woman may want to go to her rural community hospital for rehabilitation after a stroke, but the services that she needs are not available in that community. The rehabilitation team works to help the person access support services and find the most appropriate environment for the rehabilitation process.

Restorative nursing care is related to rehabilitation. It has the same goal—to assist older people to reach their highest functional ability. The major difference is the intense involvement of the whole health-care team. Because of the direct involvement of therapies and other health-care professionals, rehabilitation is an expensive service. Restorative care is initiated after an older person has reached the rehabilitative goal or has not demonstrated any further improvement. The whole health-care team is involved in designing restorative care plans but is not directly involved in the implementation. For example, an older person who is in a rehabilitation program after a stroke would have the benefits of a physical therapist to learn exercise, safe walking, and transferring techniques. The older adult continues to need assistance with exercises and walking, but a nurse or a nursing assistant encourages the person to do as much as possible independently and assists him or her only if necessary.

Rehabilitation provides individuals with intensive short-term strengthening and retraining, whereas restorative care continues the process over time. It is unfortunate when an older adult has a major health crisis and goes through intensive therapy and training only to move to an environment where everything is done for him or her, and the benefits of the therapy are lost. Examples of restorative programs are ambulation, personal care, feeding, and toileting. The challenge for the nursing team is to continue to promote high levels of independent function. It is faster to transfer a person into a wheelchair and push the person to the dining room for breakfast but that is not promoting independence. Restorative care demands that the nursing staff assist the older adult to walk to the dining room. Unfortunately, this same concept of needing to hurry is associated with high incidences of incontinence. It is often perceived as faster to change an older adult's briefs and bedclothes than to anticipate the need for voiding and then walk the person to the bathroom. With rehabilitative and restorative nursing care, "faster" is not the goal.

The same principle applies to eating and personal care. Have you ever watched someone struggle to put on a shirt on to a paralyzed arm? Watching that struggle is uncomfortable because the nurses know they could help that person get the shirt on faster and without as much stress and strain. It is very difficult to watch someone try to eat independently and see the stress and frustration that can occur. Yet, that older person deserves the right to feel the satisfaction of accomplishing a task or meeting a personal goal.

The concepts of rehabilitation and restorative care are critical to promoting an older adult's optimal level of function. The focus of rehabilitative and restorative care is to maximize the abilities and functions of older adults to ensure the highest level of independence and quality of life. Rehabilitation and restorative care are not isolated treatments with limited application. They embody a broad set of principles to incorporate into every facet of nursing care in all settings.

Within the context of the interdisciplinary team (IDT) effort and after clinical conferences with the team to determine what plan is to be designed, licensed practical nurses (LPNs), working cooperatively with the registered nurse (RN), prepare the goals and the nursing care plan. In this capacity, the nurse's role becomes one of practitioner, educator, counselor, case manager, researcher, and consultant.

▶ NURSING ROLES

BEDSIDE CAREGIVER

As caregivers, LPNs provide direct care to older adults until the skills necessary for self-care have been developed by the individual. Nurses need to give older adults positive reinforcement, encouragement, hope, and an opportunity to develop and use both their physical and social skills.

EDUCATOR

When serving in the role of educator, nurses provide older people and their families with information related to the disability, and its treatment and management. Included in the education plan should be health measures to obtain and retain function and to prevent further disability. The nurse must realize that effective outcomes are more likely to occur when older adults and their families are included in the process of determining the goals of rehabilitation and restoration of function and treatment. It is important for older adults and the family or other caregivers to recognize that they are responsible for the decisions made and actions that result from those decisions. That is a predominant principle of rehabilitative and restorative care.

COUNSELOR

As counselors, nurses assist elderly people to describe, analyze, and respond to the current situation that makes rehabilitation or restorative care necessary. Counseling is the process of helping people solve and effectively cope with their problems. Counseling disabled

POINT OF INTEREST

Refer back to the chapter on End-of-Life issues. Review Kubler-Ross's five stages of grief again. The older adult and the family will be going through these stages because of the loss that has brought them to the IDT for rehabilitation and restorative care.

people and their families is an ongoing progress that requires supportive behaviors from the entire IDT. LPNs, after establishing trust and rapport with the older adult and the family, need to focus on assisting them to deal with their grief over the losses imposed by the older person's current disability. The opportunity to express personal feelings assists the elderly person in developing coping skills related to the event of trauma that made rehabilitation and restoration therapy necessary. The LPN should counsel disabled, elderly persons and their families to respond to the feelings of loss, frustration, and anger that they generally feel. It is important to express and deal with such feelings as a family.

ADVOCATE

When assuming the role of advocate, LPNs use their influence and power as health professionals to bring about necessary changes for both the older person and the family's well-being. That allows the rehabilitation and restorative care to have maximum effect. Such interventions aid the older adult and the family members in obtaining necessary community-based services. Such services assist to maintain older disabled adults as fully functioning, independent individuals within the constraints of the limitations imposed by the disability. Such interventions may include the use of assistive or adaptive devices like crutches, a walker, a plate guard, and a padded spoon.

CASE MANAGER

Generally an RN is the case manager for disabled persons. However, in some situations the LPN is asked to serve in that role. The case manager role places the nurse as a central figure working with the total health-care team throughout the entire episode of illness. The major focus for a case manager is to resolve actual problems and prevent potential problems for the aging person. The treat-

ment plan, once agreed on by the IDT, is under the supervision of the licensed nurses (RNs and LPNs) working in conjunction with each older adult and family. Once the plan is agreed on, a contract is entered into by the individual, family members, and the nurse so that the plan can be implemented with clear communication with each person involved. This management may take place in a hospital or nursing home and continue into the community where home-based care is provided.

RESEARCHER

Many LPNs work in conjunction with RNs and a qualified nurse researcher to gather data on the rehabilitation and restorative care of older adults. Many questions remain unanswered regarding rehabilitative and restorative care of older adults in a number of areas. Each area provides a rich arena for research. Some of the research interests are given in the following list:

- The management of behavioral symptoms
- Feelings about placing disabled family members outside the home and into an institution for care on a permanent basis
- Barriers that prevent the use of respite and day-care services
- Accurate measures of caregiver burden
- Effective coping strategies used by caregivers
- Types of educational and support programs needed to assist caregivers
- Services needed to individualize care at different stages of an illness or injury

All of these clinical questions need to be raised when older individuals suffer a traumatic episode and require nursing care. The nurse is responsible for raising questions regarding the specific needs of older individuals and seeking systematic answers through research. A research approach helps build a body of knowledge regarding rehabilitation and restorative care.

▶ GOALS OF REHABILITATION AND RESTORATIVE CARE

A goal is defined as a written statement of desired behavioral outcomes from which steps or strategies may be designed to achieve that desired end. Goals provide direction. They are the measuring tool for an effective plan of care. For example, "I will buy a car today" is a statement of the desired outcome. A defined series of steps needs to be taken before the accomplishment of that goal such as establishing a means to pay for the car, deciding what type of car to buy, finding out the selling price of cars at various car dealers, checking on insurance, and so forth.

From the time of injury or disability, the efforts of all health-care professionals involved in the older adult's care are to be focused on the ultimate goal: the highest level of personal independence possible within the limitations imposed by the injury. In setting goals, LPNs assess the older person to determine what assets of mind, body, and spirit are present that will aid in the accomplishment of the goal. For instance, can the person ambulate sufficiently to make trips to the bathroom, dining room, and physical therapy department? The LPN might ask a number of questions:

- Is the person able to communicate needs verbally?
- Can the person feed himself or herself?
- What are the goals of the older adult?

The information derived from the assessment is important in determining realistic and achievable goals for each individual. For lifelong quality of living, the components of a successful rehabilitation and restorative program must include the following goals, which should be individualized toward increasing the function and performance of the individual:

- Independence and self-care
- Mobility
- Involvement in activities—social, civic, family, church, and recreation
- Fulfillment of life's goals
- Holistic approach to living with a disability

You must be knowledgeable in evaluating the current holistic status of the older adult. For older adults, major changes in three areas are critical to the success of a rehabilitation and restorative care program. Changes must be noted in physical, functional, and psychological status. Each of these areas can greatly affect the ability of the older adult to carry out the goals identified in the plan of care.

PHYSICAL CHANGES AFFECTING RESTORATIVE CARE

A number of physical changes may be present when an older adult sustains an injury or trauma necessitating rehabilitation. Existing health problems must be considered in planning rehabilitative and restorative care.

- Musculoskeletal changes due to old fractures, osteoporosis, arthritis, osteoarthritis, muscular dystrophy, or loss of strength in arms and legs can create mobility difficulties. Such situations can occur because of muscle atrophy, decreased bone mass, loss of subcutaneous fat, and decreased flexibility of the joints and limbs.
- Cardiovascular changes due to diminished cardiac output, irregular heart rate, and increased blood pressure readings can result in diminished circulation that does not bring sufficient oxygen to the body. Such conditions often cause a lack of activity because of fatigue. Cardiac changes may be the result of thickening of heart valves, thickening of blood vessels, or delayed response to stress.
- Respiratory changes related to diminished respiratory rates can create ventilation chal-

Goal assessment on a daily or weekly basis is essential to good care.

lenges for the older person and may be caused by long-standing asthma, obstructive lung disease, emphysema, tuberculosis, upper respiratory illnesses, limited rib cage expansion, atrophy of respiratory muscles, decreased arterial oxygen tension, decreased vital capacity, and diminished cough.

- Renal and digestive tract changes create elimination difficulties that may impair the proper implementation of a restorative program. These changes may include decreased peristalsis of the intestinal tract that results in constipation or diarrhea, decreased intestinal enzyme levels that reduce the ability to properly digest foods, diminished glomerular filtration in the kidney, and decreased bladder capacity resulting in incontinence or retention of residual urine. The latter may create edematous lower limbs that make it difficult for the older person to ambulate in a comfortable manner.
- Consciousness and mental status changes may result in short-term memory loss, slower thought processing, and decreased pain threshold.

- Perceptual changes may be demonstrated by loss of visual acuity, diminished hearing, decreased sense of taste, lower sensitivity to touch, and decreased proprioception (spatial sensitivity or awareness of where things are in the available space).

FUNCTIONAL CHANGES AFFECTING REHABILITATIVE AND RESTORATIVE CARE

Changes in function in older adults may result from the impact of social and environmental situations. These changes can include the following:

- Inability to negotiate stairs in the home
- Functional implications of acute or chronic disease processes
- Physical factors such as limited range of motion, strength, and endurance
- Inability to consume sufficient nutrients to maintain optimum health
- Inability to cook food, clean a home, or complete the laundry and other critical chores

These functional changes need to be assessed by a nurse so that the realistic goals can be established.

PSYCHOLOGICAL CHANGES AFFECTING REHABILITATIVE AND RESTORATIVE CARE

The psychological status of an older adult is a critical component of any rehabilitation and restorative care program. When the older person enjoys psychological well-being, there is a strong motivation to work toward the highest possible level of function. When older people feel needed and wanted by family, friends, and associates, they generally possess self-esteem and a positive self-image, which are two critical factors in developing a high degree of motivation to proceed with the restorative care program.

▶ DEVELOPING GOALS FOR REHABILITATIVE AND RESTORATIVE CARE

When developing goals for rehabilitative and restorative care, LPNs need to complete a full

- Nursing history that includes the older adult's past medical conditions, psychological impairments, hospitalizations, and previous injuries (see Chapter 9)
- Physical assessment of all bodily systems (see Chapter 9)
- Functional assessment to check for functional ability and mobility (see Chapter 9)
- Mental status and psychological parameters that may be present, for example, depression, anxiety (see Chapter 12)
- A spiritual assessment to determine any spiritual needs or deficits that may be a deterrent to good rehabilitation progress

Following the assessment, the LPN and RN work together as a team to analyze the data and prioritize rehabilitative and restorative goals for the older person. The following principles of holistic nursing care should be the guidelines for identifying such goals:

- When the older adult enters the hospital or nursing facility, rehabilitation must begin immediately.
- Proper body alignment is to be maintained at all times.
- Pressure ulcers are to be prevented on all body parts.
- Rehabilitation is to be implemented concurrently with the illness, whether chronic or acute, temporary or permanent, or disabling or nondisabling.
- All joints must be kept free through proper exercise/range of motion.
- Convalescence is a gradual process and may extend over a considerable period for the older person.
- Nurses must understand the person's self-concept and feelings of dependency and isolation if they exist.
- The time period for rehabilitation depends on the person's psychological acceptance of the condition.
- People born with disabilities usually have less difficulty accepting their condition than those who acquire disabilities later in life.
- More severe emotional reactions are produced when accidents are traumatic.
- Loss and its meaning vary with every person.
- Any personality problems that may be exhibited are generally the result of the person's personality characteristics before disability.

nursing assessment under the guidance of a registered nurse. The nursing assessment should include a complete database with the following elements:

- The usual initial reactions to physical injury are shock, fear, disbelief, and anxiety.
- Periods of grief are produced when loss of any physical ability is experienced.
- Depression, anger, and denial may be present.
- Values are examined and limitations put in perspective over time.
- Time is essential for acceptance.
- The family needs emotional support and comfort during the acute phase of the trauma or illness.
- All information possible should be given to the family and older adult, including information about resources for rehabilitation services and economic assistance.
- The nurse or social worker should be familiar with community agencies that can help.

▶ IMPLEMENTATION OF GOALS IN REHABILITATIVE AND RESTORATIVE CARE

GOAL 1: MAINTENANCE OF JOINT FUNCTION

The implementation of planned care for older people suggests that a holistic approach should be adopted. The major concern in implementing care is the prevention of deformities through passive exercises that keep joints moveable, promote venous return and lymphatic flow, and help prevent excessive demineralization of bones. This goal and care are dependent on the physician's orders that identify the extent of the exercise program to be implemented. By means of a thorough assessment of the physical condition of the older adult, and the specific illness and prognosis for recovery, nurses assume responsibility for the passive exercise program. Such a program may include range-of-motion activities, in which each joint is put through the normal activities of which it is capable, that is, supine, prone, lateral, medial, anterior, and posterior positions. This approach maintains the wellness capability of the joints and reduces the complication of contractures, strictures, and the limitation of activity. By implementing passive range of motion, nurses are assisting the injured person to resume independence of function and perform at optimal levels.

GOAL 2: ACTIVE EXERCISE

Another group of interventions is designed to improve function and performance. This group of interventions can be referred to as active exercise. Active exercise entails transferring from bed to chair, walking and ambulating with assistive devices, proper use of crutches, knowledge of how to maneuver the wheelchair, hand-eye coordination, and the use of assistive devices that promote independent living in a normal manner. In each of these activities, nurses, in the role of teacher, help motivate the person to be as active in personal care as possible.

GOAL 3: BLADDER CONTINENCE

In some situations, it is necessary for the LPN to initiate bladder-training programs. Achievement of continence avoids the use of indwelling catheters. Bladder training aids in reducing the chance for urinary tract infections and increases self-esteem. Retraining is based on the development of clear patterns of communication between staff, the older adult, and the family regarding the schedule for toileting (usually every 2 hours). It is necessary for the bladder to be emptied at set times throughout the day. Limiting fluids after 6:00 P.M. so that the bladder can retain urine throughout the night is another strategy. At times, periodic catheterization may be employed to develop reflex emptying when the sensation for voiding is diminished or absent.

GOAL 4: BOWEL CONTINENCE

In addition to bladder training, it is important to employ bowel-training techniques if they are needed. Bowel training requires the establishment of a routine for emptying the bowel daily. This occurs most normally in the morning approximately 20 minutes after breakfast. The intake of breakfast stimulates the duodenocolic reflex, which assists in bowel elimination. A diet consisting of whole-grain breads, cereals, fresh fruits, fluids, and whole bran, along with increased fluid intake is helpful in providing both the bulk and fluid needed for effective bowel training. This approach also reduces the complication of constipation in the older adult. If constipation does occur, it may be necessary to provide medication to soften the stool and allow the bowel contents to move into the lower colon area for elimination. It also is helpful in bowel-training programs to request that the older adult assume the squatting position (use the toilet instead of the bed pan) to facilitate bowel elimination. This is not always possible. Rectal suppositories are useful when initiating a bowel-training program. Enemas are rarely used as part of a bowel-training program.

GOAL 5: APPROPRIATE SEXUAL EXPRESSION

The implementation of a holistic plan of care means that the LPN must be aware of the older adult's sexual needs. It is important to implement nursing care that allows each person to meet personal sexual needs. This means building in time during the rehabilitation and restorative care process for partners to have privacy. It also can include offering the sense of touch by holding hands with the elderly in appropriate ways and, when given permission, for squeezing the shoulder or forearm with a firm but gentle touch.

GOAL 6: PSYCHOSOCIAL AND SPIRITUAL WELL-BEING

It is extremely important to include interventions that address the psychosocial and spiritual needs of older adults. Communication, increased self-concept and self-esteem, treating the person with dignity and respect, as well as meeting spiritual needs are essential to holistic nursing care. Examples could include uninterrupted time to pray, arrangements for visits from the local clergy, and allowing religious artifacts in the room.

In implementing rehabilitation and restorative care, nurses follow the plan of care outlined by the IDT. Such information comes from the database of information collected during the admission assessment and periodically throughout the course of the care. The nurse must be alert to changes that need to be made in the plan of care.

The implementation of care measures should focus on previous coping skills of the older adult. It is important that older adults become partners in the care regimen by sharing knowledge and adaptability. The goals are established by the older person, the family, and the nurse, as a member of the IDT, based on the assessment data. When the goal is stated in specific, measurable terms, then evaluation of the progress and outcome of care is easily measured. The terms of the goal are to be put in the framework of self-care and self-responsibility.

▶ ASSESSMENT OF GOALS

Goals are assessed at intervals—sometimes daily, sometimes weekly, sometimes monthly—depending on the goal to be accomplished. When the goals have been stated in observable, measurable terms, then the assessment of their achievement is relatively easy. In the course of the disease or traumatic injury, in-depth documentation is extremely important for noting the progress of the person. A systematic approach to fulfill all the stated goals assures the patient, family, and health-care team that a holistic approach has been incorporated into the older adult's care. This approach reassures both the older adult and the nurse that custodial care will be avoided, and that rehabilitation and restorative nursing from a holistic perspective is in place.

GOALS SPECIFIC TO THE ELDERLY POPULATION

Restorative nursing goals specific to older adults include:

• Improvement of function

- Delay of deterioration
- Accommodation to dysfunction
- Comfort in the dying process

IMPROVEMENT OF FUNCTION

Functionality is defined as the ability to continue to live one's preferred lifestyle without disruption. To put that concept into different terms, it means that each older adult can live independently, do activities of daily living (ADLs) and instrumental ADLs (IADLs), be mobile, and have self-care ability. To live independently suggests that there is no need for physical assistance or supervision from another person. Goal assessment on a daily or weekly basis is essential to good care.

To improve function, it is necessary to take into account the impact of the older person's social and environmental situation, functional implications of acute or chronic disease processes, and the physical factors that may influence function. By combining these factors, a picture of the capability of older adults to live and function should emerge for the health-care team.

Range of motion is a series of exercises performed on a regular basis to preserve the function of the joints and muscles. It is extremely important that this maintenance function be performed correctly and on a schedule so that no deterioration of the physical status of the person occurs. The nurse, under the direction of the physical therapist, does this activity or instructs another health team member to carry out this procedure correctly.

Improving the strength of the muscles necessitates that some resistance be exerted so that the muscle works hard to maintain or improve its function. This is often accomplished through the use of weights or by pushing against an object to provide resistance. The actual testing of the muscle strength and endurance is done by the physical therapist, and a plan of exercise is identified. This plan must be carried out meticulously so that every muscle and its function is duly exercised, and strength and endurance are improved.

Mobility is identified in various stages, depending on the type of injury or disease present in the older adult. Usually, the progression is from bed mobility, through transfer activities, to wheelchair or ambulatory locomotion. Transfer includes getting from bed to chair and back to bed, on and off a toilet, and in and out of a bathtub or car. These activities involve standing, sitting, pivoting, turning, or side-slide movement (sliding from bed to chair using a transfer board). To promote function in mobility involves locomotion or moving from one point to another. Older adults may need to use a wheelchair, so the ability to propel and maneuver the wheelchair is important. Wheelchair use involves the development of arm strength with the use of weights or other forms of strength building. Other assistive devices such as crutches, braces, and splints may be needed to assist in locomotion. To help the individual reach optimal function, instruction needs to be given regarding the best approaches to maintaining balance and endurance as well as in the use of devices to prevent falls.

When the goal is to improve function, there is a positive outcome orientation. For example, if the nursing diagnosis is stated:

- Body Image Disturbance, self-esteem disturbance related to function limitations, role and lifestyle change.

Then the goal should be written:

- The older adult will verbalize positive statements about self.
- The older adult will identify and demonstrate appropriate strategies to deal with functional limitations.

Some of these strategies could be the ability to manipulate buttons and zippers, to tie shoelaces, and to put on underwear. If the older adult is unable to perform these functions, then devices such as long-handled reachers, button hooks, and elastic shoelaces may allow the person to perform more independently.

In helping older people retain functional ability and avoid deterioration, it is important to be cognizant of the disease processes that may interfere with their ability to achieve independent living. Such limiting problems most often involve cardiorespiratory, neurological, or musculoskeletal systems. Many of these conditions may impose significant functional limitations on the person. All of these factors are to be kept in mind when implementing goals for rehabilitative and restorative care for the elderly patient. Dedication to the restorative care plan helps older people keep motivated and engage in the purposeful and varied activities that promote function and performance.

DELAY OF DETERIORATION

A primary goal of rehabilitative and restorative nursing is the delay of deterioration in all functional aspects. For example, if on admission and during the course of treatment bouts of depression are noted, this factor should be documented in terms of the behaviors exhibited as well as their frequency and duration. The RN is to be notified and a psychiatric consult requested if it is determined to be appropriate for the individual. Depression signals initial deterioration of motivation. Helping the person maintain a spirit of hopefulness is one way to assist in the delay of deterioration.

Another approach to ensure delay of deterioration is to make certain that the nursing care plan calls for exercise of all mobile bodily parts, that is, legs, arms, fingers, toes, neck, hips, and knees. Movement of all of these joints is essential in the maintenance of a healthy state. No nurse should ever allow a contracture to occur. Use of pillows, a footboard to prevent foot drop, and resting splints for wrists and fingers aids in proper alignment of the body to maintain function and delay deterioration. Properly aligned and supported body parts assume their natural posture and position. As noted earlier, passive range-of-motion exercises for all joints can delay deterioration to a great extent. However, caution must be exercised. If care is not used in moving the joints, soft tissue injury can result from undue stretching of the muscles and joints; this could cause additional injury and slow the rate of recovery or cause great pain when the person becomes active once again.

Another priority concern is the prevention of pressure ulcers. Excellent skin care should be a daily part of nursing care for all persons. This is especially important for elderly people who have impaired nutritional status. Pressure ulcers may develop over any bony prominence as well as on the occiput, ear parts, sacrum, and greater trochanter. Special devices to cushion these parts need to be used as a preventive measure and include special pillows, donuts, and gauze dressings, as well as special mattresses (egg crate, circulating water, or air). Turning the patient every 2 hours is the best preventive measure that can be taken to ensure skin integrity. When turning the patient, the support of limbs and back for good body alignment is essential to keep weakened muscles from further deterioration.

Cognitively impaired elderly are in need of individualized nursing care. These people need appropriate sensory stimulation to maintain their contact with the world. Putting the person in a position where others can be seen as well as the careful use of the radio and TV can help stimulate cognitive functions and lessen the possibility of further deterioration.

To delay deterioration, older adults should participate in out-of-bed activities as soon as they have achieved a medically stable condition. First, they should dangle their feet for several minutes to gain a sense of balance. Once this activity is tolerated, the nurse should help the older adult to stand by the side of the bed with whatever assistive device needed, for example, a walker or cane. Finally, the person should be assisted to walk to a chair and sit with proper support for approximately 15 minutes at a time. Nurses are essential for providing the appropriate encouragement for the individual.

ACCOMMODATION TO DYSFUNCTION

The goal of helping elderly people accommodate to dysfunction requires a great deal of motivation on the part of the nurse. It is essential for the LPN to listen attentively and actively to the personal fears, hopes, thoughts, feelings, and values that are expressed by the person who is adjusting to the deficits left by an accident, injury, or stroke. Nurses should be aware that a rehabilitation program is primarily a learning and training process. Each person must have the ability to absorb new information on how to use personal potential and how to practice new skills. For example, if a person has sustained an injury that created a drop-foot gait, the individual must learn to accommodate walking by lifting the foot intentionally so that it remains flat as weight is shifted from one side of the body to the next. This requires major concentration until the old adage "practice makes perfect" becomes second nature to the walker. The nurse's role is to encourage the

Holistic wellness occurs when the psychological self-image of a person incorporates his limitations in a healthy and acceptable image.

person to keep working for the highest outcome possible.

Holistic wellness occurs for the restorative care older adult when:

- The psychological self-image of the person incorporates personal limitations into a healthy and acceptable image
- Social activities and interactions with friends and family continue to be a major part of the person's life
- The person exhibits acceptance of the new lifestyle with joy, peace, and gratitude for the remaining strengths of his or her personhood.

These are the elements to be found when the goal of accommodation to dysfunction is achieved. As the grief and sense of loss diminish, a healthier view of life strikes older people so that life once again is worth living for them.

COMFORT IN THE DYING PROCESS

It has been noted that 75% of deaths in older people suffering from trauma were caused by falls, thermal injury, and motor vehicle accidents. Falls, for both elderly men and women, are the leading cause of death. Falls constitute approximately 50% of all fatalities. The most common injuries are associated with fractures of the hip, femur, proximal humerus, Colles' fracture of the wrist, and head injuries. In deaths in people 65 years of age and older, 25% are from motor vehicle accidents. As the population continues to age, this percentage of deaths and injuries will undoubtedly increase. Death from thermal injury accounts for approximately 8% of all accidental deaths in those 65 years of age and older. These injuries include burns and inhalation injuries, electrical injury, and contacts with sources of heat. The most commonly reported types of thermal injuries include scalds, flame burns, and contact with hot objects.

Restorative nursing may include providing comfort measures and palliative care to those elderly patients who, because of severe injury and trauma, are in the process of dying. Palliative care means providing the care requested by the older person in terms of advance directives and a living will. The individual's decisions are to be honored by the nurse and family members. It may be that the older adult has requested that no food or water be given after it has been determined that no benefits will be derived from such comfort measures. Life-sustaining technologies such as intravenous solutions of water and saline or use of a respirator also may be requested to be terminated if no positive outcome is predictable. All of these wishes are to be followed using the Code of Ethics for Nurses.

Nurses are to be supportive of dying elderly patients and their family members. You must be accountable to the dying person for decisions that have been made and facilitate their implementation. All decisions are to be carried out in a humane and compassionate manner. The dying process is a precious approach to the end of one's life. Nurses need to approach death with reverence for the body, mind, and spirit of the older person who moves into the terminal state of life. The nurse should attend the dying person with dignity, respect, and appreciation for personal uniqueness. Refer to Chapter 6 for more information on end-of-life issues.

▶ CLINICAL IMPLICATIONS OF REHABILITATIVE AND RESTORATIVE CARE

Using the framework of the restorative care principles and guidelines cited earlier, four clinical rehabilitative programs for older adults are outlined. These programs include the following:

- Walking or ambulation programs
- Bladder and bowel continence training
- Feeding and self-feeding programs
- Self-care—ADL programs

WALKING PROGRAMS

Mobility is critical to optimal functioning for older people. To be mobile means that the individual will enjoy the satisfaction of independence in living. Nurses play a key role in providing motivation for a walking program. Depending on the type of assistive device needed by the older adult to aid in gait control, the nurse follows the directions given by the RN, physician, or the physical therapist. A key point is that excellent foot care is critical to maintaining a walking program. Also, properly fitting shoes are important to establish proper posture while walking.

The older adult may need braces or crutches to walk in a way that is beneficial. Leg and back braces are devices that are used to support body weight, limit involuntary movements, or prevent and correct deformities. Crutches are devices that may be necessary to help the person learn to walk again in a normal manner. Crutches may be used on a temporary or permanent basis, depending on the type of injury sustained during the trauma.

For successful crutch walking, it is important to strengthen the muscle groups used in this activity. This should begin as soon as the physician believes that the older adult has recovered sufficiently to consider walking.

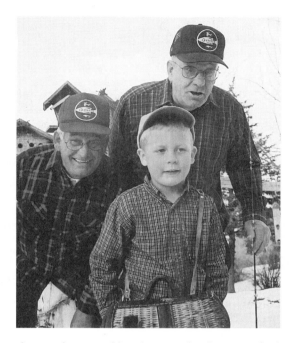

As people grow older, they need to keep moving! Even people without assistive devices need to be encouraged to keep mobile. These men are more eager to go fishing when grandchildren accompany them.

Strengthening exercises should be provided while the patient is still confined to bed. These exercises include the muscles of the arms, shoulders, chest, and back. Before ambulation, the older adult should be taught how to move from the bed to the chair and should be capable of performing this movement without assistance. Older people who need assistance to learn to stand, balance themselves, and ambulate again sometimes experience difficulty. This makes patience on the part of the nurse an important quality.

Important points in crutch walking include correct measurements for crutches so they will have a proper fit. It is important that they have heavy rubber tips to prevent the crutch from sliding. The crutches need to be moved in a rhythmical way that propels the person forward. Finally, the crutches should have padding on the underarm piece so weight is not placed on the radial nerve. The handhold on the crutches may have padding to reduce irritation there as well. The nurse should emphasize good posture for the person who is crutch walking; the head should be held high and the pelvis should be kept over the feet for excellent balance. Crutch walking is best taught in several short lessons to reduce fatigue in the older adult. When ambulation begins, it is important to have an attendant both in front and in back of the person to provide stability and to reduce anxiety about possible falls.

There are several types of gaits that may be used in crutch walking, depending on the type of injury and the physician's orders. These types are given in the following list:

- **Four-point gait:** The person bears weight on both feet and has four-point contact with the floor (both crutches and both feet).
- **Two-point gait:** There are two points of contact with the floor (crutches only).
- **Swing-to gait:** Crutches are placed ahead of the person and, with weight on the crutches, the body swings through to the crutches.
- **Three-point gait:** Partial weight bearing is permitted.

As the older adult practices the walking program outlined earlier, the person should master sufficient ADLs to be independent. This independence includes being able to get up and down steps, and in and out of cars. It is important for nurses to be very familiar with all assistive devices used in walking programs.

Walking programs also are initiated for those without assistive devices. It is recognized that walking for the older adult is an excellent physical fitness activity. It provides cardiovascular fitness as well as aerobic exercise. Walking for 20–30 minutes, three times a week, has been supported by research as a way to maintain good physical fitness and conditioning. Walking should be a lifelong program to promote wellness and joy in living.

CONTINENCE TRAINING

A second major clinical challenge is maintenance of bladder and bowel continence in the traumatized, disabled older adult. The older adult who is the recipient of good nursing care should not experience urinary or bowel incontinence. The use of an indwelling catheter is not effective bladder management. This is because urinary infection can result within 24 hours of catheter insertion. Catheter insertion also lowers the self-esteem and self-concept of the person trying to regain control of a traumatized life.

Bladder retraining is generally successful when a regular time schedule is established for emptying the bladder. Retraining of the bladder takes patience on the part of both the older adult and the nurse. A similar program for bowel training should be initiated soon after admission. As noted earlier, increasing the patient's fiber and fluid intake and a regular toileting regimen promote bowel elimination on a regular schedule. If constipation does occur, stool softeners are the treatment of choice to resolve this problem.

FEEDING AND SELF-FEEDING PROGRAMS

The clinical challenge of maintaining nutrition adequate for tissue repair and health demands a high level of skill on the part of the LPN. In the early stages of rehabilitative and restorative nursing, the older adult may need to be fed through a nasogastric tube. A specially formulated feeding prepared to caloric specifications is fed through the tube on a regular basis. The tube should be patent, and sufficient fluid should be used to keep it clear and unclogged. After each feeding, flush the tube with 30 mL of water.

As the older adult progresses in recovery, he or she may need to be placed on a feeding program in which manual assistance by the LPN or aide is needed until the person has sufficient strength for self-feeding. Older adults should be fed at regular mealtimes, and snacks also should be provided. Promoting the older person to a self-feeding program is a definite sign of progress. Encouragement is to be given by the nurse so that the older adult consumes sufficient calories to have adequate nutrition to meet the energy demands of rehabilitation.

SELF-PROMOTING BEHAVIORS AND ACTIVITIES OF DAILY LIVING

Independence in personal care is a definite challenge for older adults with disabilities that affect their range of motion, mobility, strength, coordination, and dexterity. It is important that members of the nursing care team allow older adults to have time to independently perform aspects of their own care.

Occupational therapists can provide assistive equipment that makes self-care easier. Built-up handles for tooth brushes and hair brushes are easier for older adults to hold. A chair in the tub or shower may allow a weak individual to be able to bathe independently. Lowered sinks, counters, and mirrors might allow a wheelchair bound person to sit up to the sink to wash and perform other personal care. Specially designed plastic devices with long handles are available to insert inside a person's socks, and long-handled shoe horns allow older people who are unable to bend over to put on their own socks and shoes. Clothing, with Velcro fasteners, is easier to fasten and unfasten when dressing. Adjustments in the care environment and education of all of the personal care staff is essential to the success of self-care–ADL programs.

▶ CONCLUSION

This chapter provides an overview of the principles that govern rehabilitation and restorative nursing practices for LPNs who care for older adults in various settings. Through appreciation of the uniqueness of older adults and their special needs, rehabilitative and restorative nursing care can help them achieve optimal functioning to live life to the fullest.

CASE STUDY

At the age of 60, Mr. A. suffered a severe, incapacitating stroke on the left side of his body. Mr. A. and his wife had planned to retire in 5 years and travel. The stroke created major difficulties regarding the couple's anticipated retirement. While hospitalized, Mr. A. developed a drop-foot condition that interfered with his rehabilitative program. He became despondent over his condition and refused to participate in the walking program.

Discussion

As the LPN responsible for Mr. A.'s care, you need to do an assessment of his holistic needs. What are the priorities of care?

Solution

1. Mr. A. needs assurance from the health professionals, nurses, and therapists that he will gain sufficient strength to walk with the aid of a walker and eventually to walk independently.
2. The LPN and Mr. A. contract to carry out the walking and exercise program on a daily basis to correct the drop-foot problem.
3. By setting goals, Mr. A. perceives his condition in a more positive light and is encouraged by his progress.
4. The LPN also is concerned about Mr. A's despondency. She documents Mr. A.'s behavior and informs the registered nurse about his psychological state. Together, the nurses talk with Mr. A. about his depression and seeks his approval to obtain a psychiatric consultation. This problem is then referred to the mental health professional.
5. The LPN arranges for Mr. A. and his wife to become participants in a clinical conference in which the rehabilitative team reviews Mr. A.'s case and allows him to make informed decisions on how to proceed on discharge. This may include referral to various social agencies that could assist him in obtaining medical equipment for home use, receiving nursing care in the home if his wife feels unable to take care of Mr. A., and seeking social security/pension payments if Mr. A. believes he can no longer work.
6. Mr. A. is encouraged to eat nutritious meals so that his tissue can repair. He needs sufficient energy from his nutritional intake to do his exercises and walking program properly.
7. Activities are scheduled for him so that he can regain his social skills and interact with people without embarrassment and hesitation. Mr. A. was discharged from the hospital within 2 weeks of the incident, feeling that he once again was in charge of his life and that life was worth living. He also could see that the goals he and his wife had established for retirement could indeed be accomplished. Mr. A. learned to live with his disability and, because of good nursing care, the quality of his life was not diminished.

STUDY QUESTIONS

Please select the one best answer.

1. The aim of rehabilitation for older adults is to:
   a. Engage in limited ADLs
   b. Deny function and performance that existed before the incident
   c. Keep food and fluids at a level so that energy and strength are minimized .
   d. Restore an individual to his former or best possible function and environmental status

2. Which of the following directives most closely coincides with the desired goals of a successful rehabilitation program?
   a. Keep physical changes at a minimum, and promote self-esteem.
   b. Promote independence and self-care, along with mobility and a holistic approach to living with the disability.
   c. Promote involvement in limited activities and range-of-motion exercises.
   d. Promote the fulfillment of patient's life's goals in spite of mobility problems.

3. Principles of rehabilitation include the most important step in nursing care, which is:
   a. Doing passive range of motion
   b. Understanding the patient's self-concept and encouraging feelings of dependency
   c. Beginning rehabilitation immediately on the patient's admission

   d. Giving selective information to the family

4. Rehabilitation goals specific to older adults include:
   a. Range-of-motion exercises, transfer skills from bed to chair, dependency on enema usage
   b. Improvement of function, delay of deterioration, development of codependent behavior
   c. Accommodation to dysfunction, comfort in the dying process, accommodation to an indwelling catheter
   d. Delay of deterioration, improvement of function, accommodation to dysfunction, comfort in the dying process

5. In continence training for bladder control, the nurse should:
   a. Increase fluids, especially during the evening hours, and toilet the patient every 4 hours
   b. Restrict fluids during the nighttime hours and toilet the patient at his or her request
   c. Increase fluids during the daytime hours and toilet the patient every 1000 mL
   d. Increase fluids during the daytime hours and toilet the patient every 2 hours

Pamela E. Hugie

chapter **15**

Pharmacology and Its Significance for Older Adults

Learning Objectives

After completing this chapter, the student will be able to:

1. Identify physiological changes of aging that affect pharmacotherapeutics in older adults.
2. Identify sensory changes of aging that affect pharmacotherapeutics in older adults.
3. Identify psychological changes of aging that affect pharmacotherapeutics in older adults.
4. Identify polypharmacy problems in older adults and nursing interventions to compensate for them.
5. Develop a nursing care plan to synthesize interventions to assist older persons to maintain proper pharmacotherapeutics.

▶ INTRODUCTION

One of the biggest advances in medical care has been the discovery and rediscovery of plants and chemical compounds that formulate drugs. Drugs are prescribed to manage and sometimes even cure physical and mental illnesses. Ancient civilizations used a variety of herbs and other plant and mineral substances to ward off, prevent, and treat physical and mental problems. Many modern drugs used in western medicine practice have a long history of effectiveness in healing. Some medicines that are prescribed today were originally discovered and used by medical practitioners and healers from other cultures. Quality medical care and medications are responsible for increasing life the expectancy of large populations of people. A dilemma of western medicine is the heavy dependence on the use of medications for managing and treating diseases. Many people do not consider that a medical treatment is complete unless they receive a prescription for a drug. This can be a serious issue for older adults. This chapter examines issues related to drug use and older adults. Some basic terms related to drug use are:

- *Pharmacology*—The study of medications.
- *Pharmacotherapeutics*—The use of medications to treat diseases. The benefit of a medication (desired effect) is weighed against the unwanted and dangerous effects (side effects) to measure the appropriate use of any medication.
- *Pharmacodynamics*—The effect of specific medications at the site of action. Pharmacokinetics, half-life, protein binding, disease processes, and aging affect pharmacodynamics.
- *Pharmacokinetics*—The study of how a medication moves into and through the body, and how it is excreted from the body. The processes of absorption, distribution, metabolism, and excretion, are affected by aging and diseases, and influence the pharmacodynamics of any drug.
- *Half-life*—The time required for half the medication to be excreted or inactivated by the body.
- *Protein binding*—Binding properties of proteins. Proteins in the blood stream are binding sites for many drugs. The portion of a drug that is bound to a protein is inactive

(only a free drug is available to have a desired effect). Two drugs that are both highly protein bound compete for protein binding sites. This significantly increases the level of free drug in the blood stream (drug molecules that were bound to the protein and have been released). The significant increase has an impact on the effects and adverse effects of the drug.

- *Adverse drug reactions* (ADRs)—Unwanted effects or side effects of a medication. Related to changes in pharmacokinetics, dosage amounts, timing of doses, and interactions of medications with other medications or foods

▶ AGING CHANGES THAT AFFECT PHARMACO-THERAPEUTICS

CHANGES IN VISION

Changes in vision can have a serious impact on the safe use of medications by older adults. As individuals age, they experience increased difficulty distinguishing colors, especially blue and green, because of the hardening and yellowing of the lens in their eyes. This yellowing often makes it difficult to differentiate shades of blue, purple, brown, and green, yet older people can see bright yellow, red, and black more clearly. Many older adults have difficulty distinguishing individual pills by color. When older patients are instructed to take the "pink pill in the morning and the blue one at night," they may make errors.

Reading small print is also a challenge for many older adults. Older people often have trouble reading the label on drug bottles because of the small print. Attaching a large print tag to a bottle and having a magnifying glass by drug bottles can help an older person read the medication bottle label and avoid medication errors. Using a medication box or mediplanner is a good idea for many older individuals. Medication boxes are filled with the person's ordered medication. For each time during the day that the older person has to take a medication, the box has a separate compartment. Usually, the box is filled for a week at a time, and the days of the week and times of medication doses are clearly marked in large, bold, raised initials, and symbols. Family members and friends can be taught to assist their older family member to prepare the medication box for a week at a time.

Sensitivity to glare is another visual challenge for aging eyes. Shiny surfaces like plastic tape over medication labels can be difficult for older people to read. Portions of instructions written on paper that has been laminated may be missed or difficult to read because of reflecting glare. Labels for drug bottles should be printed on paper that is not shiny. Medication instructions should be in bold, large print on white or yellow paper to ensure they can be read.

DECREASED HEARING ACUITY

Hearing changes, such as presbycusis, increase the possibility that an older person may be unable to hear and understand instructions. Often, out of habit, older adults may nod their heads or state that they understand instructions even if they did not hear them all. Asking them to repeat or demonstrate instructions are excellent ways to ensure that the instructions have been heard. Using large print instructions and following them when giving verbal instructions also helps most older people. Many people with hearing difficulties develop lip-reading skills. Make sure that the older adult can see your mouth while you are giving instructions. Wearing lipstick if you are female, and speaking slowly and intentionally, rather than louder, enhances an older person's ability to read lips. Throughout the time that you, the nurse, are giving verbal instructions, stop and ask older patients if they have any questions. Clarify information and have them restate and demonstrate the teaching that is occurring.

DECREASED TASTE ACUITY

With age, older adults experience changes in taste. It is most obvious in foods. A common complaint is that food is bland or has no taste. Changes in recognizing tastes and flavors result from changes in the taste buds and often in the sense of smell. The ability to differentiate medications by taste is inhibited, and the potential for unknowingly taking nonmedications or caustic poisons increases. Encourage older adults to throw away old prescription bottles and not to use them for storing household cleaning products and other poisons that may be mistaken for medications.

CHANGES IN TOUCH AND DEXTERITY

Older adults experience decreased touch sensitivity as they age. This can be worsened with decreased circulation and peripheral nerve deterioration in the hands and feet. Arthritic joint changes can combine with decreased touch to minimize strength seriously, which, in turn, can make it difficult to open modern packages. Childproof lids that require a person to push down and turn at the same time are very difficult for older people to open. Individual drug doses in plastic bubbles that require the plastic to be torn or the backing to be ripped off also are difficult. Pharmacists use alternative packaging for older adults if the older person requests it. Flip-top lids can replace the hard-to-twist childproof lids. Bubble-packed medications can be cut out of the packaging and placed in a pill bottle or a pill box.

COGNITIVE CHANGES

With increasing age and subsequent risk for disease, older adults may have changes in their thought patterns. It is important for the nurse to question what has caused the thought pattern changes. Are the causes pathological or drug-induced? Sometimes older adults have trouble remembering if they have taken their medications. Multiple drugs with varying dosages administered at different hours often create confusion.

Visual deficits often are a source of concern with medication management of the elderly population.

The technical language that health-care professionals frequently use can be difficult for older people to understand, and they often are unwilling to ask questions. Many older adults do not want to seem uninformed, and state they trust the doctor or nurse to do what is right.

COMPLIANCE FACTORS

Often individuals do not correctly follow their drug regimen. This can be intentional or be the result of poor understanding. If older adults do not understand how a drug works or do not like the effect of a drug, they may make mistakes in administering their medications. Common problems are taking doses at the wrong time and altering the dosage amounts.

Forgetting to take medications is a routine compliance issue. When giving older people medication instructions, ask them to describe a typical day. Instructions to take a medication everyday before breakfast rather than instructing them to take the drug at 8:00 A.M. may encourage compliance, especially if they sleep until noon or are up at five in the morning. Studies have demonstrated that more medication doses are forgotten when a drug is dosed frequently during the day rather than once a day. Simplified dosing schedules that consider the older person's daily routine and the use of medications that are dosed only once a day can help the person be compliant in taking medications.

Drugs are taken for the chemical effect that they have on the body. Unfortunately, unwanted effects or side effects are common for many medications. Individuals often choose to alter the dosages or quit taking an ordered medication because of the side effects. One of the most common side effects that older adults complain of is upset stomach. This often is caused by the medication dissolving in the stomach and irritating the stomach lining. Stomach irritation can be lessened by instructing the older adult to take the medication with food. If the medication needs to be taken on an empty stomach, encourage the person to take at least 8 oz (one cup) of water with the medication. This washes the medication through the stomach faster and, it is hoped, lessens stomach irritation. Encourage people to talk about the uncomfortable side effects of their medications. Often by simply changing the timing of a medication dosage (from morning to bedtime dosing), unwanted or bothersome side effects may decrease significantly.

It is not uncommon for people to simply stop taking a medication. News in the media and advice from neighbors or friends may make older people uncomfortable with specific drugs or even fearful of the drug's long-term effects on their body. Encourage them to discuss these concerns. Unfortunately, people who are not accurately following prescribed drug regimens are reluctant to tell their doctor. Not following orders could be interpreted as questioning the doctor's skill and knowledge, and most older people do not want to be disrespectful. Many older adults manipulate drug routines to fit their beliefs about personal medication needs. Encourage an open dialogue about medications. Allow the expression of concerns or questions. Review magazines and newspapers that older people read to keep informed regarding potential questions and concerns they may have regarding their medications.

POLYPHARMACY AND CHRONIC HEALTH CHANGES

A good rule to follow for pharmacotherapeutics in the older people is "the smallest number of drugs should be prescribed at the lowest possible dose." Two thirds of physician office visits by older adults result in the prescription of one or more new drugs. Of these prescriptions, 50% will not have the desired therapeutic action for various reasons that range from too high or too low a dosage to not getting the prescription filled. Studies have shown that many physicians who prescribe for older people do not make adjustments in dosages although the need for such adjustments related to age have been clearly established. Many physicians are not educated on dosage adjustment for older people. Most drugs are not tested for their effects on people age 65 and older. Studies on drug dosing, effects, and side effects are done most commonly with healthy middle-aged adults. The results of such studies are applied mistakenly to drug use for older adults. Such practices can lead to unanticipated drug effects and misdiagnosed drug side effects.

Older adults often have multiple chronic diseases. People with chronic health problems frequently have several drugs prescribed for each problem. The result for older adults often is a complex, which is called multiple drug medication regimen. This complexity is compounded when the older individual has multiple physicians prescribing medications. Pharmacists are skilled at identifying potential drug interactions, but their effectiveness depends on awareness of the total medication regimen. If an older person uses more than one pharmacy, a pharmacist cannot be aware of other drugs the individual is taking. Increased numbers of medications and varied dosing schedules can lead to mistakes in taking medications and serious drug interactions. For example, an older adult with Alzheimer's disease may have periods of agitated behavior. A tranquilizer may be prescribed to decrease the agitation. Unfortunately, the tranquilizer has a sedating effect that can increase drowsiness and make the older adult at a higher risk for immobility and falls. This can lead to joint pain and pain associated with injuries that may require pain medications that can further increase immobility related to drowsiness and increased risk of falls. Using drugs to treat disease symptoms and using other drugs to treat the side effects of such drugs can lead to the severe adverse drug effects of polypharmacy. A thorough assessment of drug regimens as an effort to simplify them are important steps in avoiding adverse effects of polypharmacy.

Complex prescription routines are not the only cause of polypharmacy. Many older individuals take multiple nonprescription medications, such as laxatives, herbs, vitamins, and other home remedies. These widely available, over-the-counter (OTC) medications may interfere with prescribed medications, leading to adverse drug reactions.

Older adults are significantly more prone to have undesirable drug reactions than younger adults. This potential increases in direct proportion to the number of medications being taken. Studies have shown that the potential for adverse drug reactions is 100% when an older adult is taking eight or more drugs a day. Common symptoms of adverse drug reactions or drug toxicity are changes in mood or behavior, restlessness, confusion, irritability, anxiety, insomnia, and hallucinations suggestive of mental deterioration. Many of these symptoms can be confused with acute brain problems, whereas the adverse drug reaction may go unrecognized. More medications may be prescribed to treat the symptoms of adverse drug reactions and the cycle of problems continues.

FINANCIAL CONCERNS

Medications are expensive. Sometimes older adults self-prescribe rather than pay money for an office visit and a prescription. The end result of this behavior is the use of limited financial resources on OTC, self-prescribed medication that may or may not be beneficial. Older people spend three times more on nonprescription drugs than the general public.

Many older adults experience nutritional changes related to decreased financial resources. This may mean a decreased consumption of protein, resulting in decreased serum protein levels and decreased drug-binding ability. An increased use of alcohol, with resulting liver damage, may increase the metabolism time of the drug so it circulates longer in the body.

The cost of physician office visits and getting prescriptions filled may be difficult for an older person to manage. Some people never get their prescriptions filled. Some save their prescriptions until they can get to the pharmacist with the right amount of money (this may result in not taking the medications for a month or more). Some people choose over-the-counter medications for relief of the same symptoms as the prescribed drug and never get the prescription filled. Some older persons "save" their drugs by taking only one dose a day instead of two so the medication will last longer. For the home-bound individual, filling a prescription may necessitate the added expense of hiring someone to deliver the prescription, or of being driven to the pharmacy and back home. Some people take the medications until the symptoms decrease, and then put the rest away for "later." Other people share "over-the-fence" medications and health information with their friends and neighbors to save the money of an office visit or prescription filling. "Over-the-fence" medications appear in scenarios in which Aunt Matilda has a pill that worked for her shoulder pain and a friend with shoulder pain then calls her to borrow some of the pills that helped Aunt Matilda. The friend may seem to benefit by not having to pay for and make a physician's office visit; Aunt Matilda may feel good about helping another person; but in actuality the drug may not help or may indeed be detrimental to Aunt Matilda's friend.

▶ PHARMACOKINETICS

Physiological changes related to normal aging and various disease processes affect the pharmacokinetics of many medications. When an individual takes a medication, there are certain expected events that assist the medication to get to the intended site of action or effect. Medications in pill form are usually formulated to break down in the stomach acid or the small intestine. The dissolved medication is then absorbed in the same place. If the individual has had a part of the stomach removed or has a low concentration of stomach acid, the pill may not be dissolved enough to be absorbed as expected. A good blood supply is necessary for the distribution of medication. Diminished blood supply to or from an area of the body alters the effective distribution of the medication. Most medications are metabolized by the liver. Liver disease or changes in the blood circulation to the liver change the expected metabolism of a medication. Excretion is the last step in pharmacokinetics. The kidneys have a major role in the excretion of most medications. Kidney disease or decreased blood flow to the kidneys can seriously change the intended excretion of medications. The following information is a discussion of the specific pharmacokinetic concerns for older adults.

DECREASED ABSORPTION

The overall effect of aging changes in older adults is decreased absorption. A major complaint by many older individuals is change in gastrointestinal (GI) motility, with resulting diarrhea or constipation. Drugs are absorbed poorly if they travel through the intestines at a rapid rate. Chronic diarrhea and overuse of laxatives move a medication through the intestines at a rapid rate and decrease the time that the drug is in contact with the intestinal wall to be absorbed. Drugs also are absorbed poorly if the intestine is impacted with stool, as in constipation.

Changes in the gastrointestinal tract probably interfere with normal absorption of medications. Older adults often have changes in the quality and quantity of digestive enzymes that are important for dissolving and transforming medications into a form that can be absorbed through the intestine. Gastric pH becomes less acidic, and there is an overall decrease in the number of absorbing cells in the intestinal mucosa. The smooth muscle tone and motor activity of the gastrointestinal tract decline with advancing age. These changes, along with slowed intestinal motility, decreased intestinal blood flow, and slowed gastric emptying time serve to decrease potential drug adsorption further. Atherosclerotic changes reduce the flow of blood to the major organs, resulting in slower disintegration of solid dosage forms such as tablets. Because of the changes in GI motility, drugs that are manufactured for normal adult GI motility are not suited to the slower geriatric bowel. Some drugs may be absorbed in lesser amounts; for example, acidic drugs are ionized to a greater extent, resulting in decreased absorption. Acetylsalicylic acid (aspirin), for example, is more ionized in older people because their secretion of stomach acid is decreased. Aspirin, therefore, may have decreased absorption in older adults. Some drugs may be absorbed in greater amounts. For example, drugs that are absorbed from the intestines are more thoroughly absorbed if they remain in contact with the intestinal wall for longer periods of time.

DISTRIBUTION

Drug distribution is greatly altered in older persons. As people age, the body mass becomes leaner, with decreased parenchymal tissue and increased fat content. Increased fat results in increased absorption of fat-soluble drugs. This results in decreased activity and prolonged effects for such drugs. Examples of drugs showing this effect are hypnotics, sedatives, fat-soluble vitamins, and heparin.

Changes in the cardiovascular system of the aged may result in delayed arrival of the medication at the target receptors, slow release of the drug from the storage tissue, and slowed excretion of the drug. Decreased blood flow to the specific target tissue may result in decreased drug distribution.

Older people have decreased plasma protein concentrations. Plasma protein is an important factor in drug binding in the serum. Most drug dosages are set for people with normal plasma protein levels. If the older person has less plasma protein, more of the drug is free (i.e., unbound to the protein) and, therefore, is free to act on the receptors and cause its effect. Warfarin (Coumadin), for example, is 90% bound in the average adult. Its dosage is regulated because 90% of it is bound to protein and will not be available to the person. If the person is elderly and has half the normal adult protein level, a normal dose of warfarin would be an overdose. Some researchers believe that with aging, the number and nature of drug receptors in the body change. This could result in a decreased or increased response to a normal dosage of medication.

Another factor influencing drug distribution is the chronically dehydrated state that many older adults experience. Decreased fluid consumption frequently results in a lower blood volume; this factor, in turn, decreases distribution in the blood.

METABOLISM

Older adults experience a decrease in the rates of overall metabolism, microsomal metabolism of the drug, and hepatic biotransformation of the drug, as well as a decline in the body's ability to transform active drugs into inactive drugs. The overall effect of these changes is that the drug remains for a longer time in an active form in older people. Some drugs may remain in the body twice as long as in younger adults.

EXCRETION

The altered filtration and decreased plasma volume that occur with dehydration commonly found in older people change the excretion of medications. Age-related renal changes result in slower excretion of the drug. Slowed excretion keeps drugs in the body longer and can lead to drug toxicity. Decreased respiratory and vital capacity, with increased carbon dioxide retention, results in decreased excretion of those drugs normally excreted by respiration, for example, anesthetics. Decreased and changed excretion results in an overall increased pharmacological effect of medications in older people.

The overall effect of aging changes in older adults is increased pharmacological effect. Although less medication is absorbed, it stays longer in the body and remains in the circulation for a longer time.

▶ PHARMACOLOGY PROBLEMS

Pharmacology in older adults is frequently identified as a "can of worms." Problems include misuse, overuse, underuse, erratic use, and contraindicated use of drugs. Misuse phenomena include incorrect dosing, sharing of "over-the-fence" medications between neighbors and friends, and use of the same medications for a variety of purposes. Incorrect dosing involves physicians who prescribe dosages based on guidelines for mature adults. As an individual ages, the dosage requirements for most medications decrease. Many medications given in normal adult doses to older adults result in an overdose. Another aspect of misuse occurs when a drug is taken for a variety of symptoms. "Well, this pill works for my upset stomach; it will probably work for my diarrhea."

Overuse may result from the theory that if one pill works well, then two pills will work better. People may feel that if they feel better with a vitamin supplement, two vitamin supplements will definitely improve their health. This behavior may actually poison the older person's system.

In underuse problems, the person takes less medication than prescribed to "save" pills or money if finances are a problem. Many older adults are on fixed and limited incomes, the cost of medication is high, and medication is sometimes too expensive for the person to afford. Erratic use frequently occurs with short-term memory loss or forgetfulness; for example, a person may forget to take medications for a day or two.

Contraindicated use can apply in a number of situations. For example, sometimes older adults receive several drugs from several physicians. They also may have the prescriptions filled at several pharmacies. The end result is that the older population is at a much greater risk for drug interactions, allergic reactions, and problems with polypharmacy (taking multiple medications).

SPECIFIC DRUG PROBLEMS FOR OLDER ADULTS

If all medications were carefully monitored and taken properly, and if the dosage were regulated and accompanied with instructions, the older adult would still be at greater risk than a younger adult for drug-specific problems due to aging changes in drug absorption, metabolism, and excretion. For example, if an older person is prescribed the proper dosage of digoxin, understood the medication regimen, and was in full compliance, the person

The nurse and pharmacist work together to manage every patient's and resident's medications to avoid drug interactions.

would still be at a higher risk for complications to develop. The older people simply experiences more side effects and difficulties.

Table 15.1 identifies categories of drugs that may precipitate side effects and adverse effects in older persons. It is important that you, as the LPN be aware of the possibility of potential problems and monitor for them.

▶ TABLE 15.1. SPECIFIC DRUG PROBLEMS OF ELDERLY PATIENTS

Effect	Drugs
Drugs that cause dry mouth	Analgesics, anticholinergics, antidiarrheals, antilipemics, antiemetics, antipsychotics, antiulcer medications, muscle relaxants, antihistamines, antiparkinson medications, antihypertensives
Drugs that promote gastroesophageal reflux	Anticholinergics, beta-blockers, diazepam, dopamine, theophylline
Drugs associated with ulcer formation	Adrenocorticotropic hormones, aspirin, indomethacin, iron, histamine, phenacetin, potassium
Drugs that alter absorption of nutrients	Colchicine, neomycin, cholestyramine, antacids, tricyclic antidepressants, carafate
Drugs that promote constipation	Aluminum- and calcium-containing antacids, narcotic analgesics, anticholinergics, diuretics, iron, tricyclic antidepressants
Drugs that may promote diarrhea	Analgesics, anti-inflammatory agents, antacids, antiulcer medications, antibiotics, antihypertensive medications, asthma drugs, cardiovascular drugs, diuretics, iron
Drugs that may promote hepatic damage	Acetaminophen (Tylenol), analgesics, anesthetics, antibiotics (especially penicillin and sulfa), antineoplastics, cardiovascular drugs, oral hypoglycemics, steroids
Drugs that may cause excessive depression	Antihistamines, antipsychotics, anxiolytics, cardiac glycosides, narcotics, sedative/hypnotics
Drugs that may cause dysrhythmias	Antidepressants, cardiac glycosides, phenytoin
Drugs that may damage the kidneys	Aminoglycosides, antibiotics, colchicine
Drugs that may precipitate electrolyte imbalances	Corticosteroids, diuretics
Drugs that may precipitate blood dyscrasias	Antineoplastics, antipsychotics

Another specific drug problem is the use of OTC medications. Antacids, laxatives, alcohol, and home remedies frequently interfere with the proper functioning of medication.

ANTACID ABUSE

Sometimes, antacids are consumed in large amounts by older people. Physically, a decreased amount of gastric acid has been documented with aging; paradoxically, however, antacid use usually increases with age. The antacids may be used by the elderly patient for symptoms of chest pain. Early angina attacks may be considered heartburn and treated with antacids. Other pathological processes also may be perceived as heartburn. This behavior can result in lack of care for serious health problems. Many antacids are high in sodium content. Excessive use of antacids can increase the severity of cardiovascular and renal disease, exacerbate hypertension, and result in increased fluid load for the aged body. Antacids are notorious for altering the motility of the gut, with resulting diarrhea or constipation.

Use of home remedies frequently interferes with pharmacotherapeutics. Some home remedies have actual benefits, some have only psychological benefits, and some are actually detrimental. For example, the use of bicarbonate of soda for "acid stomach" is detrimental and may result in serious acid-base imbalance. The ingredients of the home remedy need to be evaluated. The LPN must evaluate the frequency of use and the possible interactions.

LAXATIVE ABUSE

Another class of drugs sometimes abused by the older adults is laxatives. Laxatives may be taken once, twice, or more times a day. Some older people forget that they have had a bowel movement and take more laxatives to facilitate another bowel movement. Although there is no consistent alteration in frequency of bowel movements with advancing age, the ingestion of laxatives increases significantly.

Laxative abuse may result in actual damage to the intestinal mucosa. The ascending colon is often the site for this damage and may dilate and shorten, losing its typical muscular features, so there is decreased absorption of other medications (and nutrients) that are administered orally. Laxatives also inhibit the absorption of medications from the intestine; thus, there are decreased levels of drug available and frequently decreased therapeutic effect. Laxatives also result in fluid and electrolyte imbalances that may exacerbate cardiovascular or renal problems. The person who is a frequent abuser of laxatives should be assisted to develop other bowel-training methods. Psychological intervention may even be necessary.

ALCOHOL ABUSE

Alcohol abuse is a social health problem in some older people. It is the primary drug of abuse worldwide. Alcohol abuse interferes with pharmacotherapeutics and also frequently results in altered nutritional status. This may be seen in decreased serum protein levels (as discussed earlier in this chapter), decreased protein binding, and resultant overdosing of older people. Acid-base balance and fluid and electrolyte levels are adversely affected by alcohol abuse. Changes in these two homeostatic mechanisms result in changes in the pharmacotherapeutic effects of the medication regimen.

Alcohol impairs thinking, judgment, and psychomotor coordination, all of which may lead to decreased medication compliance. Alcohol increases or decreases the effects of several other drugs, and other drugs often increase or decrease the effects of alcohol. Alcohol is a central nervous system depressant that potentiates other central nervous system depressants, particularly barbiturates. When taken concurrently, these two drugs may result in central nervous system depression, coma, and death.

Alcohol has a vasodilating effect and, consequently, increases the hypotensive effects of most antihypertensive drugs. The effect of alcohol on oral anticoagulants varies. Alcohol intake decreases the effects of the anticoagulants until liver damage occurs, at which point the anticoagulant effects are increased.

▶ NURSING CARE OF OLDER ADULTS RECEIVING MEDICATIONS

When managing care of older adults receiving medications, the nurse should follow the nursing process as taught in Chapter 4 of this book. The five-stage nursing process consists of assessment, diagnosis, planning, implementation, and evaluation.

ASSESSMENT

Before administration of medication, a thorough assessment of the older adult should be completed. A thorough health history is extremely important. Ask the person about past diseases, illness, or symptoms and how they were handled. Inquire about the person's current health status. The history must include past use of drugs, present uses of drugs, prescribed drugs, OTC drugs, over-the-fence drugs, and street drugs. Specifically ask about use of laxatives and antacids. Assess the person's allergies. Did the allergic reaction cause the person to have difficulty breathing? Hives? Nausea? Vomiting?

Assess the older person's social support network and home environment. Is the person able to get prescriptions filled? Are there family or friends to help with medication compliance? Assess cognitive skills. Is the person confused or disoriented? Is this problem transitory? Is the person capable of understanding any teaching that occurs? Is depression present?

Assess the older adult's sensory status. Is vision impaired? Is hearing impaired? Is the person strong enough to open pill bottles? Assess the Individual's current understanding of therapies and medication regimen. Does the person understand the drugs, dosage, side effects, and/or adverse effects of current medications?

Assess compliance. Does the person take medications at the proper time? For what reasons would the older adult miss a medication? Is there someone to provide transportation to the doctor's office or the pharmacy?

A thorough physical examination must be performed. Watch the older adult for nutrition and fluid status. Is the person thin and emaciated? Dehydrated? Is the person's serum protein level low? This may necessitate a reduction in some drug dosages. Is the person obese? If so, the person may require increased dosages of fat-soluble vitamins and medications.

DIAGNOSIS

Many nursing diagnoses are applicable to the older adult undergoing medication therapy. Some applicable diagnoses include:

- Altered Health Maintenance related to insufficient teaching
- Ineffective Management of Therapeutic Regimen related to lack of motivation
- Noncompliance related to lack of financial resources
- Noncompliance related to inability to open bottles

PLANNING

To promote responsible medication habits in older adults, LPNs must help them become informed medication consumers. Because many older people remain in acute-care settings for only a very limited time, discharge planning and teaching must begin on admission.

Before beginning any teaching session, some preparations are important. Choose an environment with good lighting and minimal environmental distractions. Make sure that the older adult who has glasses and hearing aids is wearing them. Prepare visual aids and reading materials with strong colors and large print.

Plan the teaching session to be only 15 to 20 minutes long. Speak clearly and slowly. Use a low-pitched voice (some older people have difficulty hearing a higher pitch). Always face the person when speaking.

Whenever possible, relate the learning to prior life experiences. For example, when teaching about the thyroid drug methimazole, help the patient identify personal health problems before seeking medical treatment and relate those symptoms to how the person will feel if the medication dose is too low. Tie administration times for medications to the person's daily schedule. If the older person eats oatmeal every morning without fail, the morning dose of digoxin can be associated with the oatmeal breakfast.

Treat older adults as the mature and capable people they are. Do not be patronizing in your teaching approach. Teach a family member, friend, or neighbor at the same time. Have the older person teach the other person and observe the integration of knowledge. Provide sufficient time for review, questions, and return demonstrations.

Consider the need for assistive devices. Medication boxes come in a multitude of styles with individual slots for different days and times. Consider the need for nonchildproof caps. Medication containers can be color coded and accompanied by a wall chart with the color coding system shown. Teach the patient to turn bottles upside down once the medication is taken. Allow the older person to be responsible for taking personal medication the last few days in the hospital. The nurse should monitor these actions and review any areas of knowledge deficit.

Encourage all older adults to carry a list of medications (including prescription and nonprescription drugs) at all times. Another family member should carry the same list as well. The older person should be encouraged to share the list with all physicians and phar-macists before receiving or filling any new prescriptions. Encourage all older adults to locate a pharmacy they like and fill all prescriptions there. On all admissions to the hospital, the nurse should review all medications and refer incompatibilities to the physician or pharmacist.

IMPLEMENTATION

In administering medications to older persons, several strategies are important. When administering medications by mouth, be aware of the medication form. Time-release capsules (e.g., theophylline, cold capsules) should not be opened or crushed and mixed with food. If the person is unable to swallow the capsule, contact the physician or pharmacist for a liquid form. Enteric-coated capsules should not be crushed or dissolved. Disruption of the enteric coating allows gastric acid to come into contact with the medication and inactivate it. Offer the most important medication first. Give the person enough fluid so the medication reaches the stomach.

Parenteral injections should be given into the dorsogluteal or ventrogluteal sites. The deltoid muscle should be avoided, because in most older people, it has lost much of its mass. The vastus lateralis muscle should be avoided owing to its decreased muscle mass and decreased circulation. Avoid injections into edematous areas that have decreased circulation.

Intravenous therapy needs to be closely monitored in older people because many older adults operate in a slightly dehydrated state. Fluid overload is especially critical in the person who may have underlying cardiac and renal disease that would be exacerbated by excess fluid.

POINT OF INTEREST

You are admitting an older person to the medical unit for chest pain, shortness of breath and edema, and neither the older person nor the family member can recall the medications the older person is taking, you have a problem. A solution that is easy for the family is the "brown-bag solution." Ask the family member to go home and put all medications the older person is taking into a brown bag and bring them to you. Be sure the family member brings prescription, over-the-counter, and natural remedies. Assure the family member that all medications will be returned. This will give you the opportunity to make an accurate list of medications being taken by the older adult. It also gives you the opportunity to point out outdated medications that should be discarded.

Some older people experience visual changes with changes in a medication regimen. Recommend that the person not change prescription eyewear until the medication regimen is established.

EVALUATION

Evaluation, the final step in the nursing process, is critical in administering medication for older adults. Evaluate the person's learning curve by doing a return demonstration teaching session. Ask questions about situations the older adult may encounter in the home setting. Allow the person to ask questions of you.

Evaluation of compliance is based primarily on personal and family report. Ask the older adult if medications are being taken, then clarify how and when the medications are being consumed. Ask about the occurrence of side effects. If expected side effects do not occur, the nurse should question whether or not the medication is being taken. Blood levels (if available for a given medication) should be evaluated to determine whether the levels are commensurate with the person's report. Monitor the older adult's laboratory results to determine kidney and liver function. Ask for a personal evaluation of how the new medication is working. Does it help? What concerns does the person have?

The outcome of a successful medication plan can be evaluated by the following criteria:

- The older adult's ability to solve problems related to polypharmacy
- Communication of adverse reactions
- Adherence to regimen

▶ CONCLUSION

Pharmacology in older adults is a complex issue. The nursing care of the older person must include attention to the details of the medication regimen. The LPN needs to be familiar with the aging changes that affect pharmacotherapeutics, including pharmacokinetic changes, sensory changes, psychological changes, problems of polypharmacy, chronic health changes, and financial changes. It is important that the nurse understand the drugs likely to be misused and be aware of specific drugs of frequent misuse by the elderly population, namely antacids, laxatives, alcohol, and home remedies.

The nurse needs to be able to implement the nursing process on behalf of older adults to assist them to develop into well-informed medication consumers. The ability to teach regarding medication administration and to evaluate the impact of medications on the older person are critical skills for you, the LPN, to have.

CASE STUDY

Mr. W., 74 years of age, lives at home alone. He does fairly well on his own. He has difficulty seeing but can read soup can labels. He has arthritis in his hands and opens cans with an electric opener.

Mr. Wyatt's drug history includes:

- Digoxin 0.4 mg p.o. q.d.
- Hydrochlorothiazide 50 mg p.o. b.i.d.
- Potassium supplement daily
- Propranolol 40 mg t.i.d.

Note: p.o. = orally; q.d. = daily; b.i.d. = twice daily; t.i.d. = three times a day.

Mr. W. denies any use of street drugs and states that he "doesn't believe in that stuff." When asked about other medications, he states that he uses Mylanta "several times a day, just one tablespoon full," and Ex-Lax every day for a bowel movement. He also takes a small blue-and-white capsule that his brother gave him because it helps his brother's arthritis. He takes that capsule "once or twice, maybe three or four times a week."

Mr. W. is currently complaining of weakness, dizziness, and occasional chest pains that he treats with Mylanta. His feet and hands seem to be swelling lately.

Mr. W.'s neighbor called the home health-care agency where you work and requested that a home visit be made because Mr. W. seems to be getting thinner and thinner. The agency assigns you to go visit. You find Mr. W. sitting on the porch with his feet propped up and half asleep.

Discussion

1. What is the first step in your home visit?
2. What nursing diagnoses may apply to Mr. W. at this time?
3. While looking at his brother's blue-and-white capsule, you discover the word "indomethacin" on the side. What is your best course of action regarding this over-the-fence drug?
4. Mr. W. is wondering why his feet are swelling and he is feeling weak and dizzy. What drug interactions could be causing these symptoms?
5. What role does the Ex-Lax play in Mr. W.'s pharmacotherapeutics?
6. What referrals does the nurse need to make?
7. What should the nurse do to assist Mr. W. to become compliant?

Solution

1. Introduce yourself, explain why you have come, and begin a complete assessment. The history, drug history, and physical assessment need to be complete. View Mr. W.'s environment. Ask about support services, friends, family, and neighbors. Explore nutritional status and assess what food is available for Mr. W. Assess eyesight. Can he read drug labels? Assess compliance. Does he know when and how to take the medications?
2. Knowledge Deficit related to medication regimen

   Noncompliance related to lack of understanding

   Ineffective Management of therapeutic regimen

   Sensory Deficit related to diminished visual acuity

3. Although indomethacin is a non-narcotic analgesic and nonsteroidal anti-inflammatory drug, it has not been prescribed for Mr. W. Identify his feelings about the medication. Does it seem to help his arthritis? Does he have side effects with the drug? Explain to the patient why it is important not to use this drug unless it is prescribed by the physician. Identify interactions of indomethacin with other prescribed medications (decreases the effectiveness of diuretics and antihypertensive therapy, increases gastric irritation, increases serum levels and risk of toxicity from digoxin). Stress the importance of not taking drugs unless they are prescribed by the physician. Offer to make an appointment for him to see his physician and ask for a prescription for a medication to relieve arthritis pain.
4. Increased sodium intake from use of Mylanta could result in peripheral edema. Use of indomethacin could decrease the effect of the hydrochlorothiazide and propranolol, thereby increasing body fluid volume. With increased body fluid volume the heart could be working harder, increasing myocardial oxygen demand and causing angina.
5. Ex-Lax facilitates movement through the gut, thereby decreasing absorption of all the other medications; it probably contributes to fluid and electrolyte imbalance.
6. Refer to the physician for evaluation of chest pain (if this resembles cardiac angina,

consider emergency referral) or to social services for necessary social support. Call on family members for assistance with medications and transportation, and suggest Meals-on-Wheels.

7. Set up a scheduling plan. Draw a calendar with medications depicted. Teach Mr. W. to take medications at specific times each day.

Encourage discontinuance of Ex-Lax, Mylanta, and indomethacin. Build on the knowledge that he already has. Relate medications to events in Mr. W.'s lifestyle. If he seems unable to manage medications on his own, ask the physician for a referral for home-health nurses to administer medications as needed.

STUDY QUESTIONS

Please select the one best answer.

1. Considering the pharmacokinetics in the OLDER person, which of the following statements is true?
   a. Overall absorption is decreased.
   b. Overall distribution is enhanced.
   c. There is an increase in receptors with aging.
   d. Excretion is facilitated, resulting in a shorter duration of drug action.

2. Which of the following factors would be the strongest In influencing compliance in the older person on a fixed income?
   a. Dietary habits
   b. Cost of filling prescriptions
   c. Body fat–to–lean muscle weight ratio
   d. Family support

3. Mrs. M., age 82, lives at home alone. Her daughter visits once a day and helps her bathe. Mrs. M. cooks her own meals and works in her home and yard. Which of the following factors could place Mrs. M. at risk of making a medication error?
   a. Multiple medications
   b. Visual changes

   c. Different schedules for different drugs
   d. All of the above

4. Mrs. M.'s daughter reports that she seems to take laxatives two or three times per day. What effect would laxative abuse have on the other medications Mrs. M. is taking?
   a. Increased absorption due to clearance of the GI tract
   b. Increased absorption due to facilitation of medication through the GI tract
   c. Decreased absorption due to increased gut motility
   d. Decreased distribution due to increased fluid consumption

5. Mrs. M. seems to have difficulty remembering whether or not she has taken her pills. Which of the following would assist her in this endeavor?
   a. Medication pill boxes with compartments
   b. Turning the bottles upside down
   c. Color coding the medications with a check-off list
   d. All of the above

Yvonne A. Sehy

chapter **16**

Laboratory Values and the Older Adult

Learning Objectives

After completing this chapter, the student will be able to:

1. Identify laboratory tests that are important indicators of health and disease in the elderly patient.
2. Apply an understanding of laboratory tests to the health of elderly persons.
3. Identify at least three reference resources for understanding laboratory values.
4. Identify medications that have an influence on laboratory tests for elderly people.
5. Describe nursing actions appropriate for abnormal laboratory values.

▶ INTRODUCTION

Among the tools for health and illness measurement are laboratory tests. A battery of laboratory tests are done on admission to a hospital or nursing home and, for the elderly patient, they also are done often when visiting the physician. As a licensed practical nurse (LPN), you have studied laboratory values and their meaning in your medical and surgical nursing classes. You also use laboratory resources at the facility where you work in order to interpret correctly laboratory values of older adults. The purpose of this chapter is not to repeat that information; instead it is to provide a ready reference of significant tests for elderly people, along with specific and pertinent information that relates to the elderly.

▶ MEANING OF LABORATORY VALUES IN THE ELDERLY PERSON

Laboratory tests are a routine part of the health examination for all people. For many tests, the normal ranges are different for

It is important to remember that behind every laboratory procedure there is a human being who is anxious about the procedure itself or the results of the procedure.

elderly people than for the people younger than 65 years of age. For others, there is no change with age. Also, elderly people may have greater deviations from normal laboratory indicators when under stress, and their return to normal is often slower. Conditions such as anemia, electrolyte imbalances, and infections are common in the elderly population. They can be discovered and treatment can be monitored through the use of laboratory tests. The diagnosis and treatment of these conditions result in substantial improvement in health, even in elderly individuals with multiple health problems.

RELATIONSHIP TO CLINICAL STATUS

You, as the LPN, need to remember that all laboratory findings must be evaluated in relation to the individual's total clinical situation. The elderly person's gender, dietary pattern, activity level, use of tobacco and alcohol, current medications, and aggressive medical and nursing interventions can alter laboratory findings. Laboratory values should never be considered in isolation, especially when dealing with the often frail elderly person seen in clinical settings. For example, abnormal laboratory values may indicate a physiological stressor such as dehydration or medication side effect rather than illness. It is essential that you consider all facets of the individual's health and habits when you review the laboratory results.

ROUTINE LABORATORY EVALUATIONS

A routine laboratory evaluation generally consists of the following:

- Complete blood cell count
- Serum glucose
- Serum creatinine level
- Serum electrolytes
- Thyroid function tests
- Urinalysis
- Stool guaiac test

Other specific laboratory tests that are not part of the routine evaluation may be ordered to help diagnose illness and disease. They include:

- Chest x-ray studies for those with symptoms or at risk of pulmonary disease

- Tuberculosis testing, which is recommended for individuals in group living situations or at risk for exposure
- Baseline electrocardiograms, which should be done in all elderly patients and repeated when there is suspicion of heart rate or rhythm changes, or myocardial infarction

This chapter includes discussion of the most common laboratory tests ordered and their meaning for the elderly patient. The values shown in boxed text are normal reference values from *Harrison's Principles of Internal Medicine* (Wilson, 1991), unless otherwise indicated. As an LPN, you must refer to the reference intervals used by the clinical laboratory where you work for the most precise reference ranges.

▶ COMMON SCREENING TESTS

There are three common screening tests that should be performed on elderly clients. The physician may request additional tests, but these three are those most commonly used for general screening and are important for you to know.

TUBERCULIN SKIN TEST

Tuberculin Skin Test	
Negative result	<10 mm of induration

General Information

The tuberculin skin test, using purified protein derivative (PPD), is the screening method of choice for the detection of tuberculosis. Unfortunately, as many as 25% of older adults who are clinically ill with tuberculosis show no reaction (<10 mm of induration) to intradermal injections of 5 U of tuberculin.

Some older adults, who show no initial reaction to the test, respond after the test is repeated 1 week later. The majority of people who react positively to the test have no clinical evidence of infection. Nursing home residents, whose risk of infection is five times greater than that of nonresidents, should be screened with a tuberculin skin test on admission and annually thereafter. Although the incidence of infection is low and treatment with isoniazid is known to be effective, congregate living poses the risk of epidemic infection.

Nursing Implications

Because anergy (lack of reaction to specific antigens) is common in elderly people, some clinicians recommend that all PPDs should be placed with appropriate intradermal technique and should be done annually.

URINALYSIS

Urinalysis	
Appearance	Clear yellow/straw
Specific gravity	1.005–1.020
pH	4.5–8.0

General Information

The normal urine should test negative for glucose, ketones, blood, bilirubin, lupus erythematosus, protein nitrates, and calculi in the elderly person, although traces of protein may be present. There may be between 0 and three red blood cells (RBCs), 0 and four white blood cells (WBCs), a few epithelial cells, and a few crystals per high-power field on microscopic examination. Elderly people commonly have the presence of 0 to three hyaline casts on low-power field. In addition, between 10% and 50% of older people have asymptomatic bacteriuria.

Nursing Implications

- Usually a midstream, clean-catch specimen is requested. For this sample, the urinary meatus is cleansed with soap and water or a mild cleaning solution, voiding is initiated, then a sample is collected in midstream to allow clearing of contamination from outside the urinary meatus.
- First morning and fasting urine specimens are collected when the individual awakes and can provide the most concentrated urine of the day. Analytic values for protein, nitrite, fasting urine glucose, and urinary sediment are highest at that time.
- The 24-hour urine specimen measures the average excretion for substances eliminated in variable amounts during the day.
- Urine specimens should be sent to the laboratory within 10 minutes or refrigerated

to prevent growth of bacteria, as well as to prevent the bacteria from using the glucose.

A urinary tract infection is a specific illness that is common in the elderly population. The highest incidence of reported urinary tract infections is in long-term care facilities. This occurs because the urinary tract pathogens often become resistant to antibiotics in nursing homes.

1. Typical symptoms are:
   Frequency
   Burning
   Hematuria
2. In an older person, the only symptoms exhibited may be:
   Nocturia
   Incontinence
   Confusion
   Anorexia
   Lethargy

STOOL FOR OCCULT BLOOD

Stool for Occult Blood	
Negative result	Absence of test color

General Information

Gastrointestinal (GI) bleeding is common in older people, especially in those taking aspirin-containing medications and nonsteroidal anti-inflammatory agents (NSAIDS). Approximately 2.5 mL of blood per day normally appears in the stool. Hemorrhoids and colorectal cancer are the most common causes of minor bleeding in the elderly population.

Abnormal bleeding from the GI tract may be either occult (hidden) or obvious by observation. Minor bleeding may be accompanied by a decrease in the hemoglobin and hematocrit, as well as by symptoms of fatigue and weakness. The fecal occult blood test is useful in screening for colorectal cancer.

Nursing Implications

- There are various tests for fecal occult blood, all requiring the contact of a reagent with a stool specimen.
- A positive test result, indicated by color (usually blue), occurs when there is more than the normal amount of GI blood loss.

- Recommendations are to test at least three stool specimens and to sample from at least two areas of each stool.
- Instruct the patient to avoid red meats, vitamin C intake, iron supplements, and aspirin for 2 to 3 days before and during stool testing, to avoid invalidating the results. Check the manufacturer's directions for other restrictions.

▶ HEMATOLOGICAL INDICATORS

In addition to the three common screening tests, hematologic tests are routinely done on all clients.

COMPLETE BLOOD COUNT

The complete blood count (CBC) includes RBC count, hemoglobin, hematocrit, RBC indices, white blood cell (WBC) count, platelets, and frequently, but not always, a differential. Values for the CBC do not change with age.

Red Blood Cell Count	
Men	$5.4 \pm 0.9 \times 10^{12}/L$
Women	$4.8 \pm 0.6 \times 10^{12}/L$

General Information

The RBC count is used to compute and support other hematological tests to diagnose anemia, polycythemia, and other bone marrow abnormalities.

1. Decreased RBC count may indicate:
   Anemia
   Fluid overload
   Kidney problems
   Bone marrow invasion of other cells or tumors
   Recent hemorrhage
   Chronic illness and autoimmune diseases
2. An increased RBC count may be caused by:
   Polycythemia
   Dehydration
   Hypoxia
   Congestive heart failure
   Impaired pulmonary ventilation
   Abnormal hemoglobin

Hemoglobin	
Men	14–18 g/dL
Women	12–16 g/dL

General Information

Normal hemoglobin levels are maintained throughout life in healthy individuals. Hemoglobin concentration in whole blood correlates closely with the RBC count.

1. Increased hemoglobin levels may be caused by:
   Polycythemia
   Dehydration
2. Decreased hemoglobin levels may be caused by:
   Anemia
   Recent hemorrhage
   Fluid retention causing hemodilution
   Kidney disease

Every person needs an explanation of his or her laboratory results. When you give the explanations necessary, determine the level of understanding the older adult has and clarify any instructions.

Hematocrit	
Men	47.0 ± 5.0%
Women	42.0 ± 5.0%

General Information

Hematocrit measures the percentage by volume of packed RBC in whole blood.

1. Decreased hematocrit levels may be caused by:
   Anemia
   Hemodilution
   Bone marrow disease
   Kidney disease
2. Increased hematocrit may be caused by:
   Polycythemia

   Significant volume depletion with an associated increased blood urea nitrogen (BUN) and creatinine

Red Blood Cell Indices	
MCV	90 ± 7 fL
MCH	29 ± 2 pg
MCHC	34 ± 2%

General Information

RBC indices—mean corpuscular volume (MCV), mean corpuscular hemoglobin (MCH), and mean corpuscular hemoglobin concentration (MCHC)—aid in the diagnosis and classification of anemias by providing information about the size, hemoglobin concentration, and hemoglobin weight of an average RBC.

White Blood Cell Count
4.5–11.0 × 10^9/L

General Information

The WBC count is also known as the leukocyte count. It is used to identify infectious or inflammatory processes, to evaluate the need for further tests, and to monitor the patient's response to chemotherapy or radiation therapy. There is a decrease in the WBC count with age due to a reduction in lymphocyte counts. This results in fewer lymphocytes to resist infection.

1. A decreased WBC count (leukopenia) may be caused by:
   Bone marrow depression, due to primary disease (leukemia, myeloma, and other tumors)
   Reactions to antineoplastics or other toxins
   Viral infections (influenza, infectious hepatitis)
   Sepsis
   Radiation treatments

Drug use, including phenytoin, NSAIDS, and metronidazole

2. An increased WBC count (leukocytosis) may be caused by:
Infection
Inflammation
Tissue necrosis
Leukemia
Excessive exercise
Stress

In the elderly patient, infection may not be accompanied by a normal increase in the number of WBC (leukocytes), so that a WBC differential is required to detect and diagnose disease.

White Blood Cell Differential	
Neutrophils 1.8–7.7	$\times 10^9$/L or 30%–60%
Eosinophils 0–0.45	$\times 10^9$/L or 1%–4%
Basophils 0–0.20	$\times 10^9$/L or 0%–0.5%
Lymphocytes 1.0–4.8	$\times 10^9$/L or 25%–35%
Monocytes 0–0.8	$\times 10^9$/L or 1%–4.0%

General Information

The WBC differential is used to determine the severity of an infection, detect allergic reactions and parasitic infections, identify various leukemias, and assess the individual's capacity to resist and overcome infection.

Five types of WBCs are classified in the normal differential:

- Neutrophils
- Eosinophils
- Basophils
- Lymphocytes
- Monocytes

Platelet Count
130,000–400,000/mL

General Information

Platelets, also called thrombocytes, are necessary for the formation of the aggregate or plug necessary for clot formation and hemostasis. Platelets also supply phospholipids for the process of coagulation in the thromboplastin generation pathway. When the platelet count is below 50,000/mm^3, spontaneous bleeding may occur.

1. A decreased platelet count (thrombocytopenia) may be caused by:
Bone marrow disease
Folic acid or vitamin B_{12} deficiency
Disseminated intravascular coagulation
Drugs (antineoplastics, furosemide, indomethacin, penicillin, phenytoin, quinidine sulfate, salicylates, sulfonamides, thiazides, tricyclic antidepressants, and others)
Destruction due to immune disorders, radiation, or mechanical injury
Disseminated intravascular coagulation

2. An increased platelet count (thrombocytosis) may be caused by:
Iron deficiency anemia
Hemorrhage
Splenectomy
Polycythemia vera
Malignancies
High altitudes
Persistent cold temperature
Strenuous exercise

COAGULATION

Prothrombin Time (PT)	
Normal	9.5–11.8 s (control ± 1 s)
Therapeutic	1.5–2.0 times normal control

General Information

Anticoagulation therapy is indicated in many conditions, such as pulmonary embolus, deep vein thrombosis, chronic atrial fibrillation, and heart valve prosthesis. Warfarin (Coumadin) is used in oral anticoagulation therapy. PT is an indirect measure of prothrombin and an overall evaluation of these extrinsic coagulation factors. The PT is determined before initiation of warfarin therapy and then daily until maintenance dosage is established. Thereafter, PT determinations may be made at 1 to 4-week intervals, depending on the stability of the patient's therapeutic level.

Nursing Implications

- Risk of serious hemorrhage is high in elderly anticoagulated patients over age 70, especially those at risk for falls.
- Many drugs have a potentiating or inhibiting effect on warfarin, so that all medica-

tions being taken by an individual taking warfarin must be reviewed. Diets high in vitamin K should be encouraged.

Activated Partial Thromboplastin Time (APTT)	
Normal	25–36 s
Therapeutic	1.5–2.5 times normal control

General Information

APTT evaluates all the clotting factors of the intrinsic pathway, except for two, by measuring the time required for formation of a fibrin clot. The APTT is used to monitor heparin anticoagulation therapy aimed at increasing the APTT to a therapeutic range. The APTT is more sensitive and is often used in place of the PTT.

Nursing Implications

- If PT or APTT values are higher than the therapeutic range, or if bleeding or signs of bleeding such as hematuria, black tarry stools, hematemesis, bruising and petechiae, epistasis, hemoptysis, continuous abdominal or head pain, faintness, or dizziness occur, withhold the anticoagulant dose and notify the physician immediately.
- Periodic urinalyses as well as stool guaiac and liver function tests are carried out to detect hemorrhage or liver dysfunction.

▶ BLOOD CHEMISTRY INDICATORS

BLOOD GLUCOSE

Blood Glucose, Plasma	
Fasting:	
Normal	75–115 mg/dL
Diabetes mellitus	140 mg/dL on at least 2 occasions
Two hours after eating:	
Normal	140 mg/dL
Impaired glucose tolerance	140–200 mg/dL
Diabetes mellitus	>200 mg/dL on at least two occasions

General Information

In the elderly patient, the exact definition of abnormal glucose tolerance is unclear. Using the National Diabetes Data Group and the World Health Organization diagnostic criteria, diabetes mellitus is present when the fasting (12–14-hour fast) plasma glucose is over 140 mg/dL on two separate occasions or over 200 mg/dL 2 hours after oral glucose administration.

A number of drugs and conditions affect plasma glucose levels.

1. Decreased blood plasma glucose (hypoglycemia) is indicated by:
   Plasma blood glucose values below 100 mg/dL
   Weakness
   Restlessness
   Hunger
   Nervousness
   Sweating
   Rapidly decreasing mental alertness in the elderly patient without the common symptoms listed earlier
2. Decreased plasma glucose levels may be caused by:
   Beta-blockers
   Ethanol
   Clofibrate
   Monoamine oxidase inhibitors
   Strenuous exercise
   Failure to refrigerate the blood sample and analyze it within a few hours of collection
3. Increased blood plasma glucose (hyperglycemia) is indicated by:
   Plasma glucose levels, which usually exceed 600 mg/dL. Plasma glucose above 160–180 mg/dL is the average renal threshold, resulting in glycosuria in older persons.
   Lack of symptoms.
   Urinary frequency.
   Dehydration.
   Weakness.
4. Elevation of plasma glucose levels may be caused by:
   Chlorthalidone
   Thiazide diuretics
   Furosemide
   Oral contraceptives
   Benzodiazepines
   Phenytoin
   Phenothiazines
   Lithium

Epinephrine
Nicotinic acid
Corticosteroids
Recent illness or infection

If undetected, worsening hyperglycemia results in alterations in mental status and hyperosmolar coma in the older patient with noninsulin-dependent diabetes mellitus.

ELECTROLYTES

Normal values for electrolytes are the same for the young and old. Numerous conditions, medications, and dietary factors influence electrolyte values. Common electrolyte-related causes of weakness in the elderly patient are hypernatremia (high sodium), hyponatremia (low sodium), and hypokalemia (low potassium).

Sodium, Serum
136–145 mEq/L

General Information

The elderly population is at increased risk of serum sodium imbalance. Decreased sodium levels promote water excretion and increased levels promote retention, primarily through stimulation or depression of aldosterone secretion. Loss of body water causes concentration of serum sodium (hypernatremia), whereas an increase in body water causes dilution of serum sodium (hyponatremia). Sodium also plays a role in acid-base balance, chloride and potassium levels, and neuromuscular function.

Hyponatremia

A sodium concentration of less than 136 mEq/L occurs when there is an excess of water in relation to total sodium.

1. Symptoms may be absent or there may be:
Fatigue
Headache
Restlessness
Decreased skin turgor
Nausea
Muscle cramps and tremors
Disorientation

Confusion
Coma
Seizures
Death
2. Conditions causing hyponatremia include:
Vomiting
Diarrhea
Renal disorders
Diuretics
Congestive heart failure
Cirrhosis
Overhydration
Adrenal insufficiency
Use of nutritional support formulas without additional sodium
Syndrome of inappropriate antidiuretic hormone secretion associated with numerous drugs and diseases

Hypernatremia

A sodium concentration greater than 146 mEq/L is a result of a deficit of body water relative to total sodium content and is usually caused by dehydration.

1. Symptoms include:
Weakness
Thirst
Restlessness
Dry, sticky mucous membranes
Flushed skin
Oliguria
Diminished reflexes
2. Conditions contributing to hypernatremia include:
Inadequate fluid intake
Diarrhea
Polyuria associated with diabetes mellitus
Diuretics
Increased insensible water loss from fever and tachypnea
3. Conditions causing hypernatremia include:
Hypertension
Dyspnea
Edema
Kidney disease due to a lack of response to ADH
4. Conditions causing excess sodium concentration are:
Increased dietary intake
Aldosteronism
Intravenous infusion of normal saline for treatment of fluid loss or shock

Potassium, Serum
3.5–5.0 mEq/L

General Information

Potassium maintains cellular osmotic equilibrium and helps regulate muscle activity by maintaining electrical conduction within the cardiac and skeletal muscles. Potassium also helps regulate acid-base balance, enzyme activity, and kidney function. Potassium deficiency develops rapidly because the body has no effective way to conserve potassium.

1. Signs and symptoms commonly seen with hypokalemia (decreased serum potassium levels) include:
   Mental confusion
   Rapid, weak, irregular pulse
   Hypotension
   Anorexia
   Decreased reflexes
   Muscle weakness
   Paresthesia
2. Hypokalemia is caused by:
   Diuretics
   Diarrhea
   Vomiting
   Renal tubular acidosis
   Malnutrition
   Urinary potassium losses associated with glycosuria and ketonuria, and with hyperaldosteronism
3. Signs and symptoms of hyperkalemia (increased serum potassium) are:
   Weakness
   Malaise
   Nausea
   Diarrhea
   Muscle irritability
   Oliguria
   Bradycardia
4. Hyperkalemia is caused by:
   Renal failure
   Cell damage from burns
   Injuries
   Chemotherapy
   Acidosis
   Addison's disease
   Diabetes mellitus
5. Several drugs may increase serum potassium levels, including:
   Spironolactone
   Triamterene

NSAIDs
Beta-blockers
Angiotensin-converting enzyme inhibitors
Penicillin G
Amphotericin B
Methicillin
Tetracycline

General Information

Calcium, Plasma
9–10.5 mg/dL

Calcium absorption becomes less efficient in both men and women with age. Dietary calcium is associated with the loss of bone that begins in the 40s. Calcium helps regulate and promote neuromuscular and enzyme activity, skeletal development, and blood coagulation. Parathyroid hormone, vitamin D, calcitonin, and adrenal steroids control calcium blood levels. Almost all of the body's calcium is stored in the bones and teeth. Serum calcium varies inversely with the body's phosphorus level. The body requires ingestion of about 1 g per day of dietary calcium, because calcium is excreted in the urine and feces.

1. Signs and symptoms of hypocalcemia include:
   Circumoral and peripheral numbness and tingling
   Muscle twitching
   Facial muscle spasm
   Muscle cramping
   Seizures
   Dysrhythmias
2. The causes of hypocalcemia include:
   Insufficient activity of the parathyroid glands
   Hypomagnesemia
   Hyperphosphatemia due to renal failure
   Laxatives
   Chemotherapy
   Corticosteroids
   Malabsorption
   Acute pancreatitis
   Alkalosis osteomalacia
   Diarrhea
   Rickets (vitamin D deficiency)
3. Signs and symptoms of hypercalcemia are:
   Hypertension

Bone pain
Muscle hypotonicity
Nausea
Vomiting
Dehydration
Mental confusion
Coma
Cardiac arrest
4. The causes of hypercalcemia are:
Hyperparathyroidism
Thiazide diuretics
Cancer
Addison's disease
Hyperthyroidism
Paget's disease
Immobilization
Excessive vitamin D intake
Calcium-containing antacids
Androgens
Progestins or estrogens
Lithium carbonate

Phosphate Serum
3–4.5 mg/dL

General Information

Phosphate helps regulate calcium levels, carbohydrate and lipid metabolism, and acid-base balance. Adequate levels of vitamin D are necessary for absorption of phosphates from the intestine. About 85% of the body's phosphate is found in bone. Calcium and phosphate have a reciprocal relationship. The kidneys regulate phosphate excretion to maintain a balance with serum calcium.

Chloride, Serum
98–106 mEq/L

General Information

Chloride interacts with sodium to maintain the osmotic pressure of the blood. Chloride is important in maintaining the acid-base balance in the body and varies inversely with the bicarbonate level. Low chloride levels are usually seen with low sodium and potassium levels.

END PRODUCTS OF METABOLISM

Blood Urea Nitrogen (BUN), Serum
10–20 mg/dL

General Information

Blood Urea Nitrogen is the chief end product of protein metabolism. The BUN level reflects protein intake, liver function, and kidney excretory capacity. The normal BUN value remains unchanged with age. Because protein intake is often low in the elderly population, BUN values may be normal even with impaired renal function. Elevation of BUN levels without serum creatinine elevation suggests dehydration.

There are usually no signs or symptoms of an increased BUN level other than those associated with dehydration or other underlying renal disease. Likewise, with decreased BUN levels, the signs and symptoms are those of the underlying condition.

1. Increased BUN levels occur with:
   Renal disease
   Reduced renal blood flow
   Urinary tract obstruction
   Increased protein catabolism (starvation, burns)
   Drugs such as aminoglycosides, amphotericin B, and methicillin
2. Decreased BUN levels occur with:
   Severe liver failure
   Malnutrition
   Overhydration
   Chloramphenicol use

Creatinine, Serum
<1.5 mg/dL

General Information

Creatinine values also are unchanged with age. Yet, because lean body mass declines with age, the total daily production of creatinine also declines, staying below 1.2 mg/dL. This causes an overestimate of renal function in the elderly based on static measurements of serum creatinine.

Creatinine clearance declines by almost 10% per decade after 40 years of age and is a more reliable indicator of kidney function than the BUN and serum creatinine values. In the elderly patient, creatinine clearance is important for determining the dosage for drugs that are cleared by the kidney to avoid drug toxicity. Creatinine clearance (mL/min) is defined as a ratio. For men, the formula is:

$$\frac{[140 - \text{age (y)}] \times \text{body weight (kg)}}{\text{serum creatinine (mg/dL)} \times 72}$$

For women, multiply the result from the above formula by 0.85.

An increase in serum creatinine may be caused by:

- Renal disease
- Diabetic acidosis
- Starvation
- Muscle disease
- Hyperthyroidism
- Use of ascorbic acid
- Barbiturates
- Diuretics

A high serum creatinine level indicating renal failure may be associated with nonspecific symptoms such as weight loss and weakness. Because creatinine is easily excreted by the kidneys, with minimal tubular reabsorption, serum creatinine levels are directly related to the glomerular filtration rate (GFR).

Bilirubin, Serum	
Total	0.3–1.0 mg/dL
Direct	0.1–0.3 mg/dL
Indirect	0.2–0.7 mg/dL

General Information

Bilirubin is the major product of hemoglobin breakdown and is excreted as a pigment in bile. The excretion of bilirubin is dependent on the normal production and destruction of RBCs and a functional hepatobiliary system, whereas bilirubin is conjugated and excreted. The direct bilirubin value increases with the obstruction of the flow of bile through the biliary system because this causes uptake of direct bilirubin into the circulation. Levodopa may cause false increases in bilirubin.

Uric Acid, Serum	
Men	2.5–8.0 mg/dL
Women	1.5–6.0 mg/dL

General Information

Uric acid, the major end metabolite of dietary and endogenous purines, is excreted through the kidneys. Cell breakdown and catabolism of nucleic acids, excessive production and destruction of cells, and inability to excrete uric acid are causes of hyperuricemia. An increase in serum uric acid is found in a variety of conditions including gout, impaired renal function, congestive heart failure, hemolytic anemia, polycythemia, neoplasms, and psoriasis.

Serum uric acid levels above 8 mg/dL in men and 6 mg/dL in women are often associated with symptoms of gout. Gout is an acute inflammation of a joint, commonly the metatarsophalangeal joint of the great toe, caused by uric acid crystal accumulation.

Causes of increased serum uric acid levels include:

- Loop diuretics
- Thiazides
- Starvation
- A high-purine diet
- Stress
- Alcohol abuse
- Chemotherapy

Levodopa, acetaminophen, ascorbic acid, and phenacetin may cause false elevations in uric acid levels.

LIVER FUNCTION TESTS

Most liver function tests remain unchanged in the elderly population. The alkaline phosphatase level is frequently elevated in older patients. Total alkaline phosphatase may rise owing to Paget's disease, bone fracture, trauma, or osteoporosis. For clients taking tacrine (Cognex) for Alzheimer's disease, liver function tests are very important.

ALT (SGPT) (alanine aminotransferase, alanine transaminase, or serum glutamic-pyruvic transaminase)
0–35 U/L

General Information

Alanine aminotransferase, an enzyme necessary for tissue energy production, is present predominantly in the liver. It is also present in the kidney, heart, and skeletal muscles and is a relatively specific indicator of acute liver cell damage.

Elevated ALT levels are caused by:

- Liver disease
- Different medications
- Cholecystitis
- Intrahepatic cholestasis
- Pancreatitis
- Hepatic congestion due to heart failure
- Acute myocardial infarction
- Trauma
- Lead ingestion
- Carbon tetrachloride exposure

Falsely elevated ALT levels are caused by the use of barbiturates and narcotic analgesics.

aspartate aminotransferase, aspartate transaminase (AST), or serum glutamic-oxaloacetic transaminase (SGOT)
0–35 U/L

General Information

Aspartate aminotransferase is an enzyme found in cells of the liver, heart, muscles, kidneys, pancreas, and RBCs. Serum levels are highest during acute cellular damage and decrease during tissue repair. The AST level is useful in monitoring the progress of myocardial infarction and acute liver disease.

Elevations are found in:

- Myocardial infarction
- Liver disease
- Extensive surgery
- Hemolytic anemia
- Pulmonary emboli
- Delirium tremens
- Diseases of the brain, muscle, pancreas, spleen, and lungs

General Information

Alkaline phosphatase is an enzyme active in bone calcification and in lipid and metabolite transport. Serum alkaline phosphatase levels are sensitive to biliary obstruction by space-occupying hepatic lesions, such as tumors or abscesses, and to metabolic bone disease. Alkaline phosphatase isoenzymes may be identified to differentiate hepatic and skeletal diseases.

Increases in alkaline phosphatase are found in:

- Gallbladder disease associated with obstruction
- Paget's disease
- Bone metastasis
- Hyperparathyroidism
- Liver disease
- Osteomalacia

Lactic Dehydrogenase (LDH), Serum
60–100 U/mL

General Information

Lactic Dehydrogenase is most useful in diagnosing myocardial infarction but also is elevated in hepatic disease, pulmonary infarction, and anemias. It is present in almost all body tissues. Five tissue-specific isoenzymes may be measured: of these, LDH4 and LDH5 are found in the liver and the skeletal muscles. Elevated LDH values are diagnostic in hepatitis, active cirrhosis, and hepatic congestion.

▶ NUTRITIONAL INDICATORS

Elderly persons require and consume fewer total calories per day than younger adults. Carbohydrate intake may increase slightly (40% of total calories), whereas fat and protein intakes generally decline in older people. Lean body mass and total body protein decrease, whereas the percentage of body fat increases with age.

It is critical that you, as an LPN, recognize that the elderly persons are often at risk for malnutrition. This is due to conditions such as decreased mobility, cognitive and sensory deficits, chewing and swallowing difficulties, and loss of appetite due to medications, illness, or the environment. The increased occurrence of wounds, infection, and dehydration creates additional nutritional demands on the elderly, yet the most significant causes of poor nutrition in older people are poverty and chronic illness.

Because of these physiological and societal factors, it is important to have baseline laboratory values for several indices of nutritional status and to understand their significance:

- Total serum proteins measures visceral protein stores.

- Serum albumin is the most widely used indicator of protein status.
- Serum transferrin is an indicator of protein stores.
- Serum cholesterol indicates lipid mass.
- Serum creatinine indicates lean body mass.

The hemoglobin, hematocrit, and lymphocyte count included in the CBC reflect the body's ability to transport nutrients and resist disease. Other common nutritional indicators are iron and micronutrients such as vitamins and minerals.

Nutritional deficiencies are often identified only when an associated problem such as weight loss, poor wound healing, or weakness occurs. Treating an underlying cause such as medication use or an illness may correct the deficiency. Otherwise, an increased dietary intake of the nutrient, or vitamin and mineral supplements, may be indicated.

PROTEIN INDICATORS

Total Serum Protein
5.5–8.0 g/dL

GENERAL INFORMATION

The major blood proteins are serum albumin and the globulins, which together equal the total serum protein value. The measurement of total protein is performed by protein electrophoresis and aids in the diagnosis of protein deficiency, blood dyscrasias, and hepatic, GI, renal, and neoplastic diseases.

1. Symptoms commonly seen with low serum protein values are:
   Dermatitis
   Hair thinning
   Muscle wasting
   Weakness
   Poor wound healing
2. Total protein values are increased with:
   Dehydration
   Diabetic acidosis
   Infections
   Multiple myeloma
   Monocytic leukemia
   Chronic alcoholism
   Chronic inflammatory disease
3. Common causes are:
   Edema
   Tissue breakdown

Poor wound healing
4. Total protein values decrease with:
   Malnutrition
   Hepatic disease
   Renal disease
   GI disease
   Hodgkin's disease
   Trauma such as burns, hemorrhage, and shock
   Hyperthyroidism
   Congestive heart failure

Albumin, Serum
3.5–5.5 g/dL

General Information

Albumin values of less than 3.5 g/dL indicate protein malnutrition and are accompanied by an increased incidence of morbidity and mortality. Albumin maintains oncotic pressure and transports substances such as bilirubin, fatty acids, hormones, and drugs that are insoluble in water.

1. Albumin is increased only in multiple myeloma.
2. Albumin is decreased in:
   Malnutrition
   Liver and renal disease
   Collagen diseases
   Rheumatoid arthritis
   Metastatic carcinoma
   Hyperthyroidism
   Essential hypertension
   The use of cytotoxic agents

Globulins, Serum
2.0–3.0 g/dL

General Information

The four types of globulins identified by protein electrophoresis are found in differing quantities in various conditions. Alpha$_1$, alpha$_2$, and beta-globulin are carrier proteins that transport lipids, hormones, and metals through the blood. Gamma globulin is an important component of the immune system.

Globulins are increased in:

- Tuberculosis
- Chronic syphilis

- Subacute bacterial endocarditis
- Myocardial infarction
- Multiple myeloma
- Collagen diseases
- Rheumatoid arthritis
- Diabetes mellitus
- Hodgkin's disease

Nursing Implications

Because a consistent relationship between protein intake and serum albumin levels has not been established, a high-protein diet is not advised except for individuals with evidence of protein calorie malnutrition. Protein allowance is the same for older people as for younger ones: 0.8 g/kg body weight. Protein should provide at least 12% of total calories for the healthy older person. The proteins from animal sources such as beef, poultry, fish, and dairy products are the most complete, whereas complementary vegetable proteins have less biological value. Some patients may need nutritional supplementation through oral, enteral, or parenteral routes if malnutrition is severe.

IRON INDICATORS

Iron, Serum	
Men	80–180 mg/dL
Women	60–160 mg/dL

General Information

Iron appears in the plasma bound to the glycoprotein transferrin. Iron is essential in the production and function of hemoglobin as well as other compounds. Dietary iron is absorbed by the intestine and distributed in the body for synthesis, storage, and transport. The body has no mechanism for eliminating excessive iron; therefore, total body and bone marrow iron stores increase with advancing age, although serum iron may be depleted. Serum iron values should be interpreted, together with the total iron-binding capacity (TIBC) and the serum ferritin. It may be necessary to seek bone marrow and liver biopsy as well as iron absorption or excretion studies to obtain a definitive diagnosis in iron-related disease. A decrease in serum iron with an increased TIBC occurs in iron deficiency anemia, which is most commonly caused in the elderly person by GI blood loss or malabsorption.

Ferritin, Serum
15–200 ng/mL

General Information

Ferritin is an iron-storage protein. Serum ferritin level indicates the amount of available iron stored in the body. It is measured to distinguish between iron deficiency (decreased ferritin level) and chronic infection or inflammation (increased or normal ferritin level).

1. Serum ferritin is increased in:
   Hepatic disease
   Iron overload
   Leukemia
   Hodgkin's disease
   Chronic renal disease
   Hemolytic anemias
   Acute or chronic infection and inflammation
2. Ferritin is decreased in chronic iron deficiency.

Total Iron-Binding Capacity (Transferrin), Serum
250–460 mg/dL

Total iron-binding capacity decreases with age and reflects the transferrin content of the serum. Transferrin, a beta-globulin protein, transports circulating iron that is stored in various forms in the bone marrow, liver, and spleen. In protein-energy malnutrition, the TIBC is less than 250 mg/dL (see discussion under serum iron above).

LIPOPROTEINS

Total Plasma Cholesterol	
Desired	<200 mg/dL
Borderline	200–239 mg/dL
High	240 mg/dL

High-Density Lipoprotein (HDL) Cholesterol	
Desired	>35

Low-Density Lipoprotein (LDL) Cholesterol	
Desired	130 mg/dL
Borderline	130–159 mg/dL
High	160 mg/dL
Triglycerides	160 mg/dL

General Information

Blood lipid and lipoprotein cholesterol levels that are influenced by heredity, diet, and obesity are directly related to atherosclerotic heart disease in the elderly population. Higher HDL cholesterol, lower LDL cholesterol, and a decreased level of plasma triglycerides are all associated with decreased incidence of coronary heart disease.

In women, the increase in plasma total cholesterol with age is due primarily to an increase in LDL cholesterol. HDL cholesterol increases slightly in men over 65 years of age but decreases in women of the same age. Without intervening therapy, the risk for coronary heart disease in the elderly population gradually increases.

Both total cholesterol and HDL cholesterol should be measured in screening tests for the elderly population. The findings of a high initial cholesterol value should be followed by two subsequent evaluations because there may be significant daily variations in values. Older persons may have a total cholesterol of less than 200 to 240 mg/dL but have elevated LDL cholesterol and decreased HDL cholesterol and so have an increased risk of coronary heart disease. Conversely, the HDL cholesterol may be high, accounting for a total cholesterol level greater than 200 mg/dL, so that there is a reduced risk for coronary heart disease. Total cholesterol and HDL cholesterol may be obtained from nonfasting blood samples. Triglyceride levels are only accurate after a 12-hour fast. LDL cholesterol levels may be calculated after the total cholesterol, HDL cholesterol, and triglycerides are known.

Lipid abnormalities are often familial, but secondary causes are common in the elderly population. They include the following:

- Diets high in saturated fat or cholesterol
- Excessive alcohol intake
- Estrogen supplements
- Thiazide diuretics
- Beta blockers
- Smoking
- Uncontrolled diabetes
- Hypothyroidism
- Uremia
- Corticosteroid use
- Sedentary lifestyle
- Morbid obesity

Cholesterol levels less than 120 to 156 mg/dL have been associated with increased mortality in nursing home residents. Cholesterol is decreased in:

- Malnutrition
- Hyperthyroidism
- Chronic obstructive pulmonary disease

Nursing Implications for Lipid Abnormalities

- Weight control
- Increased physical activity
- Restriction of alcohol
- Cessation of smoking
- Restriction of dietary fat

Dietary restriction must be made cautiously because maintaining adequate calorie and protein intake is a major concern among elderly patients. Drug therapy to control lipid levels may be beneficial in older persons with known coronary heart disease or high risk of disease.

▶ DRUG MONITORING AND TOXICOLOGY

Drug monitoring is important when the margin of safety between therapeutic and toxic blood levels is narrow. Drug blood levels are useful guides in maintaining therapeutic levels as well as in identifying toxic levels of drugs. Not all drugs have a known therapeutic blood level even though toxic levels have been identified. Some drugs, such as amphetamines, are monitored through urine testing. Elderly persons metabolize and eliminate drugs more slowly than mature adults, a fact that heightens the importance of drug monitoring.

Three commonly monitored drugs—digoxin, theophylline, and phenytoin—are discussed, because they require close observation from you, the nurse. Numerous classes of drugs are commonly checked for therapeutic or toxic levels. Please review the list in Box 16.1. Refer to a basic laboratory manual for specific drug therapeutic and toxic values.

DIGOXIN

Digoxin (Lanoxin) level, serum	
Therapeutic	0.5–20 ng/mL
Toxic	2.5 ng/mL

General Information

Digoxin, used in the treatment of congestive heart failure and cardiac arrhythmias, has a prolonged half-life in the elderly population because of its reduced renal clearance. Serum digoxin level has a narrow therapeutic range and despite the availability of tests for serum drug levels, digitalis toxicity is relatively common in elderly patients.

The most common side effects of digitalis toxicity are:

- Visual changes
- Headache
- Nausea and vomiting
- Weakness and fatigue

Weakness and fatigue are sometimes the only indicators of digitalis toxicity in elderly people.

Quinidine significantly increases the serum level of digoxin. Consequently, the digoxin dose must be reduced when both of these drugs are prescribed. Also, a change from tablet to elixir preparation of digoxin increases the absorption and serum level, so that the digoxin dose again needs to be reduced. Both low-serum potassium level and high-serum calcium level increase the risk of serious arrhythmias in persons on digoxin therapy.

Nursing Implications for Digoxin Blood Levels

- Draw blood samples for determining serum digoxin levels at least 5 to 6 hours after the daily dose and preferably just before the next scheduled daily dose.
- Check the apical pulse for 1 full minute.
- Suspect digitalis toxicity when there is a sudden change in heart rhythm or pulse (especially a decrease).
- Withhold the medication and report to the patient's physician when there is a sudden change in pulse or rhythm.
- Monitor the serum potassium level, especially if the patient is taking diuretics.

THEOPHYLLINE

Theophylline, Serum	
Therapeutic	10–20 µg/mL
Toxic	20 µg/mL

General Information

Theophylline, a bronchodilator, may or may not be associated with improved respiratory effort on spirometry testing. Nevertheless, theophylline improves mucocilliary clearance of the lungs and may improve myocardial contractility, stimulate respirations, and act as a mild diuretic.

Wide variations in the rate and extent of absorption and rate of metabolism for theophylline result in peak-to-trough fluctuations in serum concentrations and subsequent subtherapeutic or toxic responses.

1. Indications of possible toxicity include:
   Anorexia
   Abdominal discomfort
   Nausea
   Vomiting
   Dizziness
   Shakiness
   Restlessness
   Irritability
   Palpitations
   Tachycardia
   Hypotension
   Heart arrhythmias and seizures
2. Dizziness is a common side effect at the initiation of theophylline use in elderly patients.
3. Elimination of the drug is reduced in persons with:
   Heart failure
   Kidney or liver dysfunction
   Alcoholism
   Fever
4. Smoking and phenytoin increase the elimination of theophylline so that an increase in dosage is required. The macrolide antibiotics (e.g., erythromycin), as well as others, may increase serum theophylline levels and cause toxicity.

▶ NURSING IMPLICATIONS

- Regular monitoring of serum concentrations of theophylline is necessary to determine therapeutic dosage.
- The serum level must be checked when signs or symptoms of toxicity develop or when medications affecting serum levels are added or discontinued.

BOX 16.1. COMMONLY MONITORED DRUGS

Alcohol
ethanol
isopropanol (rubbing alcohol)
methanol (antifreeze)
Amphetamines (urine testing)
amphetamine
dextroamphetamine
methamphetamine (Desoxyn)
phenmetrazine (Preludin)
Antiarrhythmics
disopyramide (Norpace)
lidocaine (Xylocaine)
procainamide (Pronestyl)
propranolol (Inderal)
quinidine (Quinaglute and others)
verapamil (Calan, Isoptin)
Antibiotics
amikacin (Amikin)
gentamicin (Garamycin)
kanamycin (Kantex)
netilmicin (Netromycin)
tobramycin (Nebcin)
Anticonvulsants
cabamazepine (Tegretol)
ethosuximide (Zarontin)
phenobarbital (Luminal)
phenytoin (Dilantin)
primidone (Mysoline)
Antidepressants
amitriptyline
nortriptyline (Pamelor, Aventyl)
desipramine (Norpramin)
doxepin (Sinequan and others)
imipramine (Tofranil)
lithium (Lithobid)
Barbiturates and Hypnotics
amobarbital (Amytal)
glutethimide (Doriden)
pentobarbital (Nembutal)
phenobarbital (Luminal)
secobarbital (Seconal)
Bronchodilators
aminophylline
theophylline (Theo-Dur and others)
Cardiac Glycosides
digitoxin (Crystodigin)
digoxin (Lanoxin)
Hemoglobin Derivatives
carboxyhemoglobin (Hg = CO)
methemoglobin
sulfhemoglobin
Non-narcotic Analgesics
acetaminophen (Tylenol and others.)
salicylates (aspirin)
Phenothiazines
chlorpromazine (Thorazine)
prochlorperazine (Compazine)
thioridazine (Mellaril)
trifluoperazine (Stelazine)

PHENYTOIN

Phenytoin (Dilantin), Serum	
Therapeutic	10–20 µg/mL
Toxic	30 µg/mL

General Information

Phenytoin, an anticonvulsant that also has antiarrhythmic properties, is metabolized by the liver and excreted in the bile and partially by the kidneys. Unfortunately, phenytoin has a number of potentially serious adverse reactions and side effects that necessitate monitoring of several parameters, including liver, kidney, thyroid, and hematological functioning.

1. Potential adverse reactions and side effects are:
   Drowsiness
   Mental confusion
   Tremors
   Bradycardia
   Hypotension
   Photophobia
   Blurred vision
   Nausea
   Vomiting
   Epigastric pain
   Abnormal blood counts
   Fever
   Skin eruptions
   Pneumonitis
2. Acute kidney or liver dysfunction results in toxic drug levels.
3. Decreased phenytoin serum levels may result from:
   Chronic alcohol abuse
   Antacids
   Antihistamines
   Antineoplastics
   Barbiturates
   Excess of folic acid
   Rifampin
4. Increased serum levels may result from:
   Acute intake of alcohol
   Anticoagulants
   Aminosalicylic acid
   Benzodiazepines
   Cimetidine
   Dexamethasone
   Estrogens
   Isoniazid
   Methylphenidate
   Phenothiazines
   Salicylates
   Sulfonamides
   Phenylbutazone

Nursing Implications

- Liver and thyroid function tests, blood counts, and urinalysis are recommended before the initiation of therapy, at monthly intervals during early therapy, and at regular intervals thereafter.
- Lower doses are given to geriatric patients and those with liver or kidney impairment.
- When phenytoin is given intravenously, vital signs and cardiac function must be monitored closely.
- Serum concentrations of magnesium, folic acid, vitamin D, and vitamin K may be decreased with phenytoin therapy and should be monitored.
- Symptoms of low serum magnesium may mimic those of phenytoin toxicity.

▶ CONCLUSION

The use and interpretation of laboratory values are important in substantiating clinical judgment and providing comprehensive health assessment in the elderly. Physiological changes in older persons, presence of disease, use of medications, variance in diets, and even exercise affect laboratory values. Therefore, it is necessary to monitor changes in an individual's laboratory values, as well as to compare an individual's values with those of other older adults in similar situations.

Understanding laboratory values in the elderly population is a continuing endeavor for all health-care practitioners. It is important to refer consistently to comprehensive laboratory manuals and individual laboratory reference intervals used in a particular locality, as well as to specialized geriatric references. As new information becomes available, the interpretation of laboratory data will become more useful in determining care for older people.

CASE STUDY

Mr. K. is an 85-year-old resident of a small, independent group home where he has been caring for himself but sharing provided meals with the other residents. He underwent a transurethral resection of the prostate 4 years ago for benign prostatic hypertrophy. He has been treated for a heart irregularity and congestive heart failure in the past. Today he is being admitted to your intermediate care facility by his daughter because of several recent falls. Mr. K. reports that he has been nauseated and has not been eating well for the past few days. He also complains of wetting before reaching the rest-room and blames this on his slow movement due to severe degenerative arthritis of his joints. Medications include:

- furosemide (Lasix) 40 mg in the morning
- digoxin 0.125 mg in the morning
- ibuprofen (Motrin) 600 mg twice a day
- acetaminophen (Tylenol) 500 mg every 4 hours as needed

On physical assessment you find the following:

- Height 5 ft 10 in
- Weight 135 lb
- Blood pressure sitting 120/70 and pulse irregular at 80/min
- Blood pressure standing 90/60 and pulse irregular at 90/min
- Respirations 20/min and unlabored
- Temperature 98.8ºF (36ºC)
- Lungs are clear
- Skin is warm and dry, with dry mucous membranes

Laboratory values available are:

- Potassium 3.2 mEq/L
- Sodium 132 mEq/L
- Chloride 106 mEq/L
- BUN 30 mg/dL
- Creatinine 1.4 mg/dL
- Glucose 130 mg/dL
- Urinalysis 3 to 5 WBCs, 0 to 3 RBCs, positive bacteria, specific gravity 1.022

Discussion

1. What problems have you identified based on the resident's history and physical assessment?
2. What other laboratory tests would be helpful?
3. What nursing actions will you take immediately?

Solutions

1. Underweight with risk of malnutrition
   Heart arrhythmia with possible orthostatic hypotension
   Probable urinary tract infection with urinary incontinence
   Anorexia and nausea possibly related to medications or urinary tract infection
   Recurrent falls with several possible causes, including weakness due to decreased food and fluid intake, hypokalemia and hyponatremia, difficulty ambulating due to degenerative arthritis, orthostatic hypotension due to dehydration, and infection
2. CBC to assess for anemia and infection
   Digoxin level to check for toxicity as a cause of anorexia and nausea
   Urine culture and sensitivity to identify and quantify the urine bacteria and determine antibiotic sensitivity
   Total protein to evaluate nutritional status
3. Safety measures to prevent falls, such as having the patient call for assistance before getting up to go to the rest room. Advise the patient to change positions slowly from lying to sitting, then from sitting to standing. Consider a bedside commode because the patient has urinary incontinence and difficulty ambulating.
   Provide fluids and simple, easily digested foods in frequent small amounts.
   If nausea occurs, notify the physician.
   Withhold digoxin until the level value is obtained. Report to the physician.
   Withhold the Lasix because the resident is dehydrated and has hypokalemia and hyponatremia, probably as a result of the diuretic. Report to the physician.
   Check any stools for occult blood because ibuprofen (an NSAID) is often the cause of GI bleeding. If the CBC indicates an iron deficiency anemia, the physician will probably discontinue this medication. Acetaminophen (Tylenol) may be used on a regular schedule to control arthritic pain.

STUDY QUESTIONS

Please select the one best answer.

1. All laboratory test results for elderly patients should be:
   a. Evaluated against younger clients
   b. Evaluated against the other older clients on the unit
   c. Evaluated against the client's total clinical situation
   d. Evaluated against the client's CBC results

2. With tuberculosis on the increase among the elderly population, it is critical for the LPN to know that:
   a. Tuberculosis (TB) skin tests are inaccurate on people over the age of 65
   b. When there is no initial reaction to the TB skin test in elderly clients, it should be given again 1 week later
   c. It is unnecessary and expensive to do TB screening on nursing home residents
   d. Isoniazid is not an effective TB drug of choice for the elderly

3. The PT test is a measure of the overall coagulation factors. The risk of serious hemorrhage is high in the elderly when:
   a. Warfarin is used
   b. Medication reviews on all medications are done
   c. PTs are drawn daily until the therapeutic dose is determined
   d. They are at risk for falls and subsequent bleeding

4. Potassium deficiency develops:
   a. Slowly in elderly patients
   b. In the kidneys
   c. Rapidly because there is no way to conserve it
   d. Only when using diuretics

5. Every elderly person with a low-serum albumin level should be:
   a. Put on a high-protein diet
   b. Put on bed rest
   c. Put on a diet of 12% complete proteins
   d. Put on vitamin supplements

Unit Resources

UNIT 1

AARP. (2000). *A profile of older Americans*. Washington, DC:AARP.

American Hospital Association. (1992). *A patient's bill of rights*. New York: American Hospital Association

American Heart Association (2001). *Eat well but eat wisely*. New York: American Heart Association.

Anderson, M. A. (2001). *Nursing leadership, management, and professional practice for the LPN/LVN*. Philadelphia: F. A. Davis Company.

Bandman, E., & Bandman, B. (2002). *Nursing ethics through the life span* (4th ed.) New Jersey: Prentice Hall.

Butler, R. M. (1969). Ageism: Another form of bigotry. *Gerontologist*, 9, 243–246.

Cruzan v. Director, Missouri Department of Health, 110 U.S. 2841 (1990).

Eliopoulos, C. (2001). *Gerontological nursing* (5th ed.). Philadelphia: J. B. Lippincott.

Health Care Financing Administration. (2002). *Interpretative guidelines to OBRA*. (No. 263-H). Washington, DC: U.S. Government Printing Office.

Kemper, D. W., Deneen, J. E., & Guiffre, J. V. (1992). *Growing younger handbook* (2d ed.). Boise, ID: health wise.

Nightingale, F. (1946). *Notes on nursing, replica edition: What it is, and what it is not*. Philadelphia: Lippincott-Raven Publishers.

Staab, A. S., & Hodges, L. C. (1996). *Essentials of gerontological nursing*. Philadelphia: Lippincott Company

U.S. Department of Health and Human Services, Public Health Services. (2001). *Healthy People 2010. National health promotion and disease prevention objectives*. (DHHS-PHS Publication No. 91-50213). Washington DC: U.S. Government Printing Office.

U.S. Department of Agriculture and U.S. Department of Health and Human Services. (1995). The Food Pyramid. Washington DC: U.S. Government Printing Office.

Watson, J. (1985). *The science of human caring*. New York: National League for Nursing.

UNIT 2

Agency for Health Care Policy Research. (1992a). *Pressure ulcers in adults: Prediction and prevention. Clinical practice guidelines* (DHHS publication No. 92–0048). Rockville, MD: Department of Health and Human Services.

Agency for Health Care Policy Research. (1992b). *Urinary incontinence in adults. Clinical practice guidelines* (DHHS publication No. 92–0038). Rockville, MD: Department of Health and Human Services.

Albert, M. S. (1990). Neuropsychological testing. In C. K. Cassel, D. E. Riesenberg, L. B. Sorenson, & J. R. Walsh (Eds.), *Geriatric medicine* (Vol. 2, pp. 48–54). New York: Springer-Verlag.

Bandler, R. (1985). *Using your brain for a change*. Moab, UT: Real People Press.

Beck, A. T., Ward, C. H., & Mendelson, M. (1961). An inventory for measuring depression. Archives of General Psychiatry, 4(53), 561–571.

Carr, D. B., & Jacox, A. K. (1994). Acute pain management: Operative or medical procedures and trauma. In *Clinical geriatric medicine. Diagnostic and statistical manual of mental disorders* (4th ed.). Washington, DC: American Psychiatric Association.

CDC (2002). *www.cdc.gov/hiv*

Feil, N. (1993). *Validation: The Feil method*. Cleveland, OH: Edward Feil Productions.

Folstein, M. F., Folstein, S. E., & McHugh, P. R. (1975). Mini-mental status: A practice method for grading the cognitive state of patients for the clinician. *Journal of Psychiatric Research*, 12, 189.

Ford, R. D. (1987). *Diagnostic tests handbook*. Springhouse, PA: Springhouse Corporation.

Gilbert, R. M. (1992). *Extraordinary relationships: A new way of thinking about human interactions*. Minneapolis: Chronimed Publishing.

Gurland, B. J. (1987). The assessment of cognitive function in the elderly. *Clinical Geriatric Medicine*, 3(1), 53–63.

Hamilton, M. (1967). Development of a rating scale for primary depressive illness. *British Journal of Social and Clinical Psychology*, 6, 78–96.

Jacobs, J. W., Bernhard, M. R., Delgado, A., & Strain, J. J. (1977). Screening for organic mental syndromes in the medically ill. *Annals of Internal Medicine*, 86, 40.

Kahn, R., Goldfarb, A., Pollak, M., & Peck, A. (1960). Brief objective measures for the determination of mental status in the aged. *American Journal of Psychiatry*, 117, 326.

Kiernan, R. J., Mueller, J., Langston, J. W., & Vandyke, C. (1987). The neurobehavioral cognitive status examination: A brief but differential approach to cognitive assessment. *Annals of Internal Medicine*, 107, 481.

Pfeiffer, E. (1975). A short portable mental status questionnaire for the assessment of organic brain deficit in elderly patients. *Journal of American Geriatrics Society*, 23, 433.

Restak, R. M. (1988). *The mind*. New York: Bantam Books.

Squire, L. R. (1987). *Memory and brain*. New York: Oxford University Press.

Sunderland, T., Alterman, I. S., Yount, D., Hill, J. L., Tariot, P. N., Newhouse, P. A., Mueller, E. A., Mellow, A. M., & Cohen, R. M. (1988). A new scale for the assessment of depressed mood in demented patients. *American Journal of Psychiatry*, 8, 145.

Wilson, J. D. (1991). *Harrison's principles of internal medicine*, vol. 2. New York: McGraw Hill.

Yesavage, J., Brink, T., Rose, T., Lum, O., Huang, O., Adey, V., & Leirer, V. (1983). Development and validation of a geriatric depression screening scale: A preliminary report. *Journal of Psychiatric Research*, 17, 37–49.

Zung, W. K. (1983). A self-rating depression scale. *Archives of General Psychiatry*, 12, 63–70

Appendix A

Introduction to Your Pennsylvania Advance Directive*

This packet contains a legal document that protects your right to refuse medical treatment you do not want, or to request treatment you do want, in the event you lose the ability to make decisions yourself.

The **Pennsylvania Declaration** is your state's living will. It lets you state your wishes about medical care in the event that you develop a terminal condition or enter a state of permanent unconsciousness and can no longer make your own medical decisions. The Declaration becomes effective when your doctor receives a copy of it and determines that you are incompetent and in a terminal condition or a state of permanent unconsciousness. On page 2 of your Declaration you can name another person, called a surrogate, to make decisions about your medical care—including decisions about life support—when you can no longer speak for yourself.

Partnership for Caring recommends that you complete all sections of your Pennsylvania Declaration, including the appointment of a surrogate, to best ensure that you receive the medical care you want when you can no longer speak for yourself.

Note: This document will be legally binding only if the person completing it is an individual of sound mind who is 18 years or older, or if a minor, is married or a high school graduate.

HOW DO I MAKE MY PENNSYLVANIA DECLARATION LEGAL?

In order to make your Declaration legally binding, you must sign it, or direct another to sign it, in the presence of two witnesses, who must also sign the document to show that you knowingly and voluntarily signed the document. Both of your witnesses must be 18 years or older and, if you are unable to sign your Declaration, neither witness can be the person who signed the Declaration on your behalf.

Note: You do not need to notarize your Pennsylvania Declaration.

WHOM SHOULD I APPOINT AS MY SURROGATE?

Your surrogate is the person you appoint to make decisions about your medical care if you become unable to make those decisions yourself. Your surrogate should be an adult, and can be a family member or a close friend whom you trust to make serious decisions. The person you name as your surrogate should clearly understand your wishes and be willing to accept the responsibility of making medical decisions for you. (A surrogate may also be called an "agent," "attorney-in-fact," or "proxy.")

You can appoint a second person as your alternate surrogate. The alternate will step in if the first person you name as surrogate is unable, unwilling, or unavailable to act for you.

CAN I ADD PERSONAL INSTRUCTIONS TO MY DECLARATION?

Yes. You can add personal instructions in the part of the document called "Other directions." For example, it is unclear when you would be considered "terminal" under Pennsylvania law. Partnership for Caring rec-

* Reproduced with permission from Partnership for Caring, inc.

ommends that you add the statement "I do not want life support if my death is imminent without its use, and there is no reasonable expectation that I will regain the ability to make decisions and express my wishes." You may also want to emphasize pain control by adding instructions such as, "I want to receive as much pain medication as necessary to ensure my comfort, even if it may hasten my death."

If you have appointed a surrogate, it is a good idea to write a statement such as, "Any questions about how to interpret or when to apply my Declaration are to be decided by my agent."

It is important to learn about the kinds of life-sustaining treatment you might receive. Consult your doctor or order the Partnership for Caring booklet, "Advance Directives and End-of-Life Decision."

WHAT IF I CHANGE MY MIND?

You may revoke your Pennsylvania Declaration at any time and in any manner. Your revocation becomes effective when you, or a witness to your revocation, notify your doctor or other health care provider. Once your doctor is notified, he or she must then make the revocation a part of your medical record.

WHAT OTHER IMPORTANT FACTS SHOULD I KNOW?

A pregnant patient's Pennsylvania Declaration will not be honored, due to restrictions in the state law, unless life-sustaining treatment will not permit the development and live birth of the unborn child, will be physically harmful to the pregnant woman, or will cause her pain that cannot be alleviated by medication. If this issue concerns you, contact Partnership for Caring for more information.

1. Your Pennsylvania Declaration is an important legal document. Keep the original signed document in a secure but accessible place. Do not put the original document in a safe deposit box or any other security box that would keep others from having access to it.
2. Give photocopies of the signed original to your surrogate and alternate surrogate, doctor(s), family, close friends, clergy, and anyone else who might become involved in your health care. If you enter a nursing home or hospital, have xerox copies of your Declaration placed in your medical records.
3. Be sure to talk to your surrogate and alternate, doctor(s), clergy, and family and friends about your wishes concerning medical treatment. Discuss your wishes with them often, particularly if your medical condition changes.
4. If you want to make changes to your Declaration after it has been signed and witnessed, you must complete a new document.
5. Remember, you can always revoke your Pennsylvania Declaration.
6. Be aware that your Pennsylvania document will not be effective in the event of a medical emergency. Ambulance personnel are required to provide cardiopulmonary resuscitation (CPR) unless they are given a separate order that states otherwise. These orders, commonly called "nonhospital do-not-resuscitate orders," are designed for people whose poor health gives them little chance of benefiting from CPR. These orders must be signed by your physician and instruct ambulance personnel not to attempt CPR if your heart or breathing should stop. Currently, not all states have laws authorizing nonhospital do-not-resuscitate orders. Partnership for Caring does not distribute these forms. We suggest you speak to your physician.

If you would like more information about this topic contact Partnership for Caring or consult the Partnership for Caring booklet "Cardiopulmonary Resuscitation, Do-Not-Resuscitate Orders and End-Of-Life Decisions."

Appendix B

Answers to Chapter Study Questions

CHAPTER 1

1. b
2. a
3. a
4. d
5. b

CHAPTER 2

1. c
2. a
3. a
4. b
5. c

CHAPTER 3

1. c
2. d
3. a
4. d
5. b

CHAPTER 4

1. b
2. c
3. c
4. d
5. a

CHAPTER 5

1. a
2. d
3. b
4. c
5. a

CHAPTER 6

1. a
2. b
3. a
4. b
5. d

CHAPTER 7

1. d
2. c
3. a
4. d
5. d

CHAPTER 8

1. d
2. d
3. c
4. t
5. t

CHAPTER 9

1. c
2. a
3. b
4. d
5. b

CHAPTER 10

1. b
2. c
3. c
4. d
5. d

CHAPTER 11

1. b
2. c
3. d
4. d
5. b

CHAPTER 12

1. d
2. c
3. d
4. c
5. d

CHAPTER 13

1. b
2. d
3. a
4. d
5. d

CHAPTER 14

1. d
2. b
3. c
4. d
5. d

CHAPTER 15

1. a
2. b
3. d
4. c
5. d

CHAPTER 16

1. c
2. b
3. d
4. c
5. c

INDEX

Note: Page numbers followed by *f* refer to illustrations; numbers followed by *t* refer to tables; and numbers followed by *b* refer to boxed material.